AF863055

Laboratory Animal Science and Medicine

Volume 1

Series Editors

Aurora Brønstad, Laboratory Animal Science, University of Bergen, Bergen, Norway

José M. Sánchez Morgado, Comparative Medicine, Trinity College Dublin, The University of Dublin, Dublin, Ireland

This book series aims at providing an easily accessible and complete toolbox for researchers, Veterinarians and technicians who design animal studies or/and work with research animals. The series equips the readers with the theoretical and practical knowledge to successfully run an animal facility, to monitor and maintain animal health and wellbeing in compliance with international ethical guidelines, to proof the genetic status of laboratory rodents and furthermore it profoundly introduces on how to design reproducible animal experiments. In a unique way, each volume focuses on a distinct topic which is always explored in a comprehensive manner.

This series is endorsed by the European Society for Laboratory Animal Veterinarians (ESLAV). As a leading voice in European Laboratory Animal Medicine, ESLAV's objectives are to promote and disseminate expert veterinary knowledge within the field of laboratory animal science, with a special focus on advancing skills in subjects connected with the breeding, health, welfare and use of laboratory animals.

More information about this series at http://www.springer.com/series/16673

José M. Sánchez Morgado •
Aurora Brønstad
Editors

Experimental Design and Reproducibility in Preclinical Animal Studies

Springer

Editors
José M. Sánchez Morgado
Comparative Medicine
Trinity College Dublin
The University of Dublin
Dublin, Ireland

Aurora Brønstad
University of Bergen
Laboratory Animal Science University of Bergen
Bergen, Norway

ISSN 2730-7859 ISSN 2730-7867 (electronic)
Laboratory Animal Science and Medicine
ISBN 978-3-030-66146-5 ISBN 978-3-030-66147-2 (eBook)
https://doi.org/10.1007/978-3-030-66147-2

© Springer Nature Switzerland AG 2021
This work is subject to copyright. All rights are reserved by the Publisher, whether the whole or part of the material is concerned, specifically the rights of translation, reprinting, reuse of illustrations, recitation, broadcasting, reproduction on microfilms or in any other physical way, and transmission or information storage and retrieval, electronic adaptation, computer software, or by similar or dissimilar methodology now known or hereafter developed.
The use of general descriptive names, registered names, trademarks, service marks, etc. in this publication does not imply, even in the absence of a specific statement, that such names are exempt from the relevant protective laws and regulations and therefore free for general use.
The publisher, the authors, and the editors are safe to assume that the advice and information in this book are believed to be true and accurate at the date of publication. Neither the publisher nor the authors or the editors give a warranty, expressed or implied, with respect to the material contained herein or for any errors or omissions that may have been made. The publisher remains neutral with regard to jurisdictional claims in published maps and institutional affiliations.

This Springer imprint is published by the registered company Springer Nature Switzerland AG.
The registered company address is: Gewerbestrasse 11, 6330 Cham, Switzerland

Contents

Part I

The Animal and Its Environment

An Introduction to Reproducibility in the Context of Animal Research

José M. Sánchez-Morgado and Aurora Brønstad

1 An Introduction to Reproducibility in the Context of Animal Research

This book's aim is to improve animal research, so they are used only when needed, provide reliable information and are not wasted. This is not a book about fraud in science.

Russel and Burch published their 3Rs concept in a book in 1959 [1]. More than 70 years later, we are still trying to embrace the 3Rs in animal research, and an important part in embracing them is to improve the reproducibility of animal experiments. Thus, we propose to add a fourth R to their original piece of work, that is, reproducibility.

The reason is that there is a reproducibility problem across all experimental sciences. Experiments are difficult to reproduce even in the same lab or in external labs. Also conclusions from preclinical studies fail to be translated into human patients. Some claim this is the nature of the scientific endeavour. We search for answers and make mistakes that lead to others not being able to reproduce our results and, in the process, coming out with different solutions. The consequence of this disparity has been leapt in knowledge that have allowed what is sometimes referred to as paradigm shifts. Some illustrations of these are:

- Ramon y Cajal's neuron theory [2–7] contrary to the then prevalent reticular theory proposed by Joseph von Gerlach and Camillo Golgi [8].
- Rosalind Franklin, James Watson, Francis Crick and Maurice Wilkins work on the DNA structure [9–12], which proved to be the correct one, contrary to the 1953 proposed one by Linus Pauling and Robert Brainard Corey [13].

However, we shall acknowledge that there is a public "trust crisis" in scientific claims based on scientific results [14].

1.1 Reproducibility

There is a lack of agreement on the meaning for the term "reproducibility". For Goodman and collaborators [14], reproducibility, replicability and repeatability have a nearly identical common language interpretation. In 2010, in an *In-*

J. M. Sánchez-Morgado (✉)
Comparative Medicine, Trinity College Dublin, The University of Dublin, Dublin, Ireland
e-mail: Jose.Sanchez-Morgado@tcd.ie

A. Brønstad
Department of Clinical Medicine, University of Bergen, Bergen, Norway
e-mail: Aurora.Bronstad@uib.no

© Springer Nature Switzerland AG 2021
J. M. Sánchez Morgado, A. Brønstad (eds.), *Experimental Design and Reproducibility in Preclinical Animal Studies*, Laboratory Animal Science and Medicine 1,
https://doi.org/10.1007/978-3-030-66147-2_1

fection and Immunity editorial [15], Casadevall and Fang said that "for most types of experiment, there is an unstated requirement that the work be reproducible, at least once, in an independent experiment, with a strong preference for reproducibility in at least three experiments". Casadevall and Fang also stated that "... a new finding should be reproduced at least once and preferably more times ...". What most laboratories do simply replicates the experiment, without changing any of the conditions. This is an unnecessary waste of animals in experiments where animals are used and will most likely produce data that is not more robust than the single replication experiment. Both editors acknowledge the confusion that both terms, replicability and reproducibility, produce on the majority of the scientific community. Thus, Goodman instead proposes a new lexicon for research reproducibility consisting of three terms: *methods reproducibility*, *results reproducibility* and *inferential reproducibility* [14]. For them, "*Methods reproducibility* is meant to capture the original meaning of reproducibility, that is, the ability to implement, as exactly as possible, the experimental and computational procedures, with the same data and tools, to obtain the same results. *Results reproducibility* refers to what was previously described as 'replication', that is, the production of corroborating results in a new study, having followed the same experimental methods. Inferential reproducibility, not often recognized as a separate concept, is the making of knowledge claims of similar strength from a study replication or reanalysis. This is not identical to *results reproducibility*, because not all investigators will draw the same conclusions from the same results, or they might make different analytical choices that lead to different inferences from the same data".

In this book, we have tried to address concepts relevant to the internal validity of the experimental design of animal research. Thus, we have focus on the control of the known sources of variation that will have an effect on how well a particular study addresses these sources of systematic error. These sources of variation addressed the genome, the animal and its environment; the mathematics employed to design and analyse experiments; and the publication bias. However, we did not address the external validity, which is an embracing variation so conclusions can be applied to other contexts or situations, i.e., generalized. As Voelkl and collaborators [16] put it: "... within-study standardization is a major cause of poor reproducibility ...", and we totally agree with them. They found that the accuracy of effect size estimates increases with the number of participant laboratories, although this also increased the confidence intervals, i.e. uncertainty [16]. The greatest improvement observed in reproducibility was when they went from one to two laboratories [16]. Thus, addressing all the factors considered in this book chapters is of fundamental importance for the quality of any animal study it will not be sufficient to guarantee reproducibility – according to the definition of *results reproducibility*. *Results reproducibility* is depending on interpretation of results in a larger context and is relevant for the external validity.

The book has been divided in three major parts: the animal and its environment in Part I; the basics of and an explanation of different designs and tests in Part II; and systematic reviews and publishing in Part III.

Even though we have not gone into some specific fields of research in this book, we would like to call the attention of the reader regarding interpretation of histopathology. We think there is a general lack of animal pathologists involved in animal research programmes. This is very worrying, as we have seen scientists trying to interpret findings in badly fixated, sectioned or stained tissues. There is a need for well-experienced animal pathologists to become involved in interpretation of histological findings. Journals should also employ these pathologists to review manuscripts with histological findings. As Jerrold M. Ward, Paul N. Schofield and John P. Sundberg have identified, "... the problem of reliable histopathological interpretation of experimental animals is perhaps one of the most tractable sources of error ..." [17]. This might be a consequence of unconscious incompetence – a gap we try to fill by publishing this book.

2 Part I: The Animal and Its Environment

The first part of the book addresses the genetic variability of the animals we use in research. A majority of these animals are rodents, and the chapter focus on them, but the genetics' chapter can be transferred to all the other animals used in research. Fernando Benavides and Jean Louis Guénet have divided the chapter in five parts: a brief introduction to mammalian genetics, an overview of the main standardized strains of laboratory rodents, what these genetically modified animals are and how you create them, and finally two sections on genetic monitoring and rodent phenotyping. Since 1981, with the creation of the first transgenic mouse [18–20], there has been an almost exponential explosion of research being carried on these genetically modified rodents. However, one caveat of these animals is the mixed genetic background due to the technology employed to generate them, whether they are created through pronuclear microinjection, where most of them would have been created on a F2 hybrid background or by homologous recombination, where the recombined genome corresponds to one inbred strain and where they are introduced into a different strain's blastocyst to then start a series of backcrossing experiments, which unfortunately do not reach the tenth generation most of the times (see chapter "Rodent Genetics", Section 2 on genetically altered (GA) rodents). As Dobrowolski and collaborators found [21], at least 50% of these genetically modified animals have a mixed genetic background with some of them carrying a mispairing Y chromosome. Nevertheless, the creation of these animals is now easier than ever, and any molecular biology laboratory can embark themselves on the task of designing and creating their own genetically modified animal using the CRISPR-Cas system (CRISPR) [22]. These animals created with CRISPR should be better at keeping an isogenic background and, thus, reducing the reproducibility problems associated with a mixed undefined genome background. Although a promising tool to avoid the mixed genetic backgrounds, the genetic drift will still have to be controlled, which lead us to be realistic and think that we will end up in the same place we are now, unless, of course, the genetic monitoring technology and the knowledge required to support the analysis become available at a very reduced cost.

Have isogenic rodents that trait stability superiority over non-inbred stocks? This is the question Tuttle and collaborators asked themselves [23] and the conclusion that reached: "... compared with inbred mice, defined outbred stocks from heterogeneous backgrounds (even considering the fact that commercially available outbred stocks are far less genetically diverse than wild mice) are more appropriate and much more cost-effective research subjects in many biomedical research applications, except in cases where precise genotypic regulation or standardization is required..." [23]. The question remains as to what those particular cases are and how we can control that the genome remains isogenic except for the allele that has been studied. What about the effect that passenger genes could have on the data we are observing in our precious genetically modified mouse [24]. We should also consider epigenetic factors interacting with these alleles. As pointed out in Chapter 3, we cannot control all the variables that may affect our data, but we can recognize and acknowledge them.

Chapter "Animal and Environmental Factors That Influence Reproducibility", by José M. Sánchez-Morgado, Aurora Brønstad and Kathleen Pritchett-Corning, deals with general considerations intrinsic to the animal or its environment that could potentially have an impact on the data. This chapter starts with an overview on therioepistemology, which is the study of how knowledge is gained from animal research and establishes the acknowledgement of these factors we cannot control. The chapter also questions the established concept of standardisation and presents Richter's work briefly to challenge the reader on this [25–27]. Then, the chapter goes on to describe how the animal itself can affect the reproducibility of the data. Some of these factors are rarely described in the Materials and Methods section of any manuscript, mainly because, we presume, they have not been taken into account in the first place. For some of the external factors that can influence the experimental animal, there are defined standards to comply with like the Commission Recommendation of 18 June 2007 on guidelines for the accommodation and care of animals used for experimental and other scientific purposes (2007/526/EC) [28], while for others there are maybe no recognized standards, and we have to rely on the current knowledge – for example, studies on how the choice of bedding material can impact a study [29].

When we use animals in research, we tend to think everything is being taken care of by the animal facility staff, and we can just concentrate in the experiment itself. We tend to consider the animal as another reagent in our chemical's shelf. We think there is a need for a shift in thinking to start considering these animals as clinical subjects. The PREPARE guidelines described by Adrian Smith in chapter "Planning Animal Experiments" propose to include early dialogue with animal care staff early in the planning of animal experiments.

In chapter "Microbiology and Microbiome", Axel Kornerup Hansen will go through the microbiota and how changes in these microorganisms can affect the animal model in ways that may render the data not reproducible at another laboratory. We will also see how the different environments affect the composition and the frequencies of the microbiota in these animals. And we will see how to tackle this variation by introducing well-defined microbiota into our experimental animals trying to harmonize the conditions of our experiment. Another issue when trying to produce good science is the inadvertent contamination of animals with infectious organisms that may interfere with our results. Thus, laboratories opt for one of the three options when dealing with these infections:

1. Cull all the animals undergoing procedures, and start the animal experiments again with animals free from any known infectious organism.
2. Treat the infection and keep using the animals.
3. Do nothing and live with the infection.

Whatever the option chosen, we certainly lose information when data on those experiments is published. First, if we decide to cull the animals and start all over again, we will be using more animals to answer our scientific question and miss any interference that the infectious organism may cause in our experiment. Most likely, the research laboratory will be studying questions that were not even thinkable decades ago. Instead of wasting these animals, why the laboratory does not finish the experiments and analyse the data to see if there is any discrepancy between their controls and if that discrepancy could be attributed to the infectious organism. We may gain knowledge through the process that could be useful. Second, if we decide to treat the infection and use the animals, the microbiome will be modified because of the use of these treatments, and this modification could lead to different interpretations of the data. Third, if we decide to live with the infection and not report it, and laboratories do not report the health status of their experimental animals, others may not be able to reproduce our results because they may be bias by this concurrent infection. All these issues are discussed in chapter "Microbiology and Microbiome" in more detail.

Finally, this part ends with a chapter on pain, analgesia and anaesthesia, chapter "Effects of Untreated Pain, Anesthesia and Analgesia in Animal Experimentation". Recently, a new definition of pain has been issued by the International Association for the Study of Pain. The previous definition dated back to 1979 [30]: *An unpleasant sensory and emotional experience associated with actual or potential tissue damage, or described in terms of such damage.* The new definition [31], *An unpleasant sensory and emotional experience associated with, or resembling that associated with, actual or potential tissue damage*, includes for the first time a note including the experiences of pain by animals: *Verbal description is only one of several behaviours to express pain; inability to communicate does not negate the possibility that a human or a nonhuman animal experiences pain.* In this chapter, Paulin Jirkof and Heidrun Potschka review the physiology of pain and what effects pain has in animal physiology. They also discuss multimodal analgesia and the effects of analgesics, desired and unwanted, on the animals, including the concept of pre-emptive analgesia. The chapter ends touching on routes of administration and the implications of their use for study design.

3 Part II: Statistics: Basics and Explanation of Different Designs and Tests

Carlos Oscar Sánchez Sorzano and Michael Parkinson have summarized statistics for the nonmathematician in Part II.

An experimental test is a comparison of (an) experimental group(s) versus one or more control groups testing a hypothesis. A hypothesis is based on a conditional statement (an "if… then" statement) and must ask a question that can be answered by a statistical test that describes an assumed reality or truth. This is usually phrased as there is no difference between test and control. In statistical words, there is zero effect (H_0). This might cause cognitive dissonance for the average person not trained in statistical thinking because we are motivated by the assumption that there should be an effect of the treatment to be studied. It is the alternative hypothesis – i.e. that we cannot say that there is no difference (we reject the null hypothesis) that better reflects our assumptions or what we typically like to "prove" by doing the study. It is important that researchers not trained in statistics collaborate with a statistician because conclusions or "evidence" are based on statistical test results. The statistician, however, may have no knowledge about the biological model or what factors that can influence the model and study outcome – which are the topic for several chapters in this book. Last but not least, the significant size of biological interest or relevance is a question that the primary researcher must define – and it will have an impact on the calculations to be made in the study design and number of animals needed.

Statistical methods are based on assumptions that have to be met to be able to use them statistical methods. If we don't check that these assumptions are actually met – but just assume that they are – we can come to wrong conclusions. If we still use them, there is a change in the probability of making a type I or type II error – so we cannot rely on the answer. One basic assumption that must be met is the assumption of *independence* of observations. That means that none of the observations are influenced by other observations. A common mistake is to consider animals in the same group, for example, mice in a cage, as independent observations. However, because of social hierarchy and individual roles and responses in a group, the criteria of independence are not met. Also, responses in one group are not necessarily the same in another group. A very dominant individual can cause stress among cage mates, with a secondary response on the hormonal level, behaviour, etc. This does not have to be the case in another cage. It is important to be aware of such factors and how they can influence results of your experiment and be aware that a number of animals in cages do not always equal the number of independent observations (or N in the statistical calculations).

Another assumption that must be met is that there is *random assignment* to experimental groups. You might think that animals are randomly assigned, but if you always put the first animal(s), you are able to pick in the same group – you are doing a nonrandom selection. The animals that are easiest to pick might have features in common like being more calm, slower and less afraid of the handler, while the animals that are more difficult to pick may be more stressed, quicker and more afraid of the handler. You might succeed to randomize animals in groups at the beginning of the experiments, but you introduce systematic errors afterwards, for example, by placing all animals in the same group on one shelf and the other group on another different shelf, with different light distribution, or you always treat one group in the beginning of the day and then the next group. There are many good practical reasons for doing so; however you will then be introducing bias and compromise the assumption of random assignment.

The assumption of independence and random assignment must always be met. There are also more assumptions to be aware of; however they can be controlled for using alternative tests, for example, the assumption of *normal distribution*, i.e. that data are equally distributed around a mean value in a bell-shaped curve like the commonly used student t-test and ANOWA tests, which are both based on the assumption of normal distribution. The proper choice of action is to be sceptic to whether data are normally distributed and rather test for it than assume it. If they are not, there are ways around it either by transformation of data or by choosing a non-parametric (distribution-free) test. We will see this in detail in chapter "Why Do We Need a Statistical Experiment Design?" of this book.

We will also have a look at how to calculate sample sizes for different statistical tests in chapter "Statistical Tests and Sample Size Calculations". To comply with the 3R principle, especially reduction, we should aspire for the design that gives the most solid information out of the least number of animals.

4 Part III: Systematic Reviews and Publishing

Finally, we have included a section on the publication process, including here the relevant planning leading to the animal experiments. In chapter "Scholarly Publishing and Scientific Reproducibility", Arieh Bomzon and Graham Tobin thoroughly review the publication process where this process can add to publication bias and, thus, irreproducible science. The authors suggest that "scientific reproducibility can be improved by upgrading editorial vigilance to assure the quality and accuracy of the scientific record, and institutional training in writing in the sciences for research trainees and institutional adoption of existing standards of quality control in manufacturing and commercial research organizations to develop good publishing and research practices and integrity". The chapter goes through the publication process in detail, starting with how a manuscript should be organized and how data should be reported, including that coming from animal experiments, for the submission process. Then, the authors dive into the appraisal process, i.e. how this manuscript will be handled by the editors and reviewed by your peers in the field, finishing with the dissemination of the accepted manuscript. The chapter then enters the minefield of "who is competent" to handle this process and "where all this can go wrong" to make your science irreproducible by others, finishing the chapter by providing some suggestion on how to improve the Scholarly Publishing system.

Chapter "Systematic Reviews" is a concise, and easy-to-follow, version of how to do a proper systematic review. Systematic reviews are a common practice before commencing any clinical trial but unfortunately a rara avis in animal research, which usually takes place before the corresponding clinical trials, and, for that reason, has been known as preclinical research. A systematic review will help review all published evidence in a particular animal model to reach conclusions and raise unanswered questions by the model which, as Ray Greek and Andre Menache have pointed out, are poor predictors of human interventions [32].

The last chapter of this book describes the planning of animal research. In 2018, 8 years after the ARRIVE guidelines [33] were published and endorsed by more than a thousand of journals from across the life sciences, Leung and collaborators [34] reported in a PLOS One article that "no paper fully reported 100% of items on the ARRIVE checklist and measures associated with bias were poorly reported. These results suggest that journal support for the ARRIVE guidelines has not resulted in a meaningful improvement in reporting quality, contributing to ongoing waste in animal research". More recently, a 2.0 version has been published [35], but it is still very early to see whether this new version will improve reporting across life sciences or will not make much difference like its predecessor. In this chapter, Adrian Smith takes us briefly through the ARRIVE guidelines to then go deeper into the PREPARE guidelines [36], which, as he will put the case forward, are better placed to prevent bias before it happens.

References

1. Russell WMS, Burch RL. The principles of humane experimental technique. London: Methuen & Co Limited; 1959.
2. Ramón y Cajal S. Estructura de los centros nerviosos de las aves. Revista trimestral de Histología normal y patológica. 1888;1:1–10.
3. Ramón y Cajal S. Morfología y conexiones de los elementos de la retina de las aves. Revista trimestral de Histología normal y patológica. 1888;1:11–6.
4. Ramón y Cajal S. Terminaciones nerviosas en los husos musculares de la rana. Revista trimestral de Histología normal y patológica. 1888;1:16–8.
5. Ramón y Cajal S. Sobre las fibras nerviosas de la capa molecular del cerebelo. Revista trimestral de Histología normal y patológica. 1888;1:33–42.
6. Ramón y Cajal S. Extructura de la retina de las aves. Revista trimestral de Histología normal y patológica. 1888;1:42–9.
7. Ramón y Cajal S. Nota sobre la estructura de los tubos nerviosos del lóbulo cerebral eléctrico del torpedo. Revista trimestral de Histología normal y patológica. 1888;1:49–57.
8. Golgi C. The neuron doctrine – theory and facts. In: Lindsten J, editor. Nobel lectures, physiology or medicine, 1901–1921. London: World Scientific Publishing Co; 1999. p. 189–217.
9. Franklin RE, Gosling RG. Evidence for 2-chain helix in crystalline structure of sodium deoxyribonucleate. Nature. 1953;172:156–7. https://doi.org/10.1038/172156a0.
10. Franklin RE, Gosling RG. Molecular configuration in sodium thymonucleate. Nature. 1953;171:740–1. https://doi.org/10.1038/171740a0.
11. Wilkins MH, Stokes AR, Wilson HR. Molecular structure of deoxypentose nucleic acids. Nature. 1953;171:738–40. https://doi.org/10.1038/171738a0.
12. Watson JD, Crick FH. Molecular structure of nucleic acids; a structure for deoxyribose nucleic acid. Nature. 1953;171:737–8. https://doi.org/10.1038/171737a0.
13. Pauling L, Corey RBA. Proposed structure for the nucleic acids. Proc Natl Acad Sci U S A. 1953;39:84–97. https://doi.org/10.1073/pnas.39.2.84.
14. Goodman SN, Fanelli D, Ioannidis JPA. What does research reproducibility mean? Sci Trans Med. 2016;8:341ps312–341ps312. https://doi.org/10.1126/scitranslmed.aaf5027.
15. Casadevall A, Fang FC. Reproducible science. Infect Immun. 2010;78:4972–5. https://doi.org/10.1128/IAI.00908-10.
16. Voelkl B, Vogt L, Sena ES, et al. Reproducibility of preclinical animal research improves with heterogeneity of study samples. PLoS Biol. 2018;16:e2003693–e2003693. https://doi.org/10.1371/journal.pbio.2003693.
17. Ward JM, Schofield PN, Sundberg JP. Reproducibility of histopathological findings in experimental pathology of the mouse: a sorry tail. Lab Anim. 2017;46:146–51. https://doi.org/10.1038/laban.1214.
18. Brinster RL, Chen HY, Trumbauer M, et al. Somatic expression of herpes thymidine kinase in mice following injection of a fusion gene into eggs. Cell. 1981;27:223–31. https://doi.org/10.1016/0092-8674(81)90376-7.
19. Gordon JW, Ruddle FH. Integration and stable germ line transmission of genes injected into mouse pronuclei. Science. 1981;214:1244–6. https://doi.org/10.1126/science.6272397.
20. Costantini F, Lacy E. Introduction of a rabbit beta-globin gene into the mouse germ line. Nature. 1981;294:92–4. https://doi.org/10.1038/294092a0.
21. Dobrowolski P, Fischer M, Naumann R. Novel insights into the genetic background of genetically modified mice. Transgenic Res. 2018;27:265–75. https://doi.org/10.1007/s11248-018-0073-2.
22. Doudna JA, Charpentier E. Genome editing. The new frontier of genome engineering with CRISPR-Cas9. Science. 2014;346:1258096. https://doi.org/10.1126/science.1258096.
23. Tuttle AH, Philip VM, Chesler EJ, et al. Comparing phenotypic variation between inbred and outbred mice. Nat Methods. 2018;15:994–6. https://doi.org/10.1038/s41592-018-0224-7.
24. Lusis AJ, Yu J, Wang SS. The problem of passenger genes in transgenic mice. Arterioscler Thromb Vasc Biol. 2007;27:2100–3. https://doi.org/10.1161/ATVBAHA.107.147918.
25. Richter SH, Garner JP, Würbel H. Environmental standardization: cure or cause of poor reproducibility in animal experiments? Nat Methods. 2009;6:257–61. https://doi.org/10.1038/nmeth.1312.
26. Richter SH, Garner JP, Auer C, et al. Systematic variation improves reproducibility of animal experiments. Nat Methods. 2010;7:167–8. https://doi.org/10.1038/nmeth0310-167.
27. Richter SH, Garner JP, Zipser B, et al. Effect of population heterogenization on the reproducibility of mouse behavior: a multi-laboratory study. PLoS One. 2011;6:e16461–e16461. https://doi.org/10.1371/journal.pone.0016461.
28. European C. Commision recommendation of 18 June 2007 on guidelines for the accommodation and care of animals used for experimental and other scientific purposes. Off J Eur Union. 2007;2003
29. Mohamed AS, Fahmy SR, Soliman AM, et al. Effects of 3 rodent beddings on biochemical measures in rats and mice. J Am Assoc Lab Anim Sci. 2018;57:443–6. https://doi.org/10.30802/AALAS-JAALAS-18-000023.
30. Pain terms: a list with definitions and notes on usage. Recommended by the IASP Subcommittee on Taxonomy. Pain. 1979;6:249.

31. Raja SN, Carr DB, Cohen M, et al. The revised International Association for the Study of Pain definition of pain: concepts, challenges, and compromises. Pain. 2020; https://doi.org/10.1097/j.pain.0000000000001939.
32. Greek R, Menache A. Systematic reviews of animal models: methodology versus epistemology. Int J Med Sci. 2013;10:206–21. Review. https://doi.org/10.7150/ijms.5529.
33. Kilkenny C, Browne WJ, Cuthill IC, et al. Improving bioscience research reporting: the ARRIVE guidelines for reporting animal research. PLoS Biol. 2010;8:e1000412. https://doi.org/10.1371/journal.pbio.1000412.
34. Leung V, Rousseau-Blass F, Beauchamp G, et al. ARRIVE has not ARRIVEd: Support for the ARRIVE (Animal Research: Reporting of in vivo Experiments) guidelines does not improve the reporting quality of papers in animal welfare, analgesia or anesthesia. PLOS One. 2018;13:e0197882. https://doi.org/10.1371/journal.pone.0197882.
35. Percie du Sert N, Hurst V, Ahluwalia A, et al. The ARRIVE guidelines 2.0: updated guidelines for reporting animal research. PLoS Biol. 2020;18:e3000410. https://doi.org/10.1371/journal.pbio.3000410.
36. Smith AJ, Clutton RE, Lilley E, et al. Improving animal research: PREPARE before you ARRIVE. BMJ. 2018;360:k760. https://doi.org/10.1136/bmj.k760.

Rodent Genetics

Fernando Benavides and Jean-Louis Guénet

Abstract

This chapter is an overview of the current and growing knowledge of the genetics of laboratory rodents, specifically the mouse (*Mus musculus*) and the rat (*Rattus norvegicus*), the two main species used in biomedical research. We present basic information about Mendelian genetics and on the structure of the mouse and rat genomes, including the protein-coding DNA and the more intriguing non-coding DNA sequences, abundant in repetitive DNA, transposable elements and different types of genetic polymorphisms. Experiments should be performed with carefully designed and approved protocols, including the use of genetically defined animals. Thus, in this chapter we discussed the different types of genetically standardized laboratory strains and the aspects related to their genetic quality control. We also present the different types of genetically altered mice and rats, including spontaneous and chemically induced mutations, random transgenesis, targeted mutagenesis using embryonic stem cells and the novel genome editing techniques. It is very important for the veterinarians and technicians in charge of animal facilities, as well as for researchers and students using mouse and rat models that they have an available up-to-date information devoted to the genetics of these species.

Keywords

aboratory rodents · Mice · Rats · Inbred strains · Genetic polymorphisms · Quality control · Transgenesis · Genome edition

1 Introduction to Mendelian Genetics and Genomics

1.1 Genes, Alleles and Their Interactions

Several years after Gregor Mendel's seminal publication *Experiments on Plant Hybridization* was published (1866), Hugo de Vries published *Intracellular Pangenesis* (1889) in which he recommended the word *pangens* be used to specify Mendel's 'hereditary particles'. The Danish biologist Wilhelm Johannsen proposed in 1909 that the (Danish) word *gen* be used to describe the units of heredity. Almost at the same time,

F. Benavides (✉)
Department of Epigenetics and Molecular Carcinogenesis, The University of Texas MD Anderson Cancer Center, Smithville, TX, USA
e-mail: fbenavid@mdanderson.org

J.-L. Guénet
Institut Pasteur (Emeritus), Paris, France

© Springer Nature Switzerland AG 2021

J. M. Sánchez Morgado, A. Brønstad (eds.), *Experimental Design and Reproducibility in Preclinical Animal Studies*, Laboratory Animal Science and Medicine 1,
https://doi.org/10.1007/978-3-030-66147-2_2

Johannsen introduced the terms *phenotype* and *genotype*. William Bateson proposed the term *genetics* to describe the science dealing with *gens* (*genes*). Shortly after the confirmation that DNA was the molecular basis of inheritance (seminal work published by Avery, McCarty and MacLeod in 1944), the gene was defined in molecular terms as 'a segment of DNA of variable size encoding an enzyme'. This definition was revised to 'one gene, one polypeptide' when it was recognized that some proteins are not enzymes. With the completion of the first (draft) sequences of the human (2001), mouse (2002) and rat (2004) genomes and the confirmation that many genes are not translated into polypeptides, the definition of the gene changed again.

Today, a gene corresponds to a segment of DNA that is transcribed into RNA. Some RNA molecules, like messenger RNAs (mRNAs), are translated into polypeptides, whereas many others are not translated but nevertheless have important functions. Recently, information collected from the systematic analysis of a single transcriptome revealed that mammalian DNA is pervasively transcribed from both strands and that the proportion of DNA transcribed into RNA is much greater than expected. The same analysis also revealed that not all mammalian genes are easily identified in DNA; on the contrary, their limits are often difficult to delineate, with some small genes being nested inside the larger ones (e.g. inserted in the introns). Thus, it seems clear that the concept of the gene must be reconsidered and its definition reformulated. Nonetheless, we will work with the idea that a gene is a functional unit contained in a short DNA segment that is transcribed into RNA and whose inheritance can be followed experimentally generation after generation. Genes can be precisely localized on a specific chromosome using a variety of techniques, and this position defines its *locus* (plural *loci*), the Latin word for 'place'.

For decades, *genome* is referred to the collection of genes in a given species. Now, the concept includes both the genes (i.e. the coding sequences) and the sum of heterogeneous DNA intermingled with the genes. Thus, when we refer to the genome sequence, we are referring to the sequence of all nuclear DNA. The number of protein-coding genes in the mammalian genome is predicted to be 22,000 to 24,000 genes, on par with the 22,628 currently listed in the mouse GRCm38 assembly and the 22,250 in the rat Rnor_6.0 assembly. However, some genes vary in copy number across different strains, and even between individuals, with many being non-functional, whereas others are present in only some strains (or species) and absent in others. Such gene variations complicate accurately evaluating organismal gene number. Predicting gene number becomes even more difficult given that multiple RNAs (coding and non-coding) can be transcribed from the same gene via *alternative splicing*, tremendously increasing the number and diversity of molecules potentially encoded in the genome. Obviously, it is the sum of these transcripts, not the raw number of genes that is important for defining the genome.

Most genes exist in alternative forms (variants) called *alleles*. The word 'allele' is an abbreviation of the ancient word *allelomorph*, which described the different forms of a gene. Formerly, the concept of alleles was tightly associated with mutations that produce phenotypes different from wild type (i.e. the version most commonly found in wild animals), for example, a different coat colour, a heritable skeletal defect or a debilitating neurological disease. The new version of the gene was called a *mutant allele*. The concept of the allele, like the gene, has changed over time so that now any alteration of DNA sequence within a gene is defined as a new allele, regardless of whether the change produces a phenotype.

The term *polymorphism* can refer to many things, including the alleles present at a specific locus or to all loci of a strain or species. The whole collection of alleles segregating in a given population represents what geneticists call the *genetic polymorphism*. In the mouse, the gene encoding tyrosinase (*Tyr*), an enzyme that is instrumental for the synthesis of the pigment melanin, was one of the first (if not the first) genes to be identified based on a variation in coat colour. At the *Tyr* locus, the wild-type allele encodes a functional tyrosinase, but many mutant alleles encode non-functional enzymes resulting in albinism. Over

120 different mutations have been identified at the *Tyr* locus, some of them affecting coat colour (e.g. chinchilla, $Tyr^{c\text{-}ch}$; extreme dilution, $Tyr^{c\text{-}e}$; and Himalayan, $Tyr^{c\text{-}h}$).

1.1.1 Dominance, Recessivity and Co-dominance

When the alleles at a given locus are identical on both chromosomes, the animal is *homozygous* for that allele. When the two alleles are different, the animal is *heterozygous*, and the phenotype will depend upon the interactions between the two alleles. To illustrate, we will again consider the *Tyr* gene in the mouse. *Tyr* has several alleles, some of which are non-functional, like Tyr^{c}. Tyr^{c}/Tyr^{c} mice are albino, but Tyr^{c}/Tyr^{+} heterozygotes are pigmented like wild mice because the mutant Tyr^{c} allele is *recessive* to the *dominant* wild-type allele (Tyr^{+} or sometimes only +). In this case, the lack of functional tyrosinase due the presence of the Tyr^{c} allele is completely compensated for by a single copy of the wild-type allele.

Other *Tyr* alleles have less dramatic effects than Tyr^{c} on the synthesis of melanin. In many cases the mice are pigmented, although always less than or differently from the wild type. Mice homozygous for the chinchilla allele $Tyr^{c\text{-}ch}$ have a diluted coat colour, but mice homozygous for the Himalayan allele $Tyr^{c\text{-}h}$ have a remarkable pattern of pigmentation. They have light-ruby eyes and a coat that is mainly white with only the tip of the nose, tip of the ears and the tail pigmented normally, like Siamese cats. This pattern results from the $Tyr^{c\text{-}h}$ allele-encoded, thermo-labile tyrosinase being active only in the colder parts of the body, where the temperature is below 35 °C. With so many *Tyr* alleles available, one could breed a wide variety of mice heterozygous or homozygous for the different alleles to find that the normal allele (Tyr^{+}) is dominant over all other alleles. However, if the mice were graded based on decreasing coat colour intensity for all possible combinations of the Tyr^{+}, $Tyr^{c\text{-}ch}$, $Tyr^{c\text{-}e}$ and Tyr^{c} alleles, we would observe an almost continuous gradient of pigmentation from wild type to albino. Therefore, dominance and recessivity must be considered only in the context of a specific allele pair.

Semi-dominance (sometimes referred to as *incomplete dominance*) describes mutant alleles that produce heterozygotes with a phenotype that is different from and often intermediate to both kinds of homozygotes. A typical example is the $Kit^{W\text{-}f}$ allele. $Kit^{W\text{-}f}/+$ heterozygous mice have a light grey coat with a white spot on the belly and on the forehead, whereas $Kit^{W\text{-}f}/Kit^{W\text{-}f}$ homozygous mice are extensively spotted. Amazingly, the tails of these mice perfectly characterize the situation; the tail is completely pigmented from the base to the tip in wild-type mice, half-pigmented in heterozygotes and unpigmented in homozygotes.

Another type of allelic interaction common in mammals is *co-dominance*. Co-dominance occurs when the two alleles at a given locus are both expressed in the heterozygote to create a unique phenotype. Most genetics textbooks illustrate the concept of co-dominance using the AB blood groups in humans, where AB heterozygotes have a phenotype in which both the A and B antigens are expressed on red blood cells. Blood groups homologous to the human AB system do not exist in the mouse or rat, but nearly all alleles that encode forms of the same protein that vary by charge are co-dominantly expressed.

Other allelic interactions have been discovered by studying the process such as sex determination. In mammalian species, males have only one X-chromosome and therefore are *hemizygous* for all genes carried by this chromosome, and all are fully expressed. In females, X-inactivation, a mechanism of dosage compensation causes most X-linked genes to be functionally haploid; only one copy of each gene is transcribed, and the other copy is switched off. The choice of which allele to inactive is usually a random process. In mammals, a few genes in the so-called pseudo-autosomal region of the X-chromosome are not inactivated and behave as autosomal genes [1]. Notably, certain autosomal regions, sometimes reduced to one or a few genes, are also functionally haploid, expressing the allele(s) inherited from only one of the two parents, a phenomenon called genomic imprinting, also resulting from epigenetic mechanisms [2, 3].

1.1.2 Epistasis and Pleiotropy

Many phenotypic traits are controlled by more than one gene, and a single gene can contribute to the phenotypic expression of one or several other genes. *Epistasis* occurs when the phenotypic expression of gene (or allele) *A* depends on the presence of one or more specific alleles (*B*, *C*, *D*) at other loci to modify or suppress the classical phenotype of gene *A*. In other words, epistasis is an interaction between nonallelic genes in which one gene suppresses or enhances the expression of another. The gene that is expressed is *epistatic* over the other genes, which are themselves *hypostatic*. The genes that determine coat colour offer simple, didactic examples. Exploiting the variety of alleles at the five major loci governing mouse coat colour (agouti, *A*; tyrosinase, *Tyr*; brown, *Tyrp1*; dilute, *Myo5a*; and pink-eyed dilution, *Oca2*), one can generate a large collection of mice with a wide array of coat colours. However, sometimes the effects of a given mutant allele cannot be observed in the presence of another particular allele. For example, a mouse with a non-agouti brown coat colour (genotype *a/a*; $Tryp1^b/Tyrp1^b$) would appear 'chocolate', except in the presence of two copies of the Tyr^c mutant allele (homozygous) that causes the mouse to be albino. In this case, the Tyr^c allele exhibits an epistatic interaction with all other coat colour genes because without tyrosinase there is no pigment.

Pleiotropy describes a common genetic phenomenon in which a mutant allele influences multiple phenotypic traits. In fact, if we carefully analyse mutants with deleterious phenotypes, we would discover that almost all of them exhibit a range of altered phenotypes. The yellow allele (A^y) was identified because of its beautiful yellow coat colour, but these mutants are also slightly diabetic, exhibit liver hypertrophy and often become obese and sterile following the first few months of life [4]. Compared to normal mice, these mice are also more susceptible to several kinds of tumours and are more aggressive. Given that the products of most genes have multiple functions, pleiotropy is more a rule than an exception. It simply means that the gene in question codes for a product that is used by various cell types, signals to multiple targets or regulates more than one pathway, as a transcription factor might.

1.1.3 Penetrance and Expressivity

Penetrance is a term used to express the fraction (percentage) of individuals of a given genotype that effectively exhibits the expected phenotype. For example, if a particular dominant mutation has 80% penetrance, then 80% of the mice carrying the mutant allele will develop the phenotype, and 20% will look normal. A genotype exhibits variable *expressivity* when individuals with that genotype differ in the extent to which they express the phenotype. One example illustrating the concept of expressivity and differentiating it from the concept of penetrance (which is not always easy) is the case of spotting in cattle. When observing an herd of Holstein Friesian cattle, one may notice that, although all the cows are spotted (penetrance is 100%), the ratio of black/white is highly variable from one animal to the next. The spotting is highly variable in shape (no surprise) and extent (which is more surprising). Similarly, rodents can also display a large amount of phenotypic variations among individuals with the same genotype, for example, the case of a mutation in the brachyury gene (*T*) which encodes a transcription factor important for proper formation of the tail and the $Ednrb^s$ spotting mouse mutation (Fig. 1).

The causes of variable penetrance and expressivity are not well understood. In the mouse and rat, one can study the phenotypic expression of the same mutation in different genetic backgrounds and note more or less consistent differences, indicating the influence of a genetic component (modifier genes). However, one can also observe phenotypic variations in animals having exactly the same mutation in exactly the same genetic background – meaning that nongenetic factors, such as epigenetic and environmental factors, also influence penetrance and expressivity.

1.2 Genomes and Genetic Variation

The sizes of the laboratory mouse (*Mus musculus* strain C57BL/6J) and rat (*Rattus norvegicus* mixed female BN and male SHR) genomes are 2.7 Gbp and 2.8 Gbp, respectively [5, 6]. Both genomes are 14% smaller than the human genome

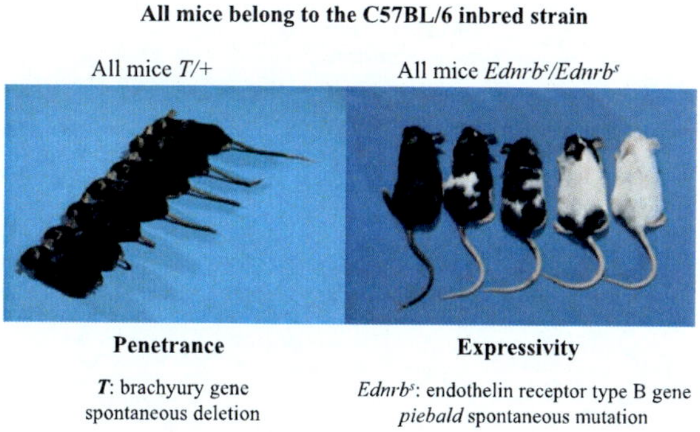

Fig. 1 Penetrance and expressivity. The picture illustrates two major characteristics of the phenotypic expression of mutant alleles in mammalian species. In the present case, all seven mice on the left panel are affected by the same mutation (*brachyury* (T), with 100% penetrance) affecting the length of the tail, but they exhibit great variations in the phenotype, with some mice (top of the picture) with a normal-looking tail. On the right-hand side, all mice exhibit a spotted coat with wide variations in expressivity (mutation *Ednrb^s*). The penetrance characterizes the fraction of individuals of a given genotype that actually shows a particular phenotype irrespective of the degree of its expression. The expressivity characterizes the phenotypic variation among individuals having the same genotype. It is now well established that modifier genes influence the phenotypic expression, but these genes cannot explain all the variations, since these deviations are also observed in inbred strains

(3.1 Gbp) likely due to a higher rate of deletions in the mouse lineage [5]. Such sequence loss indicates that the mammalian genome is a mosaic of sequences of dissimilar importance. This suggestion is supported by the decades-old observations of cytogeneticists who found that certain large chromosomal deletions (i.e. visible through the optical microscope) did not affect the phenotype of mice homozygous for the deletion. Below, we will briefly review the different kinds of DNA sequences within the mammalian genome. Besides the genome sequence of C57BL/6J, deep genome sequencing and variation analysis has been now finalized for new mouse inbred strains, including wild-derived strains [7, 8]. These new sequences show that, remarkably, genetically similar inbred strains can sometimes show divergent phenotypes and that extensive strain-specific haplotype variation still exists in these supposedly completely inbred genomes. These new genomes not only improve the mouse reference genome but also help in the discovery of unknown genes.

Approximately 5% of mammalian genome contains highly conserved sequences, of which no more than 1.5% encode proteins (one estimate is 1.27% for the mouse genome and 1.0% for the human genome) [9] (Fig. 2). The remaining 3.5% consists of sequences whose functions are only partially known but includes sequences important for regulating gene expression (e.g. DNA-binding sites), chromosome architecture and folding and binding to the mitotic spindle. Interestingly, some of these conserved non-coding sequences have been completely eliminated in mice without substantially affecting phenotype [10].

Annotation of the mouse and rat genomes (the process of identifying functional elements along the DNA sequence) is progressing thanks, in part, to the thousands of spontaneous and induced mutations. Yet, only 14,700 mouse genes have been functionally annotated based on the existence of one or more mutant alleles or through expression assays (MGI, October 2018). Because many genes are conserved in both sequence and function, genes identified in any one of the human, mouse or rat genomes may also aid in the annotation of related genes in the other species. For example, approximately 99% of mouse genes have a human orthologue. This and other examples clearly justify the 'comparative genomics' approach [11–13].

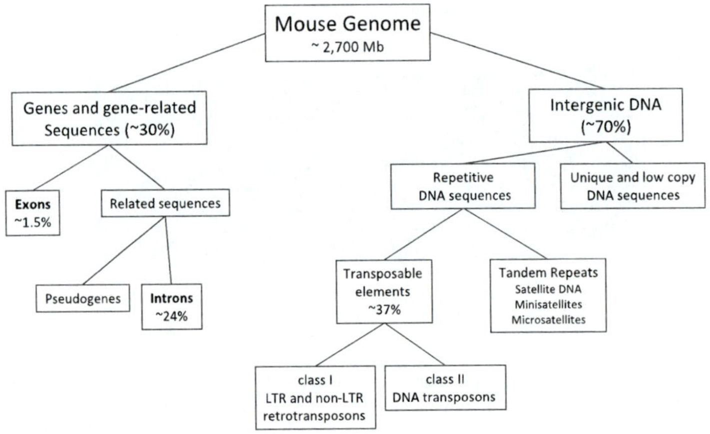

Fig. 2 Types of DNA in the mammalian genome. The graphic shows the different types of DNA sequences present in mammalian genomes, including rodents. It is estimated that only around 30% of the genome is represented by genes (protein-coding sequences) and gene-related sequences (e.g. introns, regulatory sequences and pseudogenes). On the other hand, the so-called intergenic DNA constitutes up to 70% of the genome. This non-coding DNA corresponds to different categories of repetitive and transposable sequences, together with single copy and low copy number sequences (see text for details). This DNA (inaccurately referred to as 'junk' DNA) is poorly known; however, many non-coding DNA sequences are highly conserved between mammals, most likely because they have important biological functions. At the same time, genetic variations in non-coding sequences have been widely used as tools in rodent genetics, including quality controls

1.2.1 Genes, Gene Families and Pseudogenes

Mouse and rat genes have an architecture similar to other mammalian genes, typically composed of coding exonic and non-coding intronic sequences flanked by additional canonical upstream and downstream sequences. The smallest gene known is 0.1 kbp and encodes t-RNA^{Tyr}. The biggest gene is 2.3 Mbp in mouse, rat and humans and encodes dystrophin (*Dmd*). Gene introns also vary in size, ranging from 0.5 kbp for the shortest intron to 30 kbp for the biggest *Dmd*, with an average intron size of 4.7 kbp. For exons, the average exon size is 300 bp with the shortest being only 9 bp (exon 2 of *MyoVIa*) and the longest being 7.6 kbp (exon 26 of *Apob*). The number of exons per gene varies from 1 to 314 with an average of 7.5 [14], and about 4000 genes have only one exon.

As in other species, mouse and rat genes are alternatively spliced, meaning that not all exons of a given gene are represented in all transcripts (mRNA) from that gene. Alternative splicing is a clever, evolutionarily conserved mechanism that allows more than one protein to be encoded by a single gene, based on the exons present in a particular transcript. This also means that the number of genes in an organism does not reflect the degree of genetic complexity of that organism. Instead, the total number of exons may provide a better estimate of complexity. Interestingly, interspecific comparisons indicate that although most exons in the mouse, rat and human genomes are strongly conserved, exons present only in alternatively spliced forms are less conserved and likely represent recent exon creation or loss events [15].

Interspecific comparisons of mouse and other mammalian genomes indicate that the mouse genes are *syntenic* with those of humans and rats. That is, most mouse genes are conserved in blocks, with the same linear arrangement as in the human or rat genomes. For example, when a hypothetical gene G_2 is flanked by genes G_1 and G_3 in mouse, there is a very high probability that the same linear order (G_1-G_2-G_3) is preserved in the other two species. This conservation of *synteny* (from the Greek, meaning 'on the same ribbon') helps validate candidate genes. It also aids in identifying duplications and/or deletions among species. For example, about 90% of the mouse and human genomes can be partitioned into regions of conserved synteny, reflecting the structural organization of the chromosome in the common ancestor. These genomes share about 350 segments of conserved synteny, with sizes ranging from 300 kbp to 65 Mbp.

In contrast to genes conserved across species, the mouse and rat genomes also contain rodent-specific genes. The majority of these belong to gene families associated with reproductive functions, exhibiting spermatid- or oocyte-specific expression, or with vomeronasal receptors [9, 16]. Some of these new genes originate from relatively recent duplication events in the mouse linage subsequent to its divergence from the rat, around 20 million years ago (http://www.timetree.org/). In comparison, the human genome (the primate lineage) has lost genes coding for olfactory and vomeronasal receptors [17].

The mammalian genome contains a great number of sequences that resemble protein-coding genes but are not. These *pseudogenes* may be processed or unprocessed. Processed pseudogenes originate from the retro-transcription of messenger RNAs back into the genomic DNA in more or less random locations. They lack introns and contain mutations, including frameshift mutations and premature stop codons, indicating that they are not transcribed. Unprocessed pseudogenes arise from either the tandem duplication of a gene during DNA replication or are degenerated genes that become inactive and are no longer under selection. There are roughly 12,000 pseudogenes in the mouse genome assembly (Mouse Reference GRCm38), but identifying them is often difficult. Synonymous mutations, those that will not modify the amino acid sequence, occur at the same frequency in genes and pseudogenes, whereas non-synonymous mutations are rare in functional genes. The ratio of the number of non-synonymous substitutions to the number of synonymous substitutions in orthologous genes is a strong evidence for deciding whether a 'gene' is a true gene or a pseudogene.

As mentioned, the majority of the mammalian genome consists of non-coding sequences. However, even some non-coding sequences are highly conserved between humans and rodents, likely because they have important biological functions [18]. The function of these conserved non-coding sequences is the subject of intense research, and it has been suggested that these sequences may be associated with certain diseases [19]. However, a significant portion of non-coding DNA is not conserved and therefore exhibits a higher degree of genetic variation (polymorphism) than conserved non-coding DNA.

1.2.2 Repetitive DNA Sequences

Repetitive DNA sequences are non-coding sequences present in multiple copies within mammalian genomes. Depending on the number of repeats, they are classified as moderately or highly repetitive DNA sequences. The latter include tandem and interspersed repeats. Interspersed repeats are derived from transposable elements, as explained in Sect. 1.2.3. Tandem repeats form when multiple copies of a motif are adjacent to each other in the genome. Depending on the number of nucleotides in the motif, these repeats are categorized as *satellite* DNA (between 120 and 250 nucleotides), *minisatellites* (between 10 and 60 nucleotides) and *microsatellites* (between 2 and 6 nucleotides). Polymorphisms result from variations in the number of tandem repeats within a locus and allow different alleles to be distinguished. In the mouse, satellite DNA comprises about 5% of the genome with major satellite repeats being 6 Mb long and located pericentrically and minor satellite repeats being from 500 kb to 1.2 Mb long and located in the centromere [20]. Minisatellite loci, also known as variable number tandem repeats (VNTRs), are 5–10 kb in size, extremely abundant and distributed throughout the mammalian genome [21]. These highly polymorphic loci were used as genetic markers in the late 1980s, particularly in human studies. They were also the basis for the famed DNA fingerprinting that revolutionized forensic science [22]. However, even though minisatellites were used in a few mouse linkage studies and for the genetic monitoring of inbred strains (isogenic individuals within an inbred strain share the same band pattern) [23–25], the use of DNA fingerprinting in genetic monitoring was quickly surpassed by the use of microsatellite makers. Microsatellites are very abundant (hundreds of thousands of copies per genome), extremely polymorphic and widely distributed throughout the genomes of animals and plants. Since the early 1990s, microsatellites have been ideal genetic markers because their analysis is simple, affordable and highly reliable [2]. Microsatellites are valuable for genome scans in linkage studies and background characterization of mouse and rat inbred strains [26, 27]. The use of microsatellites for genetic quality control is described in Sect. 4.

1.2.3 Copy Number Variations, Indels, Transposable Elements and SNPs

Although deletions, insertions and other large genomic rearrangements have been known since the 1980s, over the last decades, there has been an increasing interest in the study of segmental duplications and copy number variations (CNVs). CNVs are structural variants that result in copy number changes in a specific chromosomal region. As a consequence, certain large DNA segments (from 1 kb to several Mb and with more than 90% sequence conservation) can vary in copy number when compared with a reference genome, with other individuals of the same species or between inbred strains. Most importantly, CNVs are thought to affect gene expression (altering transcript dosage) and phenotypic variability in genetic diseases (e.g. affecting the penetrance of the trait) [28]. This can be particularly relevant given that the genomes of two randomly selected individuals may differ by at least 1%, mainly due to CNVs and SNPs. In the mouse, approximately 100 genomic regions harbour CNVs across the 19 autosomes, ranging in size from 20 kb to 2 Mb [29–31]. The change in gene dosage associated with these CNVs could easily explain their involvement in phenotypic variation in the mouse [32].

Transposable elements (TEs), found in virtually all eukaryotes, are genomic DNA sequences that move from location to location and exist as interspersed, repetitive DNA sequences. TEs can be inserted into different locations through DNA recombination, and after many generations, the repeated sequence can spread over various regions. There are two classes of TEs: class I, composed of long terminal repeats (LTRs) and non-LTR retrotransposons, which transpose via an RNA intermediate in a 'copy and paste' fashion, and class II, composed of DNA transposons, further divided into subclasses 1 and 2, which use a 'cut and paste' mechanism that does not involve an RNA intermediate [33, 34]. LINEs (long interspersed nuclear elements) and SINEs (short interspersed nuclear elements) are among the most studied class I non-LTR retrotransposons.

LINEs are autonomous retrotransposons and include the family of LINE-1 (L1) sequences, the most active non-LTR element identified in mammalian genomes, with 100,000 copies per haploid genome. SINEs are non-autonomous retrotransposons with repeated motifs of approximately a few hundreds of base pairs. Common examples are the Alu sequences in humans and the B1 and B2 sequences in mice, rats and other rodents [35]. In evolutionary terms, these interspersed sequences are classified as linage-specific (added to the mouse or rat genomes after the divergence from a common ancestor with other rodents) or ancestral (before the divergence). It is estimated that linage-specific sequences make up 32% of the mouse genome, compared with 24% in the human genome. In contrast, ancestral sequences represent only 5% of the mouse genome, compared with 22% of the human genome [36].

The nature of the TE-host relationship (e.g. parasitism, symbiosis or commensalism) and the role of TEs in disease and evolution have been debated extensively. There are several reports of human diseases caused by L1-driven insertional mutagenesis [35], but compared to endogenous retrovirus insertions, LINE- and SINE-related pathologies are less common in mice [37]. Even though the role of TEs in the evolution of vertebrate genomes remains controversial, these mobile elements can facilitate sequence-mediated chromosomal rearrangements that can potentially generate new gene regulatory sites [38]. Finally, these transposable elements have made pathways to new germline mutagenesis systems, such as Sleeping Beauty and PiggyBac, in the mouse and other mammals [39, 40]. This section would not be complete without mentioning endogenous retroviruses. Retroviral infections have also shaped the rodent genome. Endogenous retrovirus expression has been associated with both physiological function and disease [41]. In the mouse, a classic example of an endogenous retrovirus acting as a mutagen is the insertion into the hairless (*Hr*) gene creating the hairless (*hr*) allele [42]. Here, the insertion affects a gene splicing event and results in a hairless phenotype.

Although single nucleotide polymorphisms (SNPs) have been known for many years, their use in linkage and genome-wide association studies has rapidly expanded more recently. A SNP (pronounced 'snip') is a single nucleotide change identified by comparing the genomes of individuals of the same species or inbred strains (Fig. 3). SNPs are the most abundant genetic variation and are present in both coding and non-coding sequences. In coding sequences, non-synonymous SNPs create an amino acid change, whereas synonymous SNPs do not. Nonsense SNPs introduce a premature stop codon. Almost all SNPs are bi-allelic; only two variants segregate in a population (e.g. homozygous G/G or T/T or heterozygous G/T). In humans, the frequency of certain SNPs varies between populations, that is, a SNP allele can be common in one geographical or ethnic group and atypical in another [43]. Inbred mouse and rat strains possess long segments of DNA with either extremely high (40 SNPs per 10 kb) or extremely low (0.5 SNPs per 10 kb) levels of polymorphism, creating SNP-poor and SNP-rich genomic segments [36, 44]. Nonetheless, several SNP panels, with markers evenly distributed across the mouse and rat genome, have been developed [45–47]. The use of SNPs for genetic quality control will be presented in Sect. 4.

1.2.4 Functional Annotation of the Mouse Genome

As discussed earlier, the massive size and heterogeneous sequence structure of the mammalian genome makes it difficult to analyse. Some elements are repeated, some are unique and some are present but not essential. To make sense of the bulk of available sequence data, creating and improving the current reference gene annotation that identifies and describes gene structures are essential.

Gene annotation procedures are largely computational but are continually refined manually. We believe that annotation efforts should concentrate on the myriad of genomic transcripts (tRNA, rRNA, shRNA, miRNAs, snoRNAs, lncRNA, etc.) rather than genomic sequence per se. Both the GENCODE and FANTOM projects are essential to the process. The GENCODE project (https://www.gencodegenes.org/mouse/) produces comprehensive gene annotation for the reference mouse genome [48]. The FANTOM consortium (Functional Annotation of the Mammalian Genome), at RIKEN in Yokohama, has collected and sequenced 103,000 full-length mouse cDNAs [49]. The FANTOM project has been fundamental; it improved estimates of the total number of genes (and their alternative transcript isoforms) in the mouse, expanded our knowledge of gene families and revealed that a large fraction of the *transcriptome* is non-coding. Currently, tissue-specific expression of genes is being catalogued; consequently, it is already possible, for example, to make an exhaustive inventory of those genes that are expressed in the brain at a particular embryonic day [50] (see the Eurexpress Atlas at http://www.eurexpress.org/ee/).

Readers seeking more detailed genomic information can consult the Mouse Genome Informatics (MGI) resource [51], an international database that provides integrated genetic, genomic and biological data. The MGI consortium (http://www.informatics.jax.org) coordinates several databases and resources, including the Mouse Phenome Database (MPD), the Mouse Genome Database (MGD), the Gene Expression Database (GXD), the Mouse Tumor Biology Database (MTB), the Gene Ontology Project (GO), MouseMine, the International Mouse Strain Resource (IMSR), Cre recombinase activity data, on-line books and information regarding standard nomenclature. The MGI-LIST is a forum for topics in mouse genetics and MGI news updates. It is an active, moderated, email-

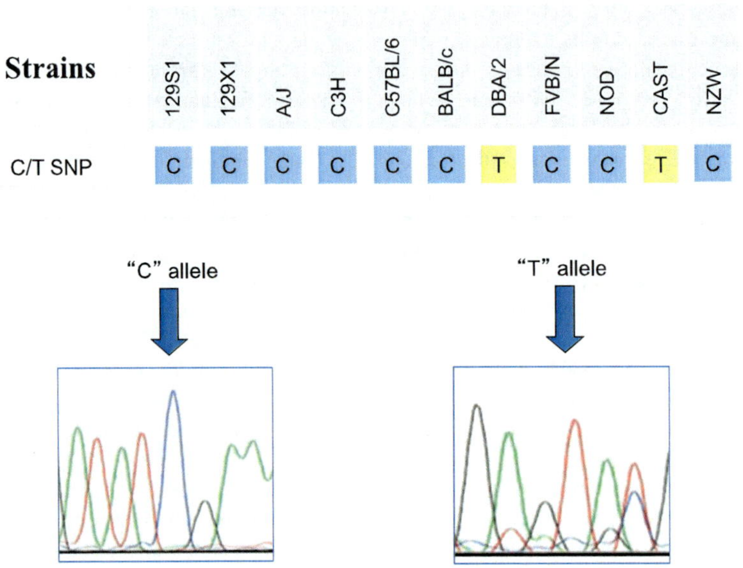

Fig. 3 Single nucleotide polymorphisms (SNPs). SNPs are discrete DNA sequence variations occurring when a single nucleotide in the genome differs between members of the same species. These SNPs are common and they are scattered throughout the genome of all species. They result from random point mutations occurring at a constant rate during evolution, either in the coding regions or in between genes, and they are inherited like a Mendelian trait. In the mouse genome, they are very unevenly distributed along the chromosomes with 'SNP-rich' and 'SNP-poor' regions depending on the phylogenetic origin of the chromosomal segment. This allows the determination of a SNP pattern, which is unique to a given strain and accordingly can be used for assessing strain purity. The upper panel represents a C/T SNP that is polymorphic between strains DBA/2 and CAST (homozygous for the 'T' allele) and other common inbred strains (homozygous for the 'C' allele). The lower panel presents DNA sequencing electropherograms showing the SNP (arrow)

based bulletin board for the scientific community supported by the MGD User Support group.

The Rat Genome Database (RGD, http://rgd.mcw.edu) provides the most comprehensive data repository and informatics platform related to the laboratory rat, one of the most important model organisms for disease studies. It includes (i) genomic variation, (ii) phenotypes and diseases, (iii) data related to the environment and experimental conditions and (iv) datasets and software tools that allow the user to explore and analyse the interactions among these and their impact on disease [52, 53].

2 Standardized Strains of Laboratory Rodents

Clarence C. Little, while at Harvard University, was the first to try to develop 'pure' mouse lines by inbreeding. Simultaneously, Helen D. King worked towards developing inbred rat lines at The Wistar Institute, eventually creating the WKA and PA inbred rat strains. The first mouse inbred strain, *dba*, was started in 1909 by Little through inbreeding mice homozygous for three recessive coat colour alleles (*d*, dilute; *b*, brown; and *a*, non-agouti). Similarly, Little established strain C57BL/6 in 1921 via a cross between two 'black' mice, female 57 and male 52, obtained from Miss Abbie Lathrop, a retired teacher and a mouse supplier from Massachusetts. A few other mouse strains were developed concurrently by other scientists, in particular Leonell C. Strong (C3H strain) at Cold Spring Harbor and Nadine Dobrovolskaia-Zavadskaia in Paris [54, 55]. In addition to these North American and European researchers, Japanese scientists established a number of colonies from fancy mice [56].

2.1 Inbred Strains and Substrains

According to the definition of the International Committee on Standardized Genetic Nomenclature for Mice, 'Strains can be termed *inbred* if they have been mated, brother × sister (sib-mating), for 20 or more consecutive generations, and individuals of the strain can be traced to a single ancestral pair at the 20th or subsequent generation'. However, it has been estimated that 24 generations of sib-mating are needed to reach a heterozygosity rate < 1% and 36 generations to reach complete fixation [57] and be regarded, for most purposes, as genetically identical (Fig. 4a). In practice, most of the mouse strains commonly used in research laboratories have undergone several tens of generations of brother × sister matings (indicated with an 'F', for filial), with some of the oldest lines surpassing 200 generations (e.g. in 2018 DBA/2 J reached F224). The definition of an inbred strain calls for some explanation. Individuals of the same inbred strain are genetically identical except for the sex-linked characters, and because of strict inbreeding, all of the individuals of a given strain have become *homozygous* at all loci that were segregating in the founder ancestors (the original or ancestral breeding pair). Each mouse is homozygous for the same allele, meaning that the maternal and paternal chromosomes are identical. This is also known as *autozygosity* because the two alleles are copies of the same ancestral allele. To describe this important characteristic, geneticists refer to the animals as being genetically identical or *isogenic*. The process leading to homozygosity by progressive allele loss (or fixation) is simply that, if an allele that was present at generation F_n is not transmitted to at least one member of the breeding pair at generation F_{n+1}, then it is permanently lost. In other words, as inbreeding progresses, alleles are constantly lost but never introduced (with the exception of de novo mutations), leading to both homozygosity and isogenicity (Fig. 4b) [2].

During inbreeding, the progression towards homozygosity is not linear. During the first few generations, many genes become homozygous, but fewer genes become homozygous in subsequent generations. Still, after 20 generations of inbreeding, no more than 2% of the loci that were heterozygous in the ancestors will still be segregating. This is because the genes becoming homozygous are linked and arranged linearly on chromosomes and the evolution towards homozygosity involves variable-sized blocks of DNA, not individual genes. This also explains why independent inbred strains carrying the same allele at a given locus have a greater chance of sharing the same short segment of neighbouring DNA (haplotype) flanking the allele in question. For example, if we analyse four classical albino strains (A, AKR, BALB/c and SJL), they are likely to be homozygous for the same short segment of chromosome 7 that flanks the albino mutation (*Tyr*^{c}), because the mutation shared by these strains results from an event that occurred well before the creation of these strains (i.e. identical by descent). In fact, all of the common albino rat strains share the same *Tyr* missense mutation, suggesting that they also share a common ancestor [58].

In most mammalian species, inbreeding of a natural population often has deleterious effects of variable intensity. These adverse manifestations are commonly referred to as *inbreeding depression*. Recent genetic studies suggest that inbreeding depression is caused predominantly by the presence of recessive deleterious mutations in natural populations that are progressively fixed in the homozygous state while inbreeding progresses. Alternative explanations, such as epistatic interactions, are also possible. Surprisingly, inbreeding depression is not a serious issue in some rodent species if the breeders stem from the same natural population of closely related individuals. Besides mice and rats, there are a few inbred strains from other rodents, like the Syrian hamster (*Mesocricetus auratus*) LSH/N strain, the guinea pig (*Cavia porcellus*) classical 2/N and 13/N strains and the gerbil (*Meriones unguiculatus*) MON/Tum strain.

The fact that all members of the same inbred strain are nearly genetically identical is the major reason why they have become so prevalent in biomedical research. Scientists working with the same inbred strain, but in different laboratories or at different time periods, can perform

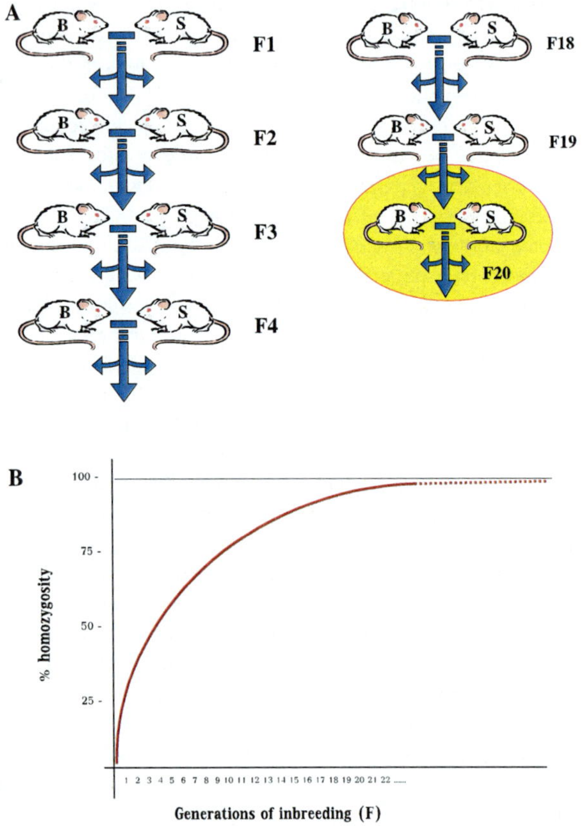

Fig. 4 Inbred strains. (**a**) This drawing represents schematically the breeding system that is commonly used to produce an inbred strain: mating a male and a female from the same litter (brother x sister) in successive generations. The uppercase letter F, followed by the number of generations, symbolizes each generation of inbreeding. When this number is not known, a question mark is often used; F? + 27, for example, would indicate that the number of brother x sister matings was not known when the strain was acquired, but 27 generations of unrelaxed inbreeding have been added since this time. According to the definition of the International Committee on Standardized Genetic Nomenclature for Mice, strains can be termed inbred if they have been mated (sib-mating) for 20 or more consecutive generations. (**b**) The curve was drawn based on the Fibonacci series and represents relatively faithfully the cumulated percentage of genes that have become fixed in the homozygous state as inbreeding progresses. From generation F5 onwards, this percentage is incremented by 19.6% at each generation

experiments where, by definition, variations in experimental results will not be due to differences in the genetic constitution of the animals. Finally, being isogenic, mice and rats of the same inbred strain are also *histocompatible* (or syngeneic). This means that they permanently accept tissue transplantations from any individual of the same strain (and sex). Researchers have used this peculiarity extensively, since it allows studying the fate of cells with an immunological function in different contexts (cellular cooperation), especially for the serial transplantation of cancer cell lines.

While inbreeding effectively eliminates a proportion of new mutant alleles, another fraction may become progressively fixed in the homozygous state (estimated between 10 and 30 mutations per generation) and replace the original allele, a process known as *genetic drift*. Genetic drift, a slow but unavoidable natural process, contributes inexorably to strain divergence and the generation of *substrains* when the same strain is propagated independently in different places [59]. Examples of mouse substrains are abundant, for example, there are 10 BALB/c substrains and 15 C57BL/6 substrains including the J and N substrains from The Jackson Laboratory and the National Institutes of Health, respectively. Some spontaneous mutations differentially segregate in these common substrains of C57BL/6, first separated in 1951. These include a retinal degeneration mutation in the *Crb1* gene (*Crb1*^{rd8}) and a non-synonymous SNP in the *Cyfip2* gene, present only in the N substrain, and a deletion in the *Nnt* gene, present only in the J substrain [60–62] (Table 1). The most comprehensive comparative phenotypic and genomic analysis of these popular substrains was recently published [63]. Notably, we can take advantage of genetic drift to accelerate the identification of causative mutations resulting in phenotypic differences between closely related substrains [62]. Considered as substrains (although we could argue that they are just related strains), the 129 family of strains is unusual for its high level of divergence, including different coat colours. For example, 129X1/SvJ and 129P3 strains are albino (or chinchilla), whereas 129S1, 129S4, 129S6 and 129S7 (*Still* group) are agouti [64] (Table 2) (for more information see http://www.informatics.jax.org/mgihome/nomen/strain_129.shtml). In the same way, many rat inbred strains present at least two substrains, for example, SHR has four substrains, including SHR/Ola and SHR/NCrl, and WKY and F344 have three substrains each. Substrain variability has been confirmed by sequencing for these rat substrains, with WKY showing the highest degree of substrain variation [65].

The insidious and unavoidable occurrence of new mutations in strains justifies the recommendation in the Guidelines for Nomenclature of Mouse and Rat Strains that inbreeding should never be relaxed. Inbreeding is inefficient in preventing mutations but helps eliminate a substantial proportion of new mutant alleles, thus preserving the genetic profile of a given strain. Similarly, the same international committee on nomenclature has stated that two strains with the same origin, but separated in different colonies for 20 or more generations (e.g. 12 generations in laboratory A and 10 in laboratory B), should be considered two different substrains and designated appropriately. The Institute of Laboratory Animal Resources (ILAR) maintains the International Laboratory Code Registry (https://www.nationalacademies.org/ilar/lab-code-database). Each lab code contains one to five letters and identifies the institute, laboratory or investigator that produced and/or maintains a particular strain [66].

Inbred strains are often described as artificial populations because their genetic constitution (isogenicity and homozygosity) has no natural equivalent. This description is supported by historical records indicating that modern mouse lines do not stem from a single subspecies of the *Mus* genus. Indeed, the polyphyletic origin (i.e. from different subspecies) of modern inbred strains has been substantiated by the complete high-resolution sequencing of the genomes of a large panel of inbred strains [45, 67]. Overall, the genomes of inbred laboratory mice are a mosaic of chromosomal regions with distinct subspecific origins. Recent estimates indicate classical inbred strains were predominantly derived from *M. m. domesticus* (94%), with variable contributions from *M. m. musculus* (5%) and *M. m. castaneus* (<1%) subspecies [68].

Over the last 30 years, a variety of strains derived from small groups of wild specimens trapped in well-defined geographical regions and belonging to well-characterized taxonomic groups, have been established in various laboratories [69]. With the increasing use of PCR amplification for the detection of genetic polymorphisms, the inbred strains derived from these wild populations have become valuable for gene mapping. Examples of theses strains are PWK/PhJ (*Mus m. musculus*), MOLD/RkJ (*Mus m. molossinus*) and CAST/EiJ (*Mus m. castaneus*). Special mention must be made of those derived from *Mus spretus* (SEG/Pas, SPRET/Ei and STF/Pas) because this species is one of the most distantly related to the laboratory strains that can still produce fertile hybrids with them. In contrast to laboratory

Table 1 Mutations present in the different C57BL/6 substrains

Substrain	Vendor	Affected Gene (mutant allele)						
		***Nnt* (*Nnt*^{B6J})**	***Crb1* (*Crb1*^{rd8})**	***Snca* (*Snca*^{del})^{1}**	***Mmrn1* (*Mmrn1*^{del})[a]**	***Nlrp12* (*Nlrp12*^{B6J})**	***Dock2* (*Dock2*^{Hsd})**	***Cyfip2* (*Cyfip2*^{B6N})**
C57BL/6J	JAX (C57BL/6J)	Mutated	Wild type (WT)	Wild type (WT)	Wild type (WT)	Mutated	Wild type (WT)	Wild type (WT)
	CRL (Europe) (C57BL/6JCrl)	Mutated	Wild type (WT)	Wild type (WT)	Wild type (WT)	Not tested	Supposedly WT	Wild type (WT)
	Janvier (C57BL/6JRj)	Mutated	Wild type (WT)	Wild type (WT)	Wild type (WT)	Not tested	Supposedly WT	Wild type (WT)
C57BL/6N	JAX (C57BL/6NJ)	Wild type (WT)	Mutated	Wild type (WT)	Wild type (WT)	Wild type (WT)	Wild type (WT)	Mutated
	CRL (C57BL/6NCrl)	Wild type (WT)	Mutated	Wild type (WT)	Wild type (WT)	Supposedly WT	Wild type (WT)	Mutated
	Envigo (C57BL/6NHsd)	Wild type (WT)	Mutated	Wild type (WT)	Wild type (WT)	Supposedly WT	Mutated	Mutated
	Taconic (C57BL/6NTac)	Wild type (WT)	Mutated	Wild type (WT)	Wild type (WT)	Supposedly WT	Wild type (WT)	Mutated
	Janvier (C57BL/6NRj)	Wild type (WT)	Mutated	Wild type (WT)	Wild type (WT)	Supposedly WT	Supposedly WT	Mutated
C57BL/6ByJ	JAX	Wild type (WT)	Wild type (WT)	Wild type (WT)	Wild type (WT)	Not tested	Not tested	Wild type (WT)
C57BL/6JEiJ	JAX	Wild type (WT)	Wild type (WT)	Wild type (WT)	Wild type (WT)	Not tested	Not tested	Wild type (WT)
C57BL/6JOlaHsd	Envigo	Wild type (WT)	Wild type (WT)	Mutated	Mutated	Not tested	Not tested	Not tested
C57BL/6JRccHsd	Envigo	Wild type (WT)	Wild type (WT)	Wild type (WT)	Wild type (WT)	Not tested	Not tested	Not tested
C57BL/6JBomTac	Taconic[b]	Wild type (WT)	Wild type (WT)	Wild type (WT)	Wild type (WT)	Not tested	Not tested	Not tested

[a]Del(6)*Snca*1Slab
[b]Y-chromosome mutation recently detected in C57BL/6JBomTac

Table 2 Current nomenclature and coat colour for the 129 families of strains

	Old nomenclature	New nomenclature	Abbreviation	Coat colour	ES cells
P (parent) group	129/ReJ	129P1/ReJ	129P1	White-bellied, pink-eyed, light chinchilla (light tan)	
	129/OlaHsd	129P2/OlaHsd	129P2	White-bellied, pink-eyed, light chinchilla (light tan)	E14, E14.1
	129/J	129P3/J	129P3	White-bellied, pink-eyed, light chinchilla or albino	EMS32
S (steel) group	129/SvImJ	129S1/SvImJ	129S1	White (or light)-bellied agouti	W9.5, CJ7
	129/SvPas	129S2/SvPas	129S2		D3, D3H
	129/SvJae	129S4/SvJae	129S4		AK7, RF8
	129/SvEvBrd	129S5/SvEvBrd	129S5		Lex-1, Lex-2
	129/SvEvTac	129S6/SvEvTac	129S6		IT2, KG1
	129/SvEvBrd	129S7/SvEvBrd	129S7		AB1, AB2.1
	129/SvEv	129S8/SvEv	129S8		
T (teratoma) group	129/Sv	129T1/Sv	129T1	White (or light)-bellied chinchilla	C1368
	129/SvEms	129T2/SvEms	129T2		
Contaminated (X)	129/SvJ	129X1/SvJ	129X1	White-bellied, pink-eyed, light chinchilla or albino	C1, C13

mice, all laboratory rat strains have been derived exclusively from *Rattus norvegicus* (no subspecies are recognized).

2.2 F1 Hybrids

F1 hybrids result from the cross of two inbred strains and are heterozygous at all loci for which the parental strains have different alleles but, like inbred strains, are genetically uniform (Fig. 5). They are also histocompatible and permanently accept tissue transplantations from either parental strain, from their littermates and from all their offspring; however, the parental strains will not

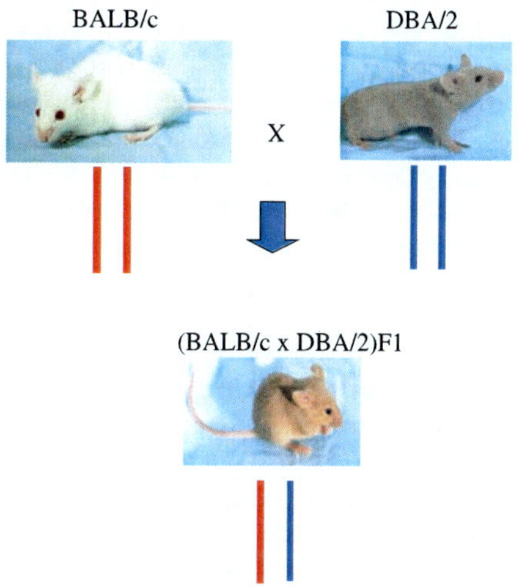

Fig. 5 Hybrid F1. This figure depicts the creation of hybrid F1 mice by intercrossing parental inbred strains BALB/c (albino, with coat colour loci AA;bb;cc;DD) and DBA/2 (diluted brown, with loci aa;bb;CC;dd). Below the mouse pictures, only one pair of chromosomes is shown as an example, with different colours representing the different backgrounds (although not all alleles will be polymorphic between the parental strains). Note that the hybrid F1 mouse obtained has the characteristic brown agouti 'cinnamon' coat colour (Aa;bb;Cc;Dd genotype). The standard nomenclature is (BALB/c x DBA/2)F1 (maternal strain listed first). Also acceptable is the abbreviated version CD2F1. Note that hybrid F1 mice are isogenic because they all receive the same maternal and paternal chromosomes. However, crossing F1 mice will generate hybrid F2 mice that are not isogenic because they will have recombinant chromosomes showing different patterns of BALB/c and DBA/2 alleles

accept a graft from the F1 hybrids. F1 mice and rats also exhibit *hybrid vigour* (heterosis), the opposite of inbreeding depression, making them the material of choice in many experimental protocols, e.g. in the protocols aimed at the production of genetically engineered animals. In this case, F1 hybrids are used because of their robust production of preimplantation embryos that are highly resistant to manipulation (e.g. DNA pronuclear microinjection). However, a major drawback is that their progeny (F2) is genetically heterogeneous when intercrossed, since the alleles at all polymorphic loci start segregating, due to meiotic recombination events, in the F1 gametes. Interstrain hybrids can also be used to generate genetically heterogeneous populations. For example, F1 hybrids between strain A and strain B (abbreviated ABF1 or AXBF1) can be crossed with F1 hybrids between strain C and strain D (CDF1 or CXDF1) to generate a four-way heterogeneous stock. In this case, the basic ingredients of the genetically heterogeneous stock (i.e. the original inbred strains A, B, C and D) are perfectly identified, and similar, but not identical stocks can be produced.

2.3 Co-isogenic, Congenic and Consomic Strains

When a mutation occurs in the breeding nucleus of an inbred strain, and the new mutant allele has replaced the original one (probability = 0.25), the new inbred strain differs from the original at only that one specific locus. If the new mutant is viable and the mutation does not impair fertility, the new strain can be propagated by mating brother to sister mutant mice or, preferably, by mating, at each generation, to a nonmutant mouse of the original inbred strain. The original strain and new mutant strain are *co-isogenic*. Co-isogenic strains are extremely useful for gene annotation because they allow a comparison of the phenotypes associated with the original and mutant alleles without the influence of genetic background. A large number of co-isogeneic strains are held in several mouse and rat repositories worldwide. Some common mouse strains, like C57BL/6, have several co-isogenic 'companion' strains segregating for a variety of allelic forms controlling, for example, coat colour. Co-isogenic C57BL/6-*Tyr*^{c} (albino) mice are commonly used to create easily recognizable chimeric mice derived from C57BL/6 ES cells injected into albino C57BL/6-*Tyr*^{c}/*Tyr*^{c} blastocysts [70]. In addition to coat colour, other mutations in co-isogenic strains may cause detrimental effects on development or metabolism. These strains have aided the analysis of developmental and metabolic pathophysiology by providing both the experimental animal and its control. However, co-isogenic strains have two major drawbacks inherent to their origin: (i) they arise mainly as a consequence of a rare mutation, and (ii), although they can emerge in any inbred strain, they generally emerge in a strain other than the one of primary interest.

Congenic strains are an alternative to co-isogenic strains with the advantage that any allele of interest may be moved (i.e. *introgressed*) into any inbred background. The *donor strain* carries the allele or chromosome region of interest (i.e. spontaneous, induced or targeted mutations, as well as transgenes) and is crossed to the *recipient* or *background* strain. The F1 offspring generated by crossing the donor and recipient strains are again backcrossed to the background strain, and the offspring that carry the allele of interest (i.e. the one originating from the donor strain) are repeatedly backcrossed to the background strain, typically for ten or more successive generations (Fig. 6), unless marker-assisted breeding is used (see Sect. 4.4). Ideally, the crosses initiate with a donor female and a recipient male. Then, the F1 mutant males will carry the correct Y-chromosome, and after mating to a recipient female, males of the N2 generation will carry the correct X- and Y-chromosomes of the recipient strain.

During the successive backcrosses, the chromosomes of the background strain progressively replace those of the donor, except for the one that carries the allele of interest. For this chromosome, the segment containing the selected allele is reduced in size only when a recombination event occurs that replaces a piece of chromosome of the donor for the homologous segment of the

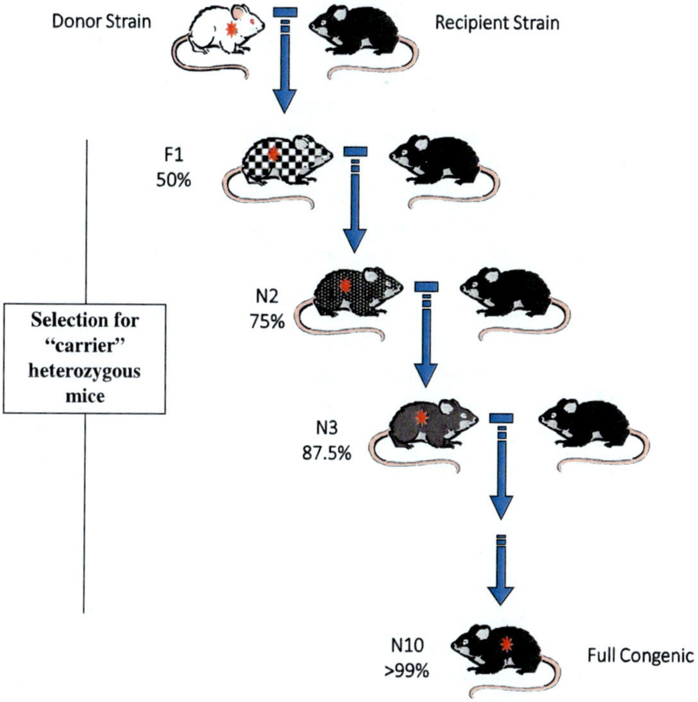

Fig. 6 Congenic strains. This scheme represents the successive steps in the establishment of a congenic strains. The first step is to cross a mouse from the donor strain (albino in the example) carrying the gene of interest (e.g. a transgene or a targeted null allele) with a mouse from the recipient inbred strain. At each generation a breeder carrying the gene of interest (*) is backcrossed to a partner of the recipient strain (black in this example). The letter 'N' is used to indicate the generation of backcross, starting with N2. The degree of grey colour is only to show how, after each backcross generation, the offspring have increasing amounts of the recipient genome. After each backcross generation, on the average, 50% of the genomic DNA of the donor strain is replaced by the equivalent proportion of genomic DNA of the (recipient) background strain

background strain. Over generations, such replacement events cause the chromosome carrying the targeted allele to gradually be 'eroded' on both sides of the allele in a nonlinear manner. Ultimately, the chromosomal segments flanking the selected locus generally remain associated with it, thus marking the basic difference between congenic and co-isogenic strains. In other words, while co-isogenic strains differ from the background strain at a single locus, congenic strains differ not only at the locus but also by a short chromosomal segment flanking the targeted locus, with the size of the flanking region being progressively reduced during backcrossing.

On average, at each generation, an equivalent proportion of the background strain replaces one half of the genome of the donor strain; thus the progression of genome substitution is given by the formula $1/2^N$, where N is the number of backcross generations. Theoretically, after ten backcross generations, only $1/2^{10}$ (1/1000) of the donor genome will remain in the congenic strain; however this is only an approximation. The actual percentage of donor genome replaced at each generation will vary. In addition, and as previously discussed, this estimate is valid only for those chromosomes lacking the allele of interest. For the chromosome bearing the allele of interest, the reduction in size is a much slower process. It is estimated that there is only a 10% chance that the segment carrying the introgressed gene will be smaller than 1 cM after a series of ten backcrosses. This is not negligible: on average, 1 cM (1.8 Mbp) of the mouse genome will contain dozens of genes, depending on the region. Congenic strains have been used extensively since the early days of mouse genetics and are still used as tools for the analysis of quantitative (complex) traits. It is precisely by developing such strains that George D. Snell and his colleagues from The Jackson Laboratory were able to elucidate the genetic determinism of histocompatibility resulting in a Nobel Prize in 1980 to G.D. Snell, J. Dausset and B. Benacerraf.

Consomic strains, also called chromosome substitution strains (CSSs), are a variation on the congenic strain concept, but the introgressed DNA is a complete chromosome, rather than a piece of chromosome flanking a given gene [71]. These strains are useful for rapidly mapping phenotypic traits to a specific chromosome and for QTL analysis. QTLs, or quantitative trait loci, are chromosomal regions that influence a particular complex, multigenic/multifactorial phenotype (e.g. resistance or susceptibility to carcinogenesis). However, in consomic strains, small fragments of donor strain chromosomes might escape the selection process.

2.4 Recombinant Inbred Strains and Recombinant Congenic Strains

Recombinant inbred strains (RISs) are developed by crossing two parental inbred strains to generate F1 hybrids followed by intercrossing these F1 to generate F2s. Then, randomly chosen F2 animals are brother-sister mated over 20 or more generations to develop a group of related inbred strains (Fig. 7) [72]. A collection of RISs derived from the same parental strains form a set (also referred to as a panel). For example, the largest RIS mouse panel is currently C57BL/6 × DBA/2 (BXD) with more than 100 strains and thousands of measured phenotypes and typed genetic markers (see GeneNetwork at http://www.genenetwork.org/webqtl/main.py). RISs are true inbred strains (an 'immortal' resource), homozygous at all loci but with a unique, fixed combination of parental alleles in a 50:50 ratio (on average). For example, each strain of the set of 33 AXB-BXA strains, derived from the initial cross of a C57BL/6 mouse with a A/J mouse, carries either the B6 allele or the A allele at each genetic locus. By typing all of these allelic forms, one can establish a strain distribution pattern (SDP) for each strain, listing the collection of alleles inherited from either parental strain A or parental strain B6. High-resolution maps of some mouse RISs and CSSs are also available [57]. Sets of rat RISs have also been created between the LE/Stm and F344 inbred strains (LEXF) [73]. Overall, RISs have proven very helpful for gene mapping, particularly for the rapid regional assignment of microsatellites on a given chromosome. They have also been used to map QTLs involved in controlling behaviour (e.g. alcohol intake, etc.) and certain immunological responses.

Recombinant congenic strains (RCSs) resemble RISs in their genomic structure except that the proportion of the parental alleles in a given strain is not 50:50 but 75:25 or 87.5:12.5, depending on the set. RCSs are established by inbreeding mice of the first or second backcross generation onto the background strain. RCSs are helpful for identifying genes associated with polygenic inheritance, especially when the number of genes is high. For example, RCSs have been very helpful for unravelling the genetic determinism of colon cancer in the mouse [74]. Interspecific recombinant congenic strains (IRCSs) have also been developed from the parental strain C57BL/6JPas and SEG/Pas (*Mus spretus*) [75]. This set of strains has proven particularly useful for describing the genetic basis of some anatomical traits [76].

2.5 The Mouse Collaborative Cross

The *Collaborative Cross* (CC) is a variation on the RIS concept but with a much higher power of resolution and level of genetic diversity segregating in the panel [77, 78]. The CC is a randomized cross of eight inbred mouse strains that have been carefully selected by a panel of mouse geneticists

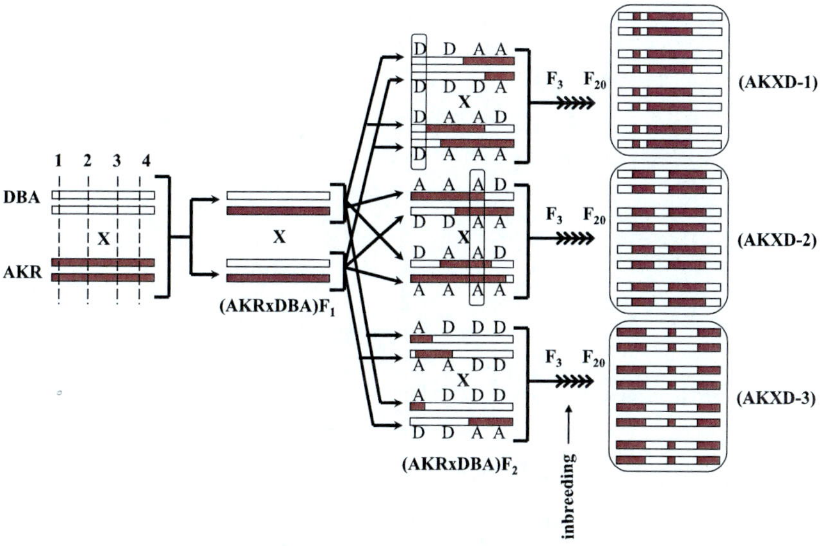

Fig. 7 Recombinant inbred strains. This diagram represents the creation of a set of three recombinant inbred strains (RIS) originated by intercrossing parental inbred strains DBA (D) and AKR (A) (only one pair of chromosomes is shown as an example). The positions of four hypothetical loci are indicated with dotted lines in the parental chromosomes (numbers 1–4). The rectangles show alleles that are already fixed (D or A) in some breeders at the F2 generation. After >20 generations of inbreeding, we obtained truly inbred strains that carry, on average, 50% of alleles from each parental strain. The boxes on the right represent the same chromosome pair showing identical patterns in four random mice from three different RIS (AKXD-1, AKXD-2 and AKXD-3). Individual RISs have a unique combination of loci derived by recombination of the alleles present in the original parental strains. Since RISs are inbred and each strain has a unique genotype, RISs have a number of advantages over F2 or backcross mouse populations as tools for mapping genes or quantitative trait loci (QTL)

(the Complex Trait Consortium). These strains consist of (i) three classical inbred strains (A/J, C57BL/6J, 129S1/SvImJ), (ii) two inbred strains afflicted by diabetes or obesity (NOD/LtJ and NZO) and (iii) three strains recently derived from wild progenitors (CAST/Ei, PWK and WSB/Ei). The eight strains are first crossed pairwise to make all (8 × 7 = 56) possible G1 parents; then all eight genomes are brought together in a series of crosses, and the offspring of these crosses are inbred for several generations (Fig. 8). Several hundreds of new inbred strains (recombinant for variable proportions of the original eight parental strains) are progressively becoming available. These strains can be used to make biologically relevant correlations among thousands of measured traits providing an unprecedented power of resolution [79, 80]. To increase mapping resolution power, investigators may also use the first-generation (F1) progeny from crosses of CC strains (designated CC-recombinant intercross or CC-RIX).

2.6 Outbred Stocks

Outbred stocks are populations of laboratory animals that are genetically heterogeneous and therefore radically different from those already discussed. Outbred stocks are 'closed populations (for at least four generations) of genetically variable animals that are bred to maintain maximum heterozygosity'. Compared with inbred strains, F1 hybrids and congenic strains, the genetic constitution of a given animal taken randomly from an outbred stock is not known a priori. Outbred

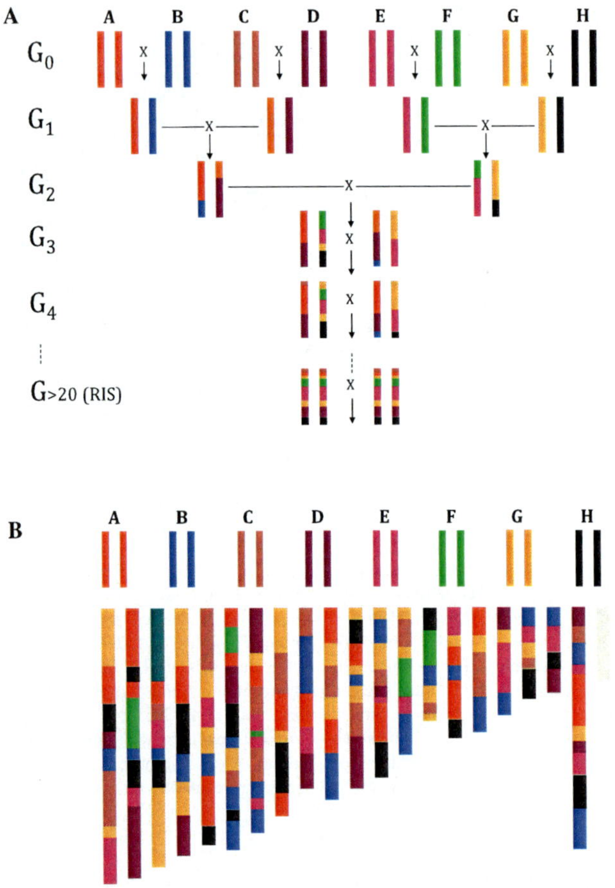

Fig. 8 The Collaborative Cross (CC). (**a**) This is a randomized cross of eight unrelated mouse inbred strains designed by members of the Complex Trait Consortium. The lines are first crossed pairwise to make all 56 possible G1 parents. A set of possible four-way crosses is performed, keeping Y-chromosome and mitochondrial balance. Finally, all eight genomes are brought together in G2:F1, and the offspring of this cross are inbred. The Collaborative Cross is a community resource that was initially designed for the purpose of mapping complex traits. (**b**) The initial previsions were to breed around 1000 inbred strains where all the alleles of the initial inbred strains would be associated in a wide and unique variety of combinations. Only one strain is represented in this illustration; other strains would be similar but with a different pattern of parental strain distribution. The pool of strains selected for the CC is constituted by five classical unrelated inbred strains (A/J, C57BL/6J, 129S1, NOD and NZO) and three wild-derived strains (CAST/Ei, PWK/PhJ and WSB/Ei)

stocks are normally bred according to a system that minimizes inbreeding and maintains a certain amount of heterozygosity in the population [81]. One frequently used outbreeding system is the 'rotational breeding' system described by Poiley [82]. Software for generating random mating schemes is freely available [83].

The degree of genetic heterogeneity in outbred colonies depends on colony history [84]. Heterogeneity can be very low, for example, as a consequence of genetic drift (or the bottleneck effect) or when the pool of breeders has been accidentally or intentionally reduced to a few individuals, as is common when starting a new breeding program with a small group of imported breeders. In contrast, genetic heterogeneity can be very high when the stock has been recently outcrossed. Although the methodology and results are not always made public, it is likely that reputable commercial breeders regularly monitor the polymorphisms segregating in their outbred stocks. Examples of outbred stocks of mice are ICR (CD-1), CFW and NMRI (all derived from the original 'Swiss' mice imported to the USA by Clara J. Lynch in 1926) and the non-Swiss CF-1 mice [84]. Examples of outbred rat stocks are Sprague Dawley (SD), Wistar (WI) and Long-Evans (LE). Outbred stocks of other laboratory rodents, including guinea pig, Syrian hamster, Chinese hamster (*Cricetulus griseus*), gerbil, cotton rat (*Sigmodon hispidus*) and sand rat (*Psammomys obesus*), are also available.

Because outbred colonies, like human populations, are heterogeneous, they are often considered the most appropriate category of laboratory animals for toxicology and pharmacology research. However, several geneticists have disputed this point and have even suggested that in many studies, outbred mice were used inappropriately, wasting animals' lives and research resources on suboptimal experiments [85]. In fact, any outbred stock can be replaced with a 'synthetic' population obtained by intercrossing classical inbred strains. As mentioned, crossing two inbred strains to produce F1 progeny followed by crossing two independent F1 individuals generates a four-way polymorphic population. This population is heterogenic, in the sense that individuals are genetically different. In addition, the population often carries a greater number of allelic forms, which is generally considered an advantage compared to a classical outbred population. Recently, however, researchers have realized that outbred stocks might be useful for refining QTL mapping experiments, because these heterogeneous stocks accumulate many recombination breakpoints that over time split their chromosomes into 'fine-grained mosaics', facilitating high-resolution mapping of complex traits [86, 87]. Other investigators recently claimed that contrary to conventional understanding, outbred mice might be better subjects for some biomedical research [88].

3 Genetically Altered (GA) Rodents

There are numerous terms used to describe genetic changes in rodents. In mice, the terms genetically engineered mice (GEM) and genetically modified mice (GMM) typically describe any genetically modified mouse. Here, we use the term genetically altered (GA) rodent to also include animals carrying spontaneous and/or chemically induced mutations and refer to 'lines' rather than 'strains' for GA rodents. GA lines are created using various genetic manipulation technologies that are summarized in several popular books and articles [89–91]. We also recommend visiting the webpage of the International Society for Transgenic Technologies (ISTT) at http://www.transtechsociety.org/.

3.1 Spontaneous and Chemically Induced Mutants

Every scientist in charge of a colony of inbred mice or rats, even if only for a few years, has almost certainly discovered a mutation segregating in a breeding nucleus. For example, dominant spotting (Kit^W), a mutant allele of the oncogene *Kit*, is very common and easy to identify on a C57BL/6, C3H or CBA background because it lightens coat colour, particularly in the tail, and often induces a white belly spot. In fact, 74 spontaneous mutations have been identified for *Kit*, with similar but not completely identical phenotypes. Other mutations are also quite common, especially those with an obvious viable phenotype (e.g. skeletal anomalies, cerebellar defects, neuromuscular syndromes, anaemia, skin defects and inner ear defects), and are generally either recessive or dominant. Since inbreeding increases the level of homozygosity in populations, it also enhances the probability of discovering recessive mutant phenotypes; however, inbreeding does not primarily increase the frequency of mutations.

It is also important to classify mutations based on their effect on the activity of their gene products. For example, an *amorphic* allele (null or loss of function) will eliminate activity completely, whereas a *hypomorphic* allele will produce a gene product with less activity than the wild-type gene product. In the same way, a *hypermorphic* allele will have increased activity, a *neomorphic* allele will have a new function and an *antimorphic* allele will have a dominant negative function.

Spontaneous mutations typically occur at low frequency, but frequency varies among loci. Some advantages of working with spontaneous mutations are that they are produced at virtually no cost and are usually freely available. In addition, they generally have an obvious phenotype, given that they are identified based on observation. Collectively, spontaneous mutations represent a great variety of molecular events, including deletions, insertions and point mutations. Such mutations generate not only loss-of-function alleles but also hypomorphs and hypermorphs. In many cases, spontaneous mutations can help establish better animal models than those produced by KO models [92–94]. Unfortunately, spontaneous mutations also have drawbacks. One major disadvantage is that the mutation's primary molecular defect is almost always unknown and therefore has unpredictable utility for gene annotation. Nonetheless, documenting spontaneous mutations is important; the Mouse Mutant Resource (MMR) at The Jackson Laboratory has been characterising (genetically and phenotypically) mice carrying spontaneous mutations for decades.

Ever since William Russell, of Oak Ridge National Laboratory, USA [95], reported that N-ethyl-N-nitrosourea (ENU) was 'the most potent mutagen in the mouse', ENU and other chemical mutagens have been used to generate mutations. ENU has numerous advantages as a mutagen, and its mode of action has been studied extensively [96, 97]. ENU is an alkylating agent producing mostly base pair changes (point mutations). In optimal conditions, ENU induces an average of 0.7–1.9 nucleotide substitutions per Mbp of DNA or one mutation at a specific locus in every 670–1000 mice of a G3 generation. Several collaborative projects aimed at the mass production of new mutant alleles were launched in the late 1990s, particularly in Europe, Japan and North America [98, 99]. In most instances, these projects were associated with downstream phenotypic screens designed to recover specific types of mutations (e.g. mutations leading to neuromuscular defects or to deafness). Interestingly, data contained in the Mutagenetix database (https://mutagenetix.utsouthwestern.edu) of mouse phenotypes and mutations induced with ENU indicates, based on over 100,000 mutations, that putative null mutations have a 61% probability of causing (phenotypically) detectable damage in the homozygous state [100].

Forward genetics is one genetic strategy used to identify the gene(s) responsible for a particular phenotype or biological process. It is a bottom-up approach that proceeds from the phenotype to the genotype. In this strategy individuals with spontaneous or induced mutations causing a phenotype of interest supply the raw material. Mapping the mutation requires subsequent breeding and a genetic map with as many informative genetic markers as possible [101]. *Positional cloning* is the process of identifying a gene based on its position in the genome, without any prior idea of its function. A good historical example of positional cloning is the identification of the gene responsible for the obese mutation (*ob*, later renamed Lep^{ob}) [102].

3.2 Classical Transgenesis by Pronuclear Microinjection (Random Insertion)

Transgenic rodents are created by the microinjection of foreign DNA fragments directly into one of the two pronuclei of one-celled embryos (zygotes), a technique widely used in the mouse and to a lesser extent in the rat [103–105]. In this process of *additive transgenesis*, the microinjected transgene randomly integrates into the genome as a concatemer with variable copy number (Fig. 9). The mouse and rat models created with this system typically overexpress a transgene placed un-

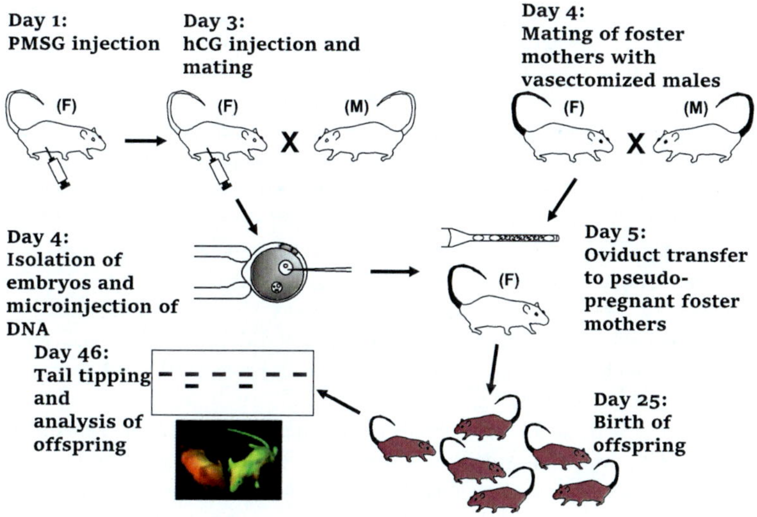

Fig. 9 Producing transgenic mice by pronuclear injection. The flowchart represents the different steps for the production of transgenic mice by pronuclear injection. One-cell embryos are flushed out of the oviduct immediately after fertilization, and then the transgene is microinjected in vitro with a glass micropipette into one of the pronucleus (typically the male pronucleus). Once injected, the embryos are kept in vitro for a few hours and then transplanted into pseudo-pregnant females (previously mated with vasectomized males). Genotyping of the G0 (presumptive) transgenic mice can be achieved at any time from birth onwards. Every pup genotyped as positive by PCR (i.e. hemizygous Tg/0 carrier) or expressing a reporter protein (e.g. GFP) should be considered a 'founder', and independent lines should be developed from each founder

der the control of a tissue-specific, developmental stage-specific or ubiquitous promoter (along with other regulatory elements), all contained in the transgene DNA construct.

The number of copies of the transgene that integrates into the host genome is not controlled and ranges from one to several tens or hundreds. DNA copies are generally arranged in head-to-tail arrays in the transgenic insertion with potential rearrangements in the flanking regions. In addition, the site of integration is random and can seriously influence transgene expression due to position effects. Position effects cause unpredictable, unexpected and somewhat erratic variations in transgene expression. For example, when an insertion occurs in a hyper-methylated region of the genome, the transgene will be weakly or not expressed. Position effects are one of the main weaknesses of pronuclear transgenesis. As it is impossible to predict either the integration site or the number of copies that will integrate, it is impossible to know how well a transgene introduced by this method will be expressed. Therefore, when developing a transgenic line, it is highly recommended to compare the offspring of several different founder mice. Likewise, it is important to avoid intercrossing mice originating from different founders; independent transgenic lines should be developed from each founder.

The recommended generic symbol for a transgenic insertion is Tg. Founder transgenic animals are hemizygous for the newly introduced DNA segment and are designated Tg/0. Establishing a transgenic line, in which the transgene is propagated by sexual reproduction, requires genotyping each generation to which the transgene was transmitted, unless the carriers have an obvious phenotype [106]. Lines are normally kept by backcrossing transgenic carriers (hemizygous Tg/0) with wild-type animals from the inbred background strain and by selecting carriers at each generation. When viability and fertility are unaffected, a transgene may be maintained by keeping transgenic lines in the homozygous state. Traditionally, to distinguish between homozygous (Tg/Tg) and hemizygous (Tg/0) mice, the mouse of interest was crossed to a non-transgenic partner, and the progeny was statistically analysed for Mendelian segregation of the transgene. Today, quantitative real-time PCR (qPCR) can be used to distinguish hemizygous from homozygous transgenic mice [107]. In order to achieve a pure genetic background, it is recommended to inject the transgene into embryos derived from an inbred strain, such as FVB/N, which is widely used because its zygotes possess large and prominent male pronuclei and the females are excellent breeders that produce large litters [108].

A later improvement on the original constructs used for transgenesis was the introduction of inducible systems allowing transgene expression to be turned on and off. Currently, the most common strategies are the Tet-on and Tet-off expression systems. In these systems, transcription of a given transgene is placed under the control of a tetracycline-controlled transactivator protein, which can be regulated, both reversibly and quantitatively, by exposing the transgenic mice to either *tetracycline* (Tc) or one of its derivatives, such as *doxycycline* (Dox). Both Tet-on and Tet-off are binary systems that require the generation of double transgenic (*bigenic*) mice. These mice carry both a responder construct, consisting of a tetracycline response element (TRE)-regulated transgene, and an effector construct (tTA or rtTA), containing a tetracycline-controlled transactivator [109].

3.3 Targeted Mutagenesis Using ES Cells

Another mouse genetic engineering technology uses pluripotent embryonic stem (ES) cell lines. ES cells are undifferentiated pluripotent embryonic cells derived from the inner cell mass of preimplantation blastocysts that can participate in the formation of the germ cell lineage of chimeric mice, an indispensable step in generating founder mice carrying the targeted mutation (Fig. 10). Most early ES cell lines were derived from embryos of the 129 families of inbred strains (129S2, 129P3, etc.). Today, ES cell lines come from a variety of strains. For example, the ES cell lines derived from C57BL/6N have become widespread and are often selected for many international projects (e.g. EUCOMM). In contrast to mice, the development of germline-competent ES cells in rats has only recently become possible [110], and their use remains limited.

Chimeras resulting from the admixture of engineered ES cells (carrying the targeted mutation in the gene of interest) with cells of the inner cell mass of a recipient blastocyst can be identified as soon as a few days after birth based on their dappled coat colour. The dappled coat is obvious when the ES cells are derived from C57BL/6N (which is non-agouti *a/a* – i.e. solid back) and the recipient blastocyst is from either a wild-type (agouti *A/A*) or albino (Tyr^c/ Tyr^c) strain. In these conditions, the chimeras exhibit a mixture of black and agouti (or albino) spots. Using coat colour as a reference, one can estimate the degree of chimerism, but a high level of chimerism does not necessarily parallel with a high rate of germline transmission. Although chimeras can be from either sex, males are generally the only sex with germline transmission because the majority of ES cell lines are XY. To avoid mixed background lines down the road, it is recommended to generate co-isogenic KO/KI lines by crossing the chimeras with wild-type mice from the same inbred background as the ES cells. For example, when C57BL/6-derived ES cells are injected into albino C57BL/6 blastocysts, the chimeric mice are easily identified because their coats exhibit white and black patches. These chimeras can then be crossed with albino C57BL/6 mice to test for germline transmission, validated by the appearance of ES cell-derived black offspring [70].

Other gene-targeting strategies have been developed to create conditional rather than constitutive KO mutations. Conditional mutations bypass

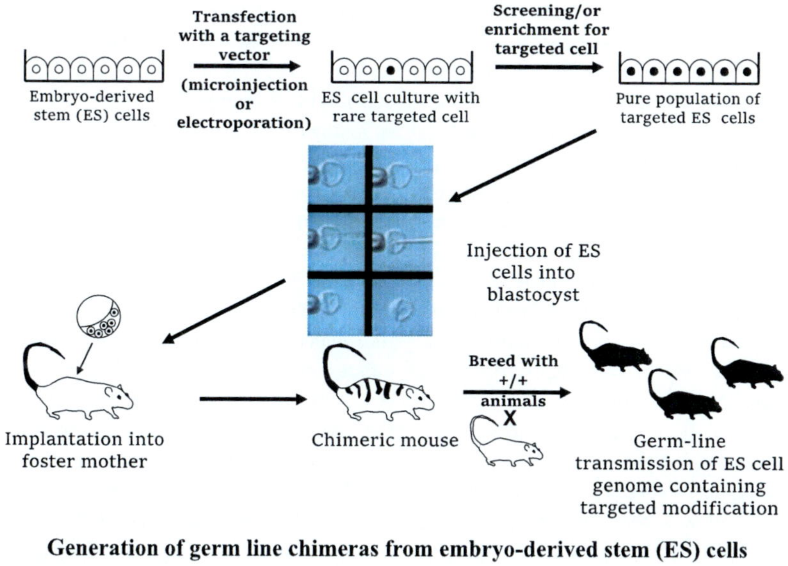

Fig. 10 Targeted mutagenesis in the mouse using engineered ES cells. The flowchart represents the different steps for the production of targeted mutants (KO and KI) using genetically modified ES cells. Pluripotent ES cells can be cultured in vitro, for several generations, remaining in an undifferentiated state. While in vitro, the ES cells can be manipulated like ordinary somatic cell lines and selected on the basis of specific criteria. ES cells are then typically injected into blastocysts (less commonly into eight-cell or morula stage) where they spontaneously merge with the inner cell mass. After embryo transfer into the uterus of a pseudo-pregnant female, and provided that the ES cells are still pluripotent, fertile chimeric mice can result from these reconstructed blastocysts. The chimeras with the best level of chimerism are then crossed with wild-type mice in order to confirm germ line transmission, basically the production of genotypically heterozygous mice carrying the targeted allele. One extra generation is necessary to observe the alteration in the homozygous state

some of the drawbacks of using constitutive null alleles of endogenous genes (e.g. pre- and postnatal lethality, fertility and welfare problems). With conditional mutations, the time and tissue in which the gene is inactivated can be controlled. Conditional KO production requires a cross between two independent lines to generate bigenic mice. The most popular conditional KO strategy is based on the Cre-*lox*P system, although a Flp-*FRT* system also exists. In the Cre-*lox*P strategy, Cre recombinase, derived from bacteriophage P1, cuts and recombines the DNA strand at specific sites called *lox*P sites (short for locus of X-ing over P1). These *lox*P sites consist of two 13-bp inverted (palindromic) repeats separated by an 8-bp asymmetric spacer region that define the orientation of the site. When the *lox*P sites are in the same orientation and on the same strand (in cis), the intervening stretch of DNA is excised as a circular loop. When two *lox*P sites are in opposite orientations and on the same chromosome, the intervening DNA segment is inverted. Finally, when the *lox*P sites are on two different chromosomes (in trans), the recombinase generates a reciprocal translocation [111].

The Cre transgene can be made inducible, adding more sophistication to the system, for example, by using Cre^{ERT2}, which can be induced by administration of tamoxifen [112]. Nowadays, many Cre-expressing lines are produced as KI mice with the Cre sequence incorporated directly into the gene of interest (rather than creating transgenic lines using pronuclear microinjection). The Cre-*lox*P strategy can also be used to control the expression of reporter genes. For example, the *lacZ* gene can be driven by a ubiquitous promoter (e.g. *Rosa 26*) with a floxed 'stop' sequence consisting of a short segment of DNA with several termination codons inserted between the promoter and the *lacZ* coding sequence, thus preventing translation of the *lacZ* gene product beta-galactosidase. When the Cre activity causes deletion of the floxed 'stop' sequence in specific cells or tissues, beta-galactosidase is produced in those cells or tissues. [113]. Because of the widespread use of this conditional targeting approach, databases cataloguing strains that synthesize Cre (designated Cre-deleters), either ubiquitously or in specific tissues, have been developed (see, for example, The Jackson Laboratory Cre Portal at https://www.jax.org/research-and-faculty/resources/cre-repository or the MGI Mouse Recombinase at http://www.informatics.jax.org/home/recombinase).

When using the Cre-*lox*P system, keep in mind the following: (i) Results may vary depending upon whether Cre is transmitted from the female or the male parent (e.g. Cre is significantly more efficient when transmitted maternally in the EIIa-Cre line). (ii) The presence of Cre alone might produce a phenotype (always include a Cre + control mouse without floxed sequences). (iii) The Cre-*lox*P system can be combined with the Tet-on or Tet-off inducible system. (iv) Cre mosaicism has been reported in some strains, resulting in variable expression. (v) Some floxed alleles are more easily recombined than others. (vi) Tamoxifen-inducible Cre lines can be leaky, that is, Cre can sometimes be active in the absence of tamoxifen.

3.4 Gene Editing Using Nucleases

Over the last 10 years, several new techniques have been developed using engineered nucleases to create targeted mutations. These techniques provide ES cell-independent approaches for the production of targeted mutations in mice, rats and other species [114].

3.4.1 Zinc-Finger Nucleases and TALEN

The production of mutations using zinc-finger nucleases (ZFNs) relies on the precise design of a chimeric protein containing a specifically designed zinc-finger DNA-binding domain and a *Fok*I endonuclease domain. Two complementary and sequence-specific multifinger peptides are designed to recognize a specific DNA sequence spanning 9–18 bp on either side of a 5–6 bp sequence, which defines the targeted region. When injected into the pronucleus or the cytoplasm of zygotes, the ZFNs bind tightly on both sides of the targeted site, one on each strand, allowing dimerization of *Fok*I which then makes double-strand breaks (DSBs) at the selected site. Once cleaved by *Fok*I, the cellular mechanisms controlling DNA integrity (DNA repair pathways) are triggered to repair the damage by either homology-dependent repair (HDR) or nonhomologous end joining (NHEJ). HDR requires a homologous sequence as a template to direct repair and accurately re-establish the original sequence. NHEJ is a much less precise mechanism that restores damaged strands incompletely, leaving behind deletions, thus creating frameshifts that commonly result in loss-of-function mutations. ZFN technology can be used to create a homozygous KO mutation faster than traditional KO strategies using ES cells and is applicable to all strains of mice and rats, allowing for the production of mutations in different inbred backgrounds. Mice and rats carrying null alleles or sequence-specific modifications have already been produced using ZFN technology [115, 116].

Like ZFN technology, transcription activator-like effector nuclease (TALEN) technology combines a nonspecific DNA endonuclease having robust cleavage activity with a DNA-binding domain that can be easily engineered to target a particular DNA sequence. In recent years, several groups have used TALENs (originally described in bacterial pathogens of crop plants) to modify endogenous genes in a wide variety of species, including zebrafish, rat, mouse, pig and cow [117, 118]. The advantages of TALENs over ZFNs are easier design and assembly, higher specificity and lower cost.

3.4.2 CRISPR-Cas System

This newly developed technology depends on small RNAs for RNA-guided cleavage of specific

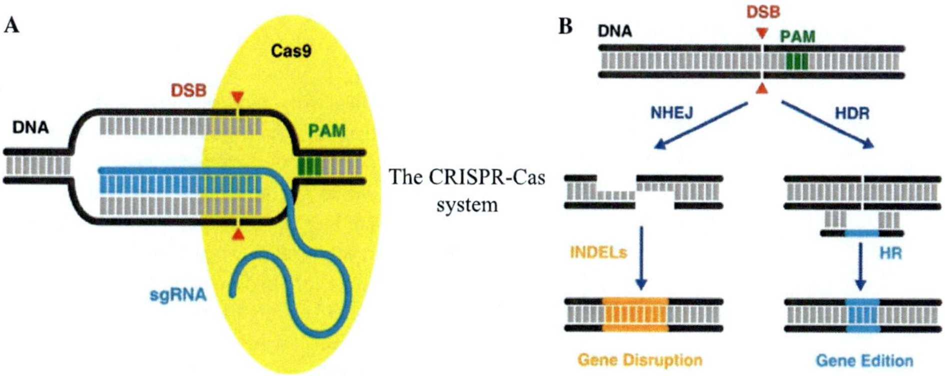

Fig. 11 Genome editing using site-specific RNA-guided DNA endonuclease (CRISPR/Cas system). (**a**) With the CRISPR strategy, Cas9 unwinds the DNA duplex and performs a double-strand break (DSB) after recognition of a specific (20 bp) target by the gRNA, provided that the correct protospacer adjacent motif (PAM) is present. (**b**) DSBs are repaired through nonhomologous end joining (NHEJ) or through homology-directed repair (HDR). In the case of DSBs repaired by NHEJ, the mechanism will induce indels and potentially produce KO alleles. For HDR to occur requires that a DNA molecule or a single-stranded synthetic DNA be added as a template. If the sequence of the template differs from the endogenous sequence by the addition or substitution of some nucleotides (light blue colour), this results in a KI allele. These methods for producing mutations at specifically targeted sites are very efficient. Figures kindly provided by Dr. Lluis Montoliu, CNB-CSIC, CIBERER-ISCIII, Centro Nacional de Biotecnología, Campus de Cantoblanco, Madrid, Spain

DNA sequences by a Cas endonuclease. The strategy was developed after the identification and characterization of a primitive bacterial/archaeal defence mechanism called CRISPR-Cas that allows these organisms to fight against infections from viruses, plasmids and phages [119, 120]. Engineered modifications to CRISPR (clusters of regularly interspaced short palindromic repeats) and the Cas enzyme (Cas9 is the most commonly used RNA-guided DNA nuclease) have led to an efficient system to produce DSBs at will. The guide RNA (gRNA or sgRNA) binds to the target DNA sequence and directs the Cas9 nuclease to create precise DSBs at the location of interest (Fig. 11).

RNA-guided endonucleases can be engineered to cleave virtually any DNA sequence by appropriately designing the gRNA, for example, to generate KO mice and rats [121–123]. CRISPR-Cas9 has several advantages over ZFNs and TALENs. It can be used to create mutations in multiple genes across the genome in a single step, by injecting multiple gRNAs targeting different sequences simultaneously. Such multiplex gene editing has proven successful not only to modify cells in vitro but also to modify mouse and rat embryos [124]. This saves substantial breeding time when several specific mutations are required in the same genome. Given the ease and speed of this method, it is clear why it is revolutionizing mammalian genetic engineering [125–128]. CRISPR-Cas also confers the possibility of producing KO lines on any inbred background because constructs are introduced either by injection into the cytoplasm or pronuclei of one-cell or two-cell stage embryos [129] or by electroporation [130, 131], thus avoiding ES cells and chimera production. However, as each indel mutation generated is unique, CRISPR-Cas-based genetic engineering requires extensive sequencing and bioinformatic analyses to characterize multiple founders (G0) to ensure against mosaicism and off-target mutations while also verifying the presence of the expected genetic change. The selected founder should then be bred with wild-type animals to evaluate transmission of the mutation to their offspring.

4 Genetic Quality Control for Mice and Rats

Genetic markers are specific DNA sequences with a known chromosomal location. The current gold standard for genetic quality control of laboratory rodents requires the analysis of polymorphic genetic markers that can distinguish between different genetic backgrounds. Historically, many of the techniques used to detect and analyse these markers have been shared with forensic DNA profiling.

4.1 Current Tools for Genetic Quality Control

Although many polymorphisms have been described in the mouse and rat, only two types are widely used in modern QA programmes: microsatellites (also known as simple sequence length polymorphisms (SSLPs) or short tandem repeats (STRs)) and/or SNPs. It is still too early to determine whether high-throughput, whole-exome sequencing (sequencing the exons of all protein-coding genes in a genome) will be useful for QA purposes, but it does provide both a robust method to discover hereditary factors contributing to rare Mendelian disorders in humans and a means to identify the precise molecular aberration underlying mutations mapped through positional cloning in mice and rats [132]. Whole-exome sequencing could also be very useful for the characterization of substrains.

4.1.1 Microsatellite (SSLP) Markers

Microsatellite markers are still used in genetic quality control programmes because they are extremely easy to type at a very low cost. Microsatellite analysis requires PCR amplification of the short, tandemly arranged, repeating DNA sequences, typically di- and tri-nucleotides (Fig. 12). The PCR products, 100–300 bp in size, are analysed on agarose or polyacrylamide gels. There are enormous numbers of microsatellite loci in the mouse and rat genomes (10^5), and identifying a set of markers whose amplification products will create a strain-specific pattern is not generally problematic. Routine analysis of DNA samples with microsatellite markers will confirm isogenicity (in the case of inbred strains) and provided the markers have been carefully selected, strain authenticity. One advantage of microsatellites is that they are multiallelic markers, meaning that, when tested in different inbred strains, a single marker can identify multiple alleles, distinguished by PCR products of different sizes. Microsatellite technology has been enhanced through the introduction of fluorescently labelled primers combined with capillary electrophoresis to provide a fast, automated system for genetic monitoring [27]. Here, PCR products are distinguished from each other by both their size and the fluorescent dye associated with them. The availability of different dyes allows multiplexing the PCR reaction (i.e. combining multiple primer sets to simultaneously amplify multiple loci in one reaction) and/or pooling several PCR reactions/products into one capillary [46]. Well-defined panels of SSLPs for mouse and rat inbred strains are available [27, 133, 134].

The MGI [51] presents comprehensive SSLP data, including primer sequences and the expected sizes of their amplified products for several mouse inbred strains (http://www.informatics.jax.org/marker). A collection of mapped SSLP markers for inbred strains of rats is available at the Rat Genome Database (RGD).

4.1.2 Single Nucleotide Polymorphisms (SNPs)

SNP genotyping is inexpensive and can be performed in most research institutions or outsourced to providers. Petkov and co-workers from The Jackson Laboratory have described the allelic distribution of 235 SNPs in 48 mouse strains and selected a panel of 28 such SNPs, enough to characterize most of the approximately 300 inbred, recombinant inbred, wild-derived, congenic and consomic strains maintained at The Jackson Laboratory [135]. This set of markers, encompassing all mouse chromosomes, is an

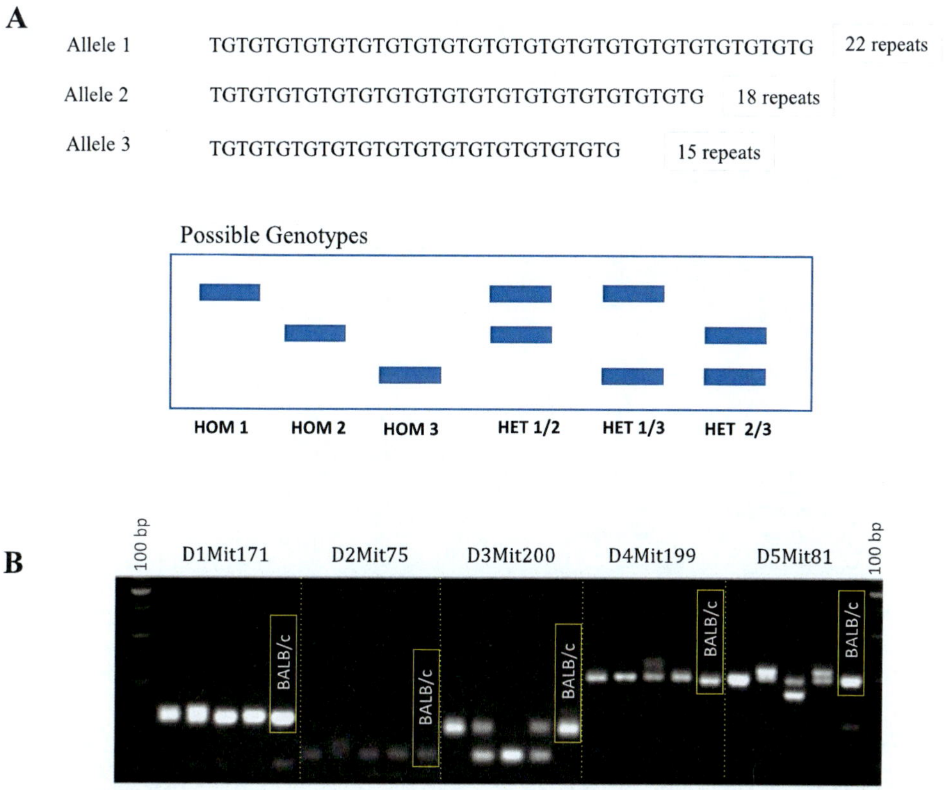

Fig. 12 Microsatellite markers. (**a**) The cartoon shows three different alleles at a hypothetical microsatellite locus composed of TG repeats (motif). Note that the number of repeats is variable, and this is the base of the polymorphism. Using specific primers flanking these repeats, we can amplify and detect the various allele combinations as shown in the schematic gel with possible genotypes. (**b**) The picture depicts the PCR products for five individual microsatellite markers (ethidium bromide-stained 4% agarose gel). These PCR products were obtained using species-specific and locus-specific primers along with genomic DNA from four different mice (genetically contaminated in this case) plus a BALB/c control DNA (last in group). The first lane of the gel shows the 100-bp ladder. The standard nomenclature for microsatellites (also known as SSLPs or STRs) is as follows: D [# of chromosome] [lab code] [ID of marker]. For example, D1Mit171 is the SSLP assigned with ID #171 on chromosome 1, identified by Massachusetts Institute of Technology (MIT)

excellent tool for detecting genetic contamination in mouse facilities. The Jackson Laboratory has also developed a set of 1638 informative SNPs, selected from publicly available databases and tested them in 102 inbred strains using Amplifluor genotyping [136]. The selected SNPs are distributed 1.5 Mb apart across the mouse genome. On average, 37% of these SNPs will be polymorphic between any two classical inbred strains. SNPs can also reveal differences between closely related substrains, for example, between C57BL/6J and C57BL/6N [63, 137–139]. Several publications have reported lists of rat SNPs: Zimdahl and colleagues described a map with more than 12,000 gene-based SNPs from transcribed regions [140]; in another study, 485 SNPs were identified in 36 commonly used inbred rat strains [141]. More recently, the STAR (rats backwards) consortium reported identifying a set of 20,000 SNPs across 167 inbred rat strains [142].

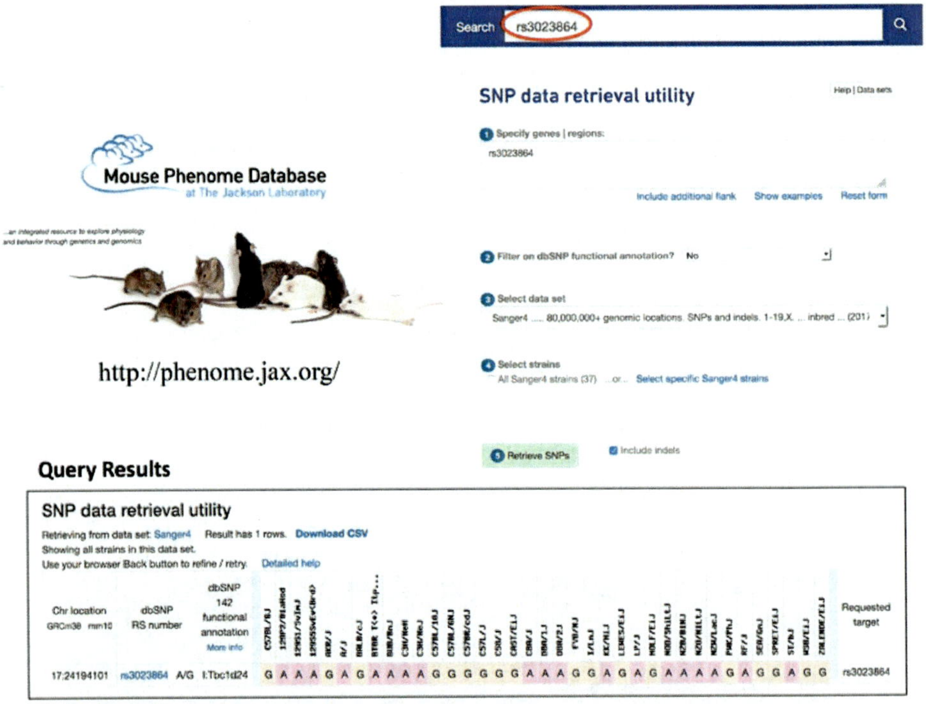

Fig. 13 SNP databases. This figure shows the results of a search using the Mouse Phenome Database seeking for polymorphism between inbred mouse strains for a SNP (ID rs3023864) located on chromosome 17. In this case, the Sanger4 set of 37 inbred strains was selected as dataset. The bottom of the figure is a screen capture of the results of the query showing the alleles (G or A) present in each of the strains (A = A/A; G = G/G). There are several other options for searching SNP data online (see text)

SNP genotyping is the current method chosen for genetic monitoring by most commercial suppliers of laboratory mice and rats. SNP genotyping assays are currently based on allele-specific PCR (including KASPar fluorescent technology) [47], real-time PCR (TaqMan®), direct sequencing and DNA arrays [101]. Another clever option is to exploit those SNPs that create a restriction fragment length polymorphism (RFLP) [143], making them easy to identify using simple technology. Databases, including the Mouse Phenome Database (MPD), the Mouse Genome Informatics (MGI), the Sanger Institute's Mouse Genomes Project and the Rat Genome Database (RGD), contain information for hundreds of thousands of SNPs for common mouse and rat inbred strains regarding their genomic locations and which alleles (C, G, A or T) to expect for a particular SNP/strain combination (Fig. 13).

4.2 Genetic Quality Control of Inbred Strains and Outbred Stocks

Historically, most techniques used to assay the genetic quality of inbred strains were based on the postulate that each inbred strain is expected a priori to be homozygous at almost all loci [144]. These techniques were designed based on the genetic tools available contemporaneously and generally consisted of analysing a few traits, controlled by a set of specific alleles, to define a unique pattern for each strain. Analysis of biochemical markers, mainly enzymatic proteins (isozymes), by electrophoresis became popular in the mid-1970s; however, this technique was expensive because each test required specific and costly reagents. Other techniques used for genetic monitoring have included immunological markers (particularly H2 haplotype), *osteometry* (mandible) traits and coat colour testcrosses [144–146].

Although genetic monitoring now relies on molecular techniques, the genetic purity of rodent populations must also be considered in a broader context that includes monitoring nonmolecular parameters, such as coat colour, behaviour, characteristics of genetic predispositions, breeding performance and/or other unique strain features [145]. For example, a sudden increase in litter sizes or elevation of the breeding index in an inbred strain is a strong indicator of possible genetic contamination. Likewise, monitoring for strain-specific pathologies is also important for quickly discovering possible genetic contamination and genetic drift.

Commercial breeders are extremely sensitized to the risk linked with genetic contamination and perform regular monitoring of their strains to detect such contamination. Most breeders monitor their nucleus colonies using SNPs, and larger vendors typically establish special programmes to tackle the issue of genetic drift. For example, The Jackson Laboratory has developed the patented Genetic Stability Program, initiated in 2003 [147]. This programme effectively limits cumulative genetic drift by rebuilding foundation stocks from cryopreserved (pedigreed) embryos every five generations. Starting in 2005, The Jackson Laboratory began selling only C57BL/6J mice descended from two chosen mice (Adam and Eve mice) through hundreds of frozen embryos of the duo's grandchildren, enough to last for 25–30 years [148]. For academic institutions, The International Council for Laboratory Animal Science (ICLAS) is promoting and helping develop genetic monitoring programmes to improve the level of QA for academically held mouse and rat models. Current ICLAS recommendations were recently reviewed by Fahey et al. [149].

4.2.1 Genetic Monitoring to Confirm Strain Identity

When inbred mice and rats are kept in-house, it is best to purchase animals from reliable vendors and refresh the colony with mice from the same vendor every 3–5 years rather than maintain independent colonies of classical inbred strains. Established vendors have excellent genetic quality programmes that allow smaller facilities to circumvent genetic monitoring altogether. As an additional benefit, acquiring animals from the same vendor prevents the formation of substrains harbouring potential mutations. Nonetheless, it is the best practice to use a small panel of SSLPs for strain authentication in those facilities that lack sophisticated equipment but wish to authenticate strains in-house. The number of markers to use has not been standardized because each situation and facility is different. However, a panel of 30–40 SSLPs, evenly distributed across the autosomal chromosomes, is generally considered adequate to rule out (recent) genetic contamination, typically resulting from accidental crosses with animals of a different inbred strain or outbred stock. Accidental crosses are more common when a facility maintains strains with the same coat colour in the same room, a particularly dangerous practice if not using individually ventilated cage (IVC) systems. The key characteristic of the SSLP panel used to detect contamination is that the markers must be polymorphic between the suspected strains.

An alternative to authenticating strains maintained in-house is to request SNP genotyping services from a commercial laboratory. Most commercial services are based on fixed DNA microarrays, so it is important to consider that only a fraction of the SNPs on any one array will be polymorphic between the strains under analysis (e.g. 40% for some classical inbred strain combinations). In addition to small-scale SNP genotyping (100–400 SNPs), there are high-density microarrays available. Although high-density arrays were designed primarily for gene mapping purposes, they may also be used to perform a complete SNP profile characterization for new or non-characterized inbred strains and substrains. For example, the Mouse Universal Genotyping Array (MUGA) in its MiniMUGA format has

11,000 SNPs, and the MegaMUGA format has 78,000 SNPs with both being built on the Illumina Infinium platform.

4.2.2 Discrimination of Substrains

The consensus is that if an inbred colony has been isolated for more than 20 generations, it should be considered a substrain, regardless of whether genetic differences between it and the parental strain have been confirmed. Opposed to standard genetic monitoring, the use of SSLPs is not recommended for identification of substrains because there are insufficient numbers of informative markers to distinguish between most of the common substrains. Instead, SNPs should be used, but the initial characterization of a substrain that has been isolated from the parent for several years requires a large set of SNPs. As an example, a pairwise comparison of sister strains using the MegaMUGA array showed that the number of polymorphic SNPs is 154 between C57BL/6J and C57BL/6N, 134 between BALB/cJ and BALB/cByJ and 827 between C3H/HeJ and C3H/HeN [150]. However, only complete exome sequencing can provide exhaustive information regarding specific mutations accumulated in protein-coding genes. Nevertheless, if the goal is only to identify to which classical substrain a colony (or an animal) is associated with, then a small number of SNPs, based on the information available in the SNP databases, can be selected for comparison. This is particularly easy for common substrains such as C57BL/6J and C57BL/6N, where small sets of markers have already been published [137–139].

4.2.3 Genetic Monitoring for Outbred Colonies

Genetic monitoring of outbred stocks is much more complex, because the essential nature of these mice and rats is that they are not genetically uniform. Outbred colonies are groups of closely related animals with common ancestors and group identity (e.g. tame, albino, prolific, etc.), but that still exhibits some level of genomic heterozygosity [81]. Outbred colonies should be treated as a population, making it difficult to establish a standard genetic monitoring programme with just a few genetic markers. However, monitoring the frequencies of different alleles present in the population with an adequate number of SNPs or SSLPs could reveal stock identity and help preserve the genetic heterogeneity (and allele pool) of a colony. This complex process requires analysing a large number of animals and access to historical allelic frequency (and level of heterozygosity) data for that particular colony.

One of the main issues with maintaining small colonies of outbred rodents with a very small number of breeders is that it reduces the number of alleles in the population and increases the inbreeding coefficient. Therefore, these colonies are neither truly outbred nor inbred. In any case, if it is not possible to keep a large number of breeders, it is better to purchase outbred rodents from vendors that maintain a very large colony and use special breeding schemes that reduce inbreeding.

4.3 Background Characterization for GA Rodents

The recent enormous increase in the number of GA lines will likely exacerbate the problem of undefined 'mixed backgrounds' in experimental rodents. This is particularly worrying in the case of inducible and conditional models that require the cross of two independent lines (e.g. Cre-expressing lines crossed with 'floxed' lines). It is well recognized that the genetic background (i.e. all genomic sequences other than the gene of interest) can influence the phenotype of an animal model. Spontaneous and induced mutations, transgenes and targeted alleles that are introgressed into a different background have been reported to exhibit altered phenotypes [151, 152]. These changes are mainly due to the influence of modifier genes in the genetic background.

One of the first cases documenting the influence of modifier genes involved the classical diabetes mutation *Lepr*^{db} that presented transient diabetes in the C57BL/6 background but overt diabetes in the C57BLKS background [153]. Later, the dominant *Apc*^{Min} (adenomatosis polyposis coli) mutation presented with an increased frequency of intestinal tumours in C57BL/6 mice but not in an AKR background. In this case, the responsible genetic modifier is an amorphic allele of *Pla2g2a* fixed in C57BL/6 [154]. Other examples include background effects on survival rate in *Egfr* (epidermal growth factor receptor) KO mice [155], effects on tumour incidence and spectrum in *Trp53* and *Pten* KO mice [156, 157] and milder phenotypes in the *Dmd*^{mdx} mouse model for Duchenne muscular dystrophy when moved to 129X1 [158]. There are also examples from rat models, like the influence of genetic background on prostate tumorigenesis in Pb-SV40 transgenic rats [159] and changes in phenotype severity in *Ednrb*^{sl} mutant rats [160].

On the other hand, mutations hidden in the genomes of introgressed strains or substrains (congenic lines) that can affect the outcome of an experiment are sometimes referred to as 'passenger mutations' [161]. There are many examples in the literature where substrains, although stemming from the same original inbred strains, have acquired new and unique phenotypes as a consequence of genetic drift [61, 162]. Mice of the C57BL/6JOlaHsd substrain, for example, are homozygous for a deletion of the *Snca* locus (encoding for α-synuclein) on chromosome 6 [163]. Alone, this deletion has modest phenotypic effects, but it could interfere unpredictably with other mutations if used as a background strain for making a knockout. Another interesting example stems from using different substrains of C57BL/6 mice as controls in acetaminophen-induced liver injury studies of *Jnk2* KOs. Researchers reported exactly opposite conclusions regarding JNK2 in helping or hurting liver health [164]. Similarly, due to the presence of a spontaneous mutation at the *Tlr4* locus (encoding for a *Toll*-like receptor) in substrain C3H/HeJ, where all mice are homozygous for the defective allele *Tlr4*$^{Lps\text{-}d}$, when C3H/HeJ mice are experimentally infected with Gram-negative bacteria, they may react very differently from mice of substrain C3H/HeN that lacks this mutation [165]. Berghe and colleagues recently reported that passenger mutations are common in most GA lines derived from 129 ES cells and that these mutations persist even after the creation of fully congenic strains [161]. This is not trivial; Berghe et al. estimate that close to 1000 protein-coding genes might be aberrantly expressed in the 129-derived chromosomal segments that are still segregating in these congenic lines. This finding emphasizes the need for proper controls to identify phenotypes due to background mutations or the combination of background mutations and the genetic modification of interest, rather than the modification itself.

Genome scans can be performed on a GA line with a mixed background to estimate the percentages of the genome contributed by different inbred origins. This process is referred to as a *background characterization* and is a service offered by some commercial enterprises and institutional core facilities. A typical background characterization requires genetic markers that are polymorphic between the most likely involved inbred strains and evenly distributed across the genome. In most mouse cases, these are C57BL/6 (the most common background strain for GA lines) and 129 substrains. The reason for the prevalence of 129 substrains is that, historically, the ES cells needed for the development of KO and KI were derived exclusively from 129 substrains [64]. The dominance of 129 substrains is now slowly changing with the availability of ES cell lines derived from other strains, particularly C57BL/6, and the arrival of genome editing techniques that create targeted alterations in any mouse or rat strain.

In any case, it is recommended to circumvent the problem of mixed background altogether by (i) injecting transgenes or nucleases (Cas9-sgRNA) into inbred embryos from the strain of choice, (ii) modifying the gene of interest in ES cells from the preferred background strain (e.g. using C57BL/6 ES cells) and (iii) crossing chimeras and KO/KI founders with mice of the same strain as the ES cells used for the targeting. Finally, if the GA is already developed (acquired from a collaborator or repository), a background characterization should be performed, and if needed, a fully congenic strain should be established through either classical backcrossing protocols or speed congenics.

4.4 Marker-Assisted Backcrossing (Speed Congenics)

Compared to traditional backcrossing schemes, *marker-assisted backcrossing*, or *speed congenics*, is a rapid and rigorous method that accelerates congenic strain development through the use of DNA markers [166, 167]. The principle that underlies the speed congenic process is based on the selection of breeders, at each generation of backcrossing, based on their percentage of donor genome as determined by analysing the presence of polymorphic genetic markers covering the whole genome. The animal with the lowest percentage of donor DNA is then selected as a breeder for setting the next backcross (Fig. 14). This process greatly reduces the number of generations necessary to reach full congenicity. Using marker-assisted crosses, we can obtain 80% recipient background at N2, 94% at N3 and 99% at N4 (instead of the classical mean values of 75.0%, 87.5% and 93.7%, respectively). It is important to note that once a marker is typed 'homozygous' for the allelic form of the background strain, it is no longer necessary to genotype the offspring of the future N generations for this marker because it is permanently fixed. Using additional markers also assists in the selection of breeders with the smallest amount of flanking DNA, helping to alleviate the 'flanking gene' concern [168, 169].

5 Mouse and Rat Phenomics

5.1 Standardized Phenotyping Protocols

Researchers now have all the means and tools to create a great variety of alterations in the mouse and rat genomes. Many of these alterations are expected to result in changes in phenotype, and the careful analysis of these phenotypic changes is fundamental for the process of genome annotation. However, even if it is relatively easy to characterize a DNA sequence, it remains difficult to unambiguously establish the link between a DNA alteration and an abnormal phenotype. The collection of physical and biochemical traits of an animal is known as the *phenome*, and *phenomics* is the discipline that deals with the measurement of these traits.

Speed Congenic Timeline (~18 months)

- **Start crossing donor (carrier) female with recipient strain male in order to generate F1 carrier males (PI).**
- **Backcross F1 males to generate ~20 N2 carrier males (~25%) (PI)**
- **Scan N2 carriers with SNPs and select the best breeders (Service)**
- **Cross best N2 males with several recipient strain females (PI)**
- **Generate ~20 N3 carrier males (~25%) (PI)**
- **Genotype N3 mice for heterozygous SNPs in N2 analysis (Service)**
- **Cross best N3 males with several recipient strain females (PI)**
- **Repeat same scheme at N4 (and if necessary at N5)**

Fig. 14 Speed Congenics Timeline. Selecting at each backcross generation, the breeder with the lowest percentage of introgressed (donor) DNA greatly accelerates the establishment of a congenic strain. It is important to note that genotyping requires many polymorphic DNA markers only for the first backcross progeny (N2). Once a marker is characterized as homozygous, it is no longer necessary to type it in the forthcoming generations. Although carrier males (heterozygous for the gene of interest) are typically recommended as 'best breeders', females can also be used, as long as they have high percentages of the recipient genome. The prediction of >98% recipient genome at N5 is based on the use of 20 best breeders (carriers) at each generation (Markel et al. [167]); however this number is not always available, and fewer breeders can be used, with disparate results, depending also on chance. *PI*, Principal Investigator

Phenotyping of rodent models has become a main concern over the last decades. Therefore, many laboratories and institutions have developed highly standardized phenotyping protocols. The range of phenotyping platforms, including dual-energy X-ray absorptiometry, electrocardiography, high-resolution imaging and FACS, ensures the recovery of phenotype data across multiple systems and disease states. In most cases the basic protocols include behaviour, neurology, clinical chemistry, development, immunology, energy metabolism, vision and hearing, pain perception and cardiovascular and gross pathology assessments. The use of standard procedures and defined protocols allows data to be comparable and shareable, even across species, which may help identify mouse and rat models of human diseases [170]. However, phenotyping loss-of-function mutations cannot predict the relevance of these alleles (and their phenotypes) to complex human diseases that are likely driven by several alleles of modest effect [171].

5.2 International Mice Phenotyping Consortiums

One of the earliest collaborative projects using standard phenotyping procedures was the European Eumorphia project. This programme also developed the Europhenome data repository and the European Mouse Phenotyping Resource for Standardized Screens [172]. The European Mouse Disease Clinical programme, together with the Sanger Mouse Genetics Program (MGP), continued the collaborative work of Eumorphia, developing protocols and phenotyping mutant mouse lines (mostly from the IKMC mutant ES cell lines) [173]. The Jackson Laboratory has developed a programme to collect baseline phenotypic data on the most commonly used inbred strains of mice through a coordinated international effort. Information collected through this programme (*The Mouse Phenome Database*) is freely available to the community through the Internet (http://phenome.jax.org/) [174]. The establishment (and updating) of this database is possible only because inbred mice are isogenic and genetically stable in the long term.

The International Mouse Phenotyping Consortium (IMPC) was established in 2011 with several goals: (i) to maintain and expand a worldwide consortium of institutions with capacity and expertise to produce germ line transmission of targeted KO mutations in ES cells, (ii) to test each mutant mouse line through a broad-based primary phenotyping pipeline, (iii) to systematically aim to discover and ascribe biological function to each gene, (iv) to maintain and expand collaborative 'networks' with specialist phenotyping consortia or laboratories and (v) to provide a centralized data centre and portal for free, unrestricted access to primary and secondary data from the scientific community [175]. The current European members of IMPC are the Medical Research Council (Harwell), the Wellcome Trust Sanger Institute (Cambridge) and the European Bioinformatics Institute (Hinxton) in the UK; the Helmholtz-Zentrum Muenchen in Germany; the PHENOMIN (Strasbourg) in France; the CNR (Monterotondo) in Italy; the Czech Centre for Phenogenomics in the Czech Republic; and the Universitat Autònoma de Barcelona in Spain [176]. Phenotyping data are accessible on the IMPC website (http://www.mousephenotype.org/). Using both gene trapping and gene targeting approaches, the IMPC has developed mutant ES cells (many with conditional mutations) for more than 18,000 genes representing more than 90% of the mouse protein-coding genes [171]. The ultimate goal is to produce a comprehensive catalogue of mouse gene functions by generating and characterizing null mutations for every mouse gene.

So far, the IMPC has used ES cells [177] to generate the mouse mutants, all on a C57BL/6N background (National Institutes of Health substrain). For example, EUCOMM and KOMP-CSD (CHORI, Sanger Institute and UC Davis) use promoter-less and promoter-driven targeting cassettes for the generation of the KO alleles [178]. This strategy relies on the identification of a critical exon common to all transcript variants that, when deleted, creates a frameshift mutation. The KO-first (*Tm1a*) allele is flexible and can produce reporter knockouts, conditional knockouts and null alleles following exposure to site-specific recombinases. For example, excising the *Tm1a* allele with Cre creates the *Tm1b* (*lacZ* tagged) allele that is a true KO because skipping over the *lacZ* cassette will no longer restore gene expression. The cassette expresses *lacZ* in tissues where the gene of interest is knocked out. Beta-galactosidase staining can be used to follow the tissue expression of the gene of interest. Finally, the *Tm1c* (conditional ready) allele has a phenotypically wild-type state where the exons are spliced together normally. However, the critical exon(s) are still flanked by *lox*P sites. Crosses with tissue-specific Cre-deleter mice can be used to create a tissue-specific KO line. Nowadays, the IMPC is starting to use CRISPR/Cas9 technology to generate the KO mutants by deleting an early critical exon.

The IMPC uses the International Mouse Phenotyping Resource of Standardised Screens (IMPReSS) phenotyping protocols, which are essential for the characterization of mouse phenotypes (see https://www.mousephenotype.org/impress). In this case, homozygous (or heterozygous in the case of embryonic lethal mutations) adult mutant mice enter a standardized pipeline [179] where cohorts of males and females undergo a wide range of phenotyping tests from 9 to 16 weeks, followed by a variety of terminal tests. The phenotyping of both male and female cohorts has allowed an in-depth analysis of the extent of sexual dimorphism. To date, the IMPC has generated over 7000 mutant lines, and phenotype data have been collected on over 5000 lines with a large number of novel phenotypes revealed [179]. More importantly, approximately 90% of the gene-phenotype annotations described by the IMPC have not been previously reported [171]. Data from the IMPC shows that around 24% of genes will not produce homozygous KO (null allele) offspring because they are homozygous lethal.

References

1. Guenet JL, Benavides F, Panthier J, Montagutelli X. Genetics of the mouse. Berlin: Springer; 2015.
2. Silver L. Mouse genetics. Concepts and applications. Oxford: Oxford University Press; 1995.
3. MacDonald WA, Mann MR. Epigenetic regulation of genomic imprinting from germ line to preimplantation. Mol Reprod Dev. 2014;81(2):126–40.
4. Michaud EJ, Bultman SJ, Klebig ML, van Vugt MJ, Stubbs LJ, Russell LB, et al. A molecular model for the genetic and phenotypic characteristics of the mouse lethal yellow (Ay) mutation. Proc Natl Acad Sci USA. 1994;91(7):2562–6.
5. Waterston RH, Lindblad-Toh K, Birney E, Rogers J, Abril JF, Agarwal P, et al. Initial sequencing and comparative analysis of the mouse genome. Nature. 2002;420(6915):520–62.
6. Gibbs RA, Weinstock GM, Metzker ML, Muzny DM, Sodergren EJ, Scherer S, et al. Genome sequence of the Brown Norway rat yields insights into mammalian evolution. Nature. 2004;428(6982):493–521.
7. Doran AG, Wong K, Flint J, Adams DJ, Hunter KW, Keane TM. Deep genome sequencing and variation analysis of 13 inbred mouse strains defines candidate phenotypic alleles, private variation and homozygous truncating mutations. Genome Biol. 2016;17(1):167.
8. Lilue J, Doran AG, Fiddes IT, Abrudan M, Armstrong J, Bennett R, et al. Sixteen diverse laboratory mouse reference genomes define strain-specific haplotypes and novel functional loci. Nat Genet. 2018;50(11):1574–83.
9. Church DM, Goodstadt L, Hillier LW, Zody MC, Goldstein S, She X, et al. Lineage-specific biology revealed by a finished genome assembly of the mouse. PLoS Biol. 2009;7(5):e1000112.
10. Nobrega MA, Zhu Y, Plajzer-Frick I, Afzal V, Rubin EM. Megabase deletions of gene deserts result in viable mice. Nature. 2004;431(7011):988–93.
11. Windsor AJ, Mitchell-Olds T. Comparative genomics as a tool for gene discovery. Curr Opin Biotechnol. 2006;17(2):161–7.
12. Liao BY, Zhang J. Null mutations in human and mouse orthologs frequently result in different phenotypes. Proc Natl Acad Sci USA. 2008;105(19):6987–92.
13. Tollis M, Schiffman JD, Boddy AM. Evolution of cancer suppression as revealed by mammalian comparative genomics. Curr Opin Genet Dev. 2017;42:40–7.
14. Sakharkar MK, Perumal BS, Sakharkar KR, Kangueane P. An analysis on gene architecture in human and mouse genomes. In Silico Biol. 2005;5(4):347–65.
15. Modrek B, Lee CJ. Alternative splicing in the human, mouse and rat genomes is associated with an increased frequency of exon creation and/or loss. Nat Genet. 2003;34(2):177–80.
16. Choi E, Lee J, Oh J, Park I, Han C, Yi C, et al. Integrative characterization of germ cell-specific genes from mouse spermatocyte UniGene library. BMC Genomics. 2007;8:256.

17. Rouquier S, Blancher A, Giorgi D. The olfactory receptor gene repertoire in primates and mouse: evidence for reduction of the functional fraction in primates. Proc Natl Acad Sci USA. 2000;97(6):2870–4.
18. Pennacchio LA, Ahituv N, Moses AM, Prabhakar S, Nobrega MA, Shoukry M, et al. In vivo enhancer analysis of human conserved non-coding sequences. Nature. 2006;444(7118):499–502.
19. Cobb J, Busst C, Petrou S, Harrap S, Ellis J. Searching for functional genetic variants in non-coding DNA. Clin Exp Pharmacol Physiol. 2008;35(4):372–5.
20. Kuznetsova IS, Prusov AN, Enukashvily NI, Podgornaya OI. New types of mouse centromeric satellite DNAs. Chromosom Res. 2005;13(1):9–25.
21. Bois PR. Hypermutable minisatellites, a human affair? Genomics. 2003;81(4):349–55.
22. Jeffreys AJ, Wilson V, Thein SL. Individual-specific 'fingerprints' of human DNA. Nature. 1985;316(6023):76–9.
23. Jeffreys AJ, Wilson V, Kelly R, Taylor BA, Bulfield G. Mouse DNA 'fingerprints': analysis of chromosome localization and germ-line stability of hypervariable loci in recombinant inbred strains. Nucleic Acids Res. 1987;15(7):2823–36.
24. Kurtz TW, Montano M, Chan L, Kabra P. Molecular evidence of genetic heterogeneity in Wistar-Kyoto rats: implications for research with the spontaneously hypertensive rat. Hypertension. 1989;13(2):188–92.
25. Benavides F, Cazalla D, Pereira C, Fontanals A, Salaverri M, Goldman A, et al. Evidence of genetic heterogeneity in a BALB/c mouse colony as determined by DNA fingerprinting. Lab Anim. 1998;32(1):80–5.
26. Benavides F, Glasscock E, Coghlan LG, Stern MC, Weiss DA, Conti CJ. PCR-based microsatellite analysis for differentiation and genetic monitoring of nine inbred SENCAR mouse strains. Lab Anim. 2001;35(2):157–62.
27. Mashimo T, Voigt B, Tsurumi T, Naoi K, Nakanishi S, Yamasaki K, et al. A set of highly informative rat simple sequence length polymorphism (SSLP) markers and genetically defined rat strains. BMC Genet. 2006;7:19.
28. Stranger BE, Forrest MS, Dunning M, Ingle CE, Beazley C, Thorne N, et al. Relative impact of nucleotide and copy number variation on gene expression phenotypes. Science. 2007;315(5813):848–53.
29. Adams DJ, Dermitzakis ET, Cox T, Smith J, Davies R, Banerjee R, et al. Complex haplotypes, copy number polymorphisms and coding variation in two recently divergent mouse strains. Nat Genet. 2005;37(5):532–6.
30. Graubert TA, Cahan P, Edwin D, Selzer RR, Richmond TA, Eis PS, et al. A high-resolution map of segmental DNA copy number variation in the mouse genome. PLoS Genet. 2007;3(1):e3.
31. She X, Cheng Z, Zollner S, Church DM, Eichler EE. Mouse segmental duplication and copy number variation. Nat Genet. 2008;40(7):909–14.
32. Watkins-Chow DE, Pavan WJ. Genomic copy number and expression variation within the C57BL/6J inbred mouse strain. Genome Res. 2008;18(1):60–6.
33. Jurka J, Kapitonov VV, Kohany O, Jurka MV. Repetitive sequences in complex genomes: structure and evolution. Annu Rev Genomics Hum Genet. 2007;8:241–59.
34. Wicker T, Sabot F, Hua-Van A, Bennetzen JL, Capy P, Chalhoub B, et al. A unified classification system for eukaryotic transposable elements. Nat Rev Genet. 2007;8(12):973–82.
35. Belancio VP, Hedges DJ, Deininger P. Mammalian non-LTR retrotransposons: for better or worse, in sickness and in health. Genome Res. 2008;18(3):343–58.
36. Wade CM, Kulbokas EJ 3rd, Kirby AW, Zody MC, Mullikin JC, Lander ES, et al. The mosaic structure of variation in the laboratory mouse genome. Nature. 2002;420(6915):574–8.
37. Ostertag EM, Kazazian HH Jr. Biology of mammalian L1 retrotransposons. Annu Rev Genet. 2001;35:501–38.
38. Sasaki T, Nishihara H, Hirakawa M, Fujimura K, Tanaka M, Kokubo N, et al. Possible involvement of SINEs in mammalian-specific brain formation. Proc Natl Acad Sci USA. 2008;105(11):4220–5.
39. Dupuy AJ, Akagi K, Largaespada DA, Copeland NG, Jenkins NA. Mammalian mutagenesis using a highly mobile somatic Sleeping Beauty transposon system. Nature. 2005;436(7048):221–6.
40. Wu SC, Meir YJ, Coates CJ, Handler AM, Pelczar P, Moisyadi S, et al. piggyBac is a flexible and highly active transposon as compared to sleeping beauty, Tol2, and Mos1 in mammalian cells. Proc Natl Acad Sci USA. 2006;103(41):15008–13.
41. Jern P, Coffin JM. Effects of retroviruses on host genome function. Annu Rev Genet. 2008;42:709–32.
42. Stoye JP, Fenner S, Greenoak GE, Moran C, Coffin JM. Role of endogenous retroviruses as mutagens: the hairless mutation of mice. Cell. 1988;54(3):383–91.
43. Hughes AL, Welch R, Puri V, Matthews C, Haque K, Chanock SJ, et al. Genome-wide SNP typing reveals signatures of population history. Genomics. 2008;92(1):1–8.
44. Zhang J, Hunter KW, Gandolph M, Rowe WL, Finney RP, Kelley JM, et al. A high-resolution multistrain haplotype analysis of laboratory mouse genome reveals three distinctive genetic variation patterns. Genome Res. 2005;15(2):241–9.
45. Frazer KA, Eskin E, Kang HM, Bogue MA, Hinds DA, Beilharz EJ, et al. A sequence-based variation map of 8.27 million SNPs in inbred mouse strains. Nature. 2007;448(7157):1050–3.

46. Bryda EC, Riley LK. Multiplex microsatellite marker panels for genetic monitoring of common rat strains. J Am Assoc Lab Anim Sci. 2008;47(3):37–41.
47. Nijman IJ, Kuipers S, Verheul M, Guryev V, Cuppen E. A genome-wide SNP panel for mapping and association studies in the rat. BMC Genomics. 2008;9:95.
48. Mudge JM, Harrow J. Creating reference gene annotation for the mouse C57BL6/J genome assembly. Mamm Genome. 2015;26(9–10):366–78.
49. Carninci P, Kasukawa T, Katayama S, Gough J, Frith MC, Maeda N, et al. The transcriptional landscape of the mammalian genome. Science. 2005;309(5740):1559–63.
50. Diez-Roux G, Banfi S, Sultan M, Geffers L, Anand S, Rozado D, et al. A high-resolution anatomical atlas of the transcriptome in the mouse embryo. PLoS Biol. 2011;9(1):e1000582.
51. Eppig JT. Mouse Genome Informatics (MGI) resource: genetic, genomic, and biological knowledgebase for the laboratory mouse. ILAR J. 2017;58(1):17–41.
52. Shimoyama M, De Pons J, Hayman GT, Laulederkind SJ, Liu W, Nigam R, et al. The Rat Genome Database 2015: genomic, phenotypic and environmental variations and disease. Nucleic Acids Res. 2015;43(Database issue):D743–50.
53. Laulederkind SJF, Hayman GT, Wang SJ, Smith JR, Petri V, Hoffman MJ, et al. A primer for the Rat Genome Database (RGD). Methods Mol Biol. 1757;2018:163–209.
54. Morse HC 3rd. Origins of inbred mice. New York: Academic Press; 1978.
55. Rader K. Making mice: standardizing animals for American Biomedical Research, 1900–1955. Princeton: Princeton University Press; 2004.
56. Moriwaki K, Shiroishi T, Yonekawa H. Genetics in wild mice: its application to biomedical research. Tokyo: Japan Scientific Societies Press; 1994.
57. Simecek P, Forejt J, Williams RW, Shiroishi T, Takada T, Lu L, et al. High-resolution maps of mouse reference populations. G3 (Bethesda). 2017;7(10):3427–34.
58. Kuramoto T, Nakanishi S, Ochiai M, Nakagama H, Voigt B, Serikawa T. Origins of albino and hooded rats: implications from molecular genetic analysis across modern laboratory rat strains. PLoS One. 2012;7(8):e43059.
59. Peters H, Reifenberg K, Wedekind, D. Substrains of inbred strains. GV-SOLAS. 2013; Specialist Information.
60. Freeman HC, Hugill A, Dear NT, Ashcroft FM, Cox RD. Deletion of nicotinamide nucleotide transhydrogenase: a new quantitative trait locus accounting for glucose intolerance in C57BL/6J mice. Diabetes. 2006;55(7):2153–6.
61. Mattapallil MJ, Wawrousek EF, Chan CC, Zhao H, Roychoudhury J, Ferguson TA, et al. The Rd8 mutation of the Crb1 gene is present in vendor lines of C57BL/6N mice and embryonic stem cells, and confounds ocular induced mutant phenotypes. Invest Ophthalmol Vis Sci. 2012;53(6):2921–7.
62. Kumar V, Kim K, Joseph C, Kourrich S, Yoo SH, Huang HC, et al. C57BL/6N mutation in cytoplasmic FMRP interacting protein 2 regulates cocaine response. Science. 2013;342(6165):1508–12.
63. Simon MM, Greenaway S, White JK, Fuchs H, Gailus-Durner V, Wells S, et al. A comparative phenotypic and genomic analysis of C57BL/6J and C57BL/6N mouse strains. Genome Biol. 2013;14(7):R82.
64. Simpson EM, Linder CC, Sargent EE, Davisson MT, Mobraaten LE, Sharp JJ. Genetic variation among 129 substrains and its importance for targeted mutagenesis in mice. Nat Genet. 1997;16(1):19–27.
65. Hermsen R, de Ligt J, Spee W, Blokzijl F, Schafer S, Adami E, et al. Genomic landscape of rat strain and substrain variation. BMC Genomics. 2015;16:357.
66. Guenet JL, Benavides FJ. Mouse strains and genetic nomenclature. Curr Protoc Mouse Biol. 2011;1(1):213–38.
67. Yalcin B, Fullerton J, Miller S, Keays DA, Brady S, Bhomra A, et al. Unexpected complexity in the haplotypes of commonly used inbred strains of laboratory mice. Proc Natl Acad Sci USA. 2004;101(26):9734–9.
68. Yang H, Wang JR, Didion JP, Buus RJ, Bell TA, Welsh CE, et al. Subspecific origin and haplotype diversity in the laboratory mouse. Nat Genet. 2011;43(7):648–55.
69. Guenet JL, Bonhomme F. Wild mice: an ever-increasing contribution to a popular mammalian model. Trends Genet. 2003;19(1):24–31.
70. Schuster-Gossler K, Lee AW, Lerner CP, Parker HJ, Dyer VW, Scott VE, et al. Use of coisogenic host blastocysts for efficient establishment of germline chimeras with C57BL/6J ES cell lines. BioTechniques. 2001;31(5):1022–4. 6
71. Nadeau JH, Singer JB, Matin A, Lander ES. Analysing complex genetic traits with chromosome substitution strains. Nat Genet. 2000;24(3):221–5.
72. Bailey DW. Recombinant-inbred strains. An aid to finding identity, linkage, and function of histocompatibility and other genes. Transplantation. 1971;11(3):325–7.
73. Shisa H, Lu L, Katoh H, Kawarai A, Tanuma J, Matsushima Y, et al. The LEXF: a new set of rat recombinant inbred strains between LE/Stm and F344. Mamm Genome. 1997;8(5):324–7.
74. Demant P. Cancer susceptibility in the mouse: genetics, biology and implications for human cancer. Nat Rev Genet. 2003;4(9):721–34.
75. Burgio G, Szatanik M, Guenet JL, Arnau MR, Panthier JJ, Montagutelli X. Interspecific recombinant congenic strains between C57BL/6 and mice of the Mus spretus species: a powerful tool to dissect genetic control of complex traits. Genetics. 2007;177(4):2321–33.

76. Burgio G, Baylac M, Heyer E, Montagutelli X. Genetic analysis of skull shape variation and morphological integration in the mouse using interspecific recombinant congenic strains between C57BL/6 and mice of the mus spretus species. Evolution. 2009;63(10):2668–86.
77. Churchill GA, Airey DC, Allayee H, Angel JM, Attie AD, Beatty J, et al. The Collaborative Cross, a community resource for the genetic analysis of complex traits. Nat Genet. 2004;36(11):1133–7.
78. Chesler EJ, Miller DR, Branstetter LR, Galloway LD, Jackson BL, Philip VM, et al. The Collaborative Cross at Oak Ridge National Laboratory: developing a powerful resource for systems genetics. Mamm Genome. 2008;19(6):382–9.
79. Aylor DL, Valdar W, Foulds-Mathes W, Buus RJ, Verdugo RA, Baric RS, et al. Genetic analysis of complex traits in the emerging collaborative cross. Genome Res. 2011;21:1213–22.
80. Srivastava A, Morgan AP, Najarian ML, Sarsani VK, Sigmon JS, Shorter JR, et al. Genomes of the mouse Collaborative Cross. Genetics. 2017;206(2):537–56.
81. Hartl DL. Genetic management of outbred laboratory rodent populations. Charles River Genetic Literature. 2001.
82. Poiley SM. A systematic method of breeder rotation for non-inbred laboratory animals colonies. Proc Anim Care Panel. 1960;10:159.
83. Schmitt AO, Bortfeldt R, Neuschl C, Brockmann GA. RandoMate: a program for the generation of random mating schemes for small laboratory animals. Mamm Genome. 2009;20(5):321–5.
84. Chia R, Achilli F, Festing MF, Fisher EM. The origins and uses of mouse outbred stocks. Nat Genet. 2005;37(11):1181–6.
85. Festing MF. Inbred strains should replace outbred stocks in toxicology, safety testing, and drug development. Toxicol Pathol. 2010;38(5):681–90.
86. Yalcin B, Nicod J, Bhomra A, Davidson S, Cleak J, Farinelli L, et al. Commercially available outbred mice for genome-wide association studies. PLoS Genet. 2010;6(9):e1001085.
87. Churchill GA, Gatti DM, Munger SC, Svenson KL. The diversity outbred mouse population. Mamm Genome. 2012;23(9–10):713–8.
88. Tuttle AH, Philip VM, Chesler EJ, Mogil JS. Comparing phenotypic variation between inbred and outbred mice. Nat Methods. 2018;15(12):994–6.
89. Jackson IJ, Abbott CM. Mouse genetics and transgenics: a practical approach. Oxford: Oxford University Press; 2000.
90. Nagy A, Gertsenstein M, Vintersten K, Behringer R. Manipulating the mouse embryo, a laboratory manual. 3rd ed. New York: Cold Spring Harbor Press; 2003.
91. Koentgen F, Suess G, Naf D. Engineering the mouse genome to model human disease for drug discovery. Methods Mol Biol. 2010;602:55–77.
92. Guenet JL. Animal models of human genetic diseases: do they need to be faithful to be useful? Mol Gen Genomics. 2011;286(1):1–20.
93. Perez CJ, Jaubert J, Guenet JL, Barnhart KF, Ross-Inta CM, Quintanilla VC, et al. Two hypomorphic alleles of mouse Ass1 as a new animal model of citrullinemia type I and other hyperammonemic syndromes. Am J Pathol. 2010;177(4):1958–68.
94. Bao J, Perez CJ, Kim J, Zhang H, Murphy CJ, Hamidi T, et al. Deficient LRRC8A-dependent volume-regulated anion channel activity is associated with male infertility in mice. JCI Insight. 2018;3(16):e99767.
95. Russell WL, Kelly EM, Hunsicker PR, Bangham JW, Maddux SC, Phipps EL. Specific-locus test shows ethylnitrosourea to be the most potent mutagen in the mouse. Proc Natl Acad Sci USA. 1979;76(11):5818–9.
96. Guenet JL. Chemical mutagenesis of the mouse genome: an overview. Genetica. 2004;122(1):9–24.
97. Gondo Y. Trends in large-scale mouse mutagenesis: from genetics to functional genomics. Nat Rev Genet. 2008;9(10):803–10.
98. Nolan PM, Peters J, Strivens M, Rogers D, Hagan J, Spurr N, et al. A systematic, genome-wide, phenotype-driven mutagenesis programme for gene function studies in the mouse. Nat Genet. 2000;25(4):440–3.
99. Hrabe de Angelis MH, Flaswinkel H, Fuchs H, Rathkolb B, Soewarto D, Marschall S, et al. Genome-wide, large-scale production of mutant mice by ENU mutagenesis. Nat Genet. 2000;25(4):444–7.
100. Wang T, Bu CH, Hildebrand S, Jia G, Siggs OM, Lyon S, et al. Probability of phenotypically detectable protein damage by ENU-induced mutations in the Mutagenetix database. Nat Commun. 2018;9(1):441.
101. Moran JL, Bolton AD, Tran PV, Brown A, Dwyer ND, Manning DK, et al. Utilization of a whole genome SNP panel for efficient genetic mapping in the mouse. Genome Res. 2006;16(3):436–40.
102. Zhang Y, Proenca R, Maffei M, Barone M, Leopold L, Friedman JM. Positional cloning of the mouse obese gene and its human homologue. Nature. 1994;372(6505):425–32.
103. Brinster RL, Chen HY, Trumbauer M, Senear AW, Warren R, Palmiter RD. Somatic expression of herpes thymidine kinase in mice following injection of a fusion gene into eggs. Cell. 1981;27(1 Pt 2):223–31.
104. Costantini F, Lacy E. Introduction of a rabbit beta-globin gene into the mouse germ line. Nature. 1981;294(5836):92–4.
105. Gordon JW, Ruddle FH. Integration and stable germ line transmission of genes injected into mouse pronuclei. Science. 1981;214(4526):1244–6.
106. Bonaparte D, Cinelli P, Douni E, Herault Y, Maas M, Pakarinen P, et al. FELASA guidelines for the

refinement of methods for genotyping genetically-modified rodents: a report of the Federation of European Laboratory Animal Science Associations Working Group. Lab Anim. 2013;47(3):134–45.
107. Ballester M, Castello A, Ibanez E, Sanchez A, Folch JM. Real-time quantitative PCR-based system for determining transgene copy number in transgenic animals. BioTechniques. 2004;37(4):610–3.
108. Taketo M, Schroeder AC, Mobraaten LE, Gunning KB, Hanten G, Fox RR, et al. FVB/N: an inbred mouse strain preferable for transgenic analyses. Proc Natl Acad Sci USA. 1991;88(6):2065–9.
109. Furth PA, St Onge L, Boger H, Gruss P, Gossen M, Kistner A, et al. Temporal control of gene expression in transgenic mice by a tetracycline-responsive promoter. Proc Natl Acad Sci USA. 1994;91(20):9302–6.
110. Li P, Tong C, Mehrian-Shai R, Jia L, Wu N, Yan Y, et al. Germline competent embryonic stem cells derived from rat blastocysts. Cell. 2008;135(7):1299–310.
111. McLellan MA, Rosenthal NA, Pinto AR. Cre-loxP-mediated recombination: general principles and experimental considerations. Curr Protoc Mouse Biol. 2017;7(1):1–12.
112. Feil S, Valtcheva N, Feil R. Inducible Cre mice. Methods Mol Biol. 2009;530:343–63.
113. West DB, Pasumarthi RK, Baridon B, Djan E, Trainor A, Griffey SM, et al. A lacZ reporter gene expression atlas for 313 adult KOMP mutant mouse lines. Genome Res. 2015;25(4):598–607.
114. Kaneko T, Mashimo T. Creating knockout and knockin rodents using engineered endonucleases via direct embryo injection. Methods Mol Biol. 2015;1239:307–15.
115. Geurts AM, Cost GJ, Freyvert Y, Zeitler B, Miller JC, Choi VM, et al. Knockout rats via embryo microinjection of zinc-finger nucleases. Science. 2009;325(5939):433.
116. Mashimo T. Gene targeting technologies in rats: zinc finger nucleases, transcription activator-like effector nucleases, and clustered regularly interspaced short palindromic repeats. Develop Growth Differ. 2014;56(1):46–52.
117. Sung YH, Baek IJ, Kim DH, Jeon J, Lee J, Lee K, et al. Knockout mice created by TALEN-mediated gene targeting. Nat Biotechnol. 2013;31(1):23–4.
118. Tesson L, Remy S, Menoret S, Usal C, Thinard R, Savignard C, et al. Genome editing in rats using TALE nucleases. Methods Mol Biol. 2016;1338:245–59.
119. Pennisi E. The CRISPR craze. Science. 2013;341(6148):833–6.
120. Fernandez A, Josa S, Montoliu L. A history of genome editing in mammals. Mamm Genome. 2017;28(7–8):237–46.
121. Horii T, Arai Y, Yamazaki M, Morita S, Kimura M, Itoh M, et al. Validation of microinjection methods for generating knockout mice by CRISPR/Cas-mediated genome engineering. Sci Rep. 2014;4:4513.
122. Guan Y, Shao Y, Li D, Liu M. Generation of site-specific mutations in the rat genome via CRISPR/Cas9. Methods Enzymol. 2014;546:297–317.
123. Shao Y, Guan Y, Wang L, Qiu Z, Liu M, Chen Y, et al. CRISPR/Cas-mediated genome editing in the rat via direct injection of one-cell embryos. Nat Protoc. 2014;9(10):2493–512.
124. Wang H, Yang H, Shivalila CS, Dawlaty MM, Cheng AW, Zhang F, et al. One-step generation of mice carrying mutations in multiple genes by CRISPR/Cas-mediated genome engineering. Cell. 2013;153(4):910–8.
125. Yoshimi K, Kaneko T, Voigt B, Mashimo T. Allele-specific genome editing and correction of disease-associated phenotypes in rats using the CRISPR-Cas platform. Nat Commun. 2014;5:4240.
126. Hsu PD, Lander ES, Zhang F. Development and applications of CRISPR-Cas9 for genome engineering. Cell. 2014;157(6):1262–78.
127. Zhang F, Wen Y, Guo X. CRISPR/Cas9 for genome editing: progress, implications and challenges. Hum Mol Genet. 2014;23(R1):R40–6.
128. Seruggia D, Fernandez A, Cantero M, Pelczar P, Montoliu L. Functional validation of mouse tyrosinase non-coding regulatory DNA elements by CRISPR-Cas9-mediated mutagenesis. Nucleic Acids Res. 2015;43(10):4855–67.
129. Gu B, Posfai E, Rossant J. Efficient generation of targeted large insertions by microinjection into two-cell-stage mouse embryos. Nat Biotechnol. 2018;36(7):632–7.
130. Chen S, Lee B, Lee AY, Modzelewski AJ, He L. Highly Efficient Mouse Genome Editing by CRISPR Ribonucleoprotein Electroporation of Zygotes. J Biol Chem. 2016;291(28):14457–67.
131. Kobayashi T, Namba M, Koyano T, Fukushima M, Sato M, Ohtsuka M, et al. Successful production of genome-edited rats by the rGONAD method. BMC Biotechnol. 2018;18(1):19.
132. Fairfield H, Srivastava A, Ananda G, Liu R, Kircher M, Lakshminarayana A, et al. Exome sequencing reveals pathogenic mutations in 91 strains of mice with Mendelian disorders. Genome Res. 2015;25(7):948–57.
133. Otsen M, Den Bieman M, Winer ES, Jacob HJ, Szpirer J, Szpirer C, et al. Use of simple sequence length polymorphisms for genetic characterization of rat inbred strains. Mamm Genome. 1995;6(9):595–601.
134. Gurumurthy CB, Joshi PS, Kurz SG, Ohtsuka M, Quadros RM, Harms DW, et al. Validation of simple sequence length polymorphism regions of commonly used mouse strains for marker assisted speed congenics screening. Int J Genomics. 2015;2015:735845.
135. Petkov PM, Ding Y, Cassell MA, Zhang W, Wagner G, Sargent EE, et al. An efficient SNP system

for mouse genome scanning and elucidating strain relationships. Genome Res. 2004;14(9):1806–11.
136. Myakishev MV, Khripin Y, Hu S, Hamer DH. High-throughput SNP genotyping by allele-specific PCR with universal energy-transfer-labeled primers. Genome Res. 2001;11(1):163–9.
137. Zurita E, Chagoyen M, Cantero M, Alonso R, Gonzalez-Neira A, Lopez-Jimenez A, et al. Genetic polymorphisms among C57BL/6 mouse inbred strains. Transgenic Res. 2011;20(3):481–9.
138. Mekada K, Abe K, Murakami A, Nakamura S, Nakata H, Moriwaki K, et al. Genetic differences among C57BL/6 substrains. Exp Anim. 2009;58(2):141–9.
139. Mekada K, Hirose M, Murakami A, Yoshiki A. Development of SNP markers for C57BL/6N-derived mouse inbred strains. Exp Anim. 2015;64(1):91–100.
140. Zimdahl H, Nyakatura G, Brandt P, Schulz H, Hummel O, Fartmann B, et al. A SNP map of the rat genome generated from cDNA sequences. Science. 2004;303(5659):807.
141. Smits BM, Guryev V, Zeegers D, Wedekind D, Hedrich HJ, Cuppen E. Efficient single nucleotide polymorphism discovery in laboratory rat strains using wild rat-derived SNP candidates. BMC Genomics. 2005;6:170.
142. Consortium S, Saar K, Beck A, Bihoreau MT, Birney E, Brocklebank D, et al. SNP and haplotype mapping for genetic analysis in the rat. Nat Genet. 2008;40(5):560–6.
143. Beckstead WA, Bjork BC, Stottmann RW, Sunyaev S, Beier DR. SNP2RFLP: a computational tool to facilitate genetic mapping using benchtop analysis of SNPs. Mamm Genome. 2008;19(10–12):687–90.
144. Wedekind D, Reifenberg K, Hedrich HJ. Genetic monitoring of inbred strains. In: Hedrich HJ, editor. The laboratory mouse. Boston: Elsevier; 2012. p. 621–37.
145. Guenet JL, Benavides F. Genetic monitoring of laboratory rodents. In: Patrinos GP, Ansorge W, editors. Molecular diagnostics. 2nd ed. Oxford: Oxford Academic Press; 2010.
146. Reifenberg K, Hedrich H, Wedekind D, Howells N. Objective and methods of genetic monitoring of isogenic mouse and rat strains. GV-SOLAS Specialist Information. 2014.
147. Taft RA, Davisson M, Wiles MV. Know thy mouse. Trends Genet. 2006;22(12):649–53.
148. Reardon S. Lab mice's ancestral 'Eve' gets her genome sequenced. Nature. 2017;551(7680):281.
149. Fahey JR, Katoh H, Malcolm R, Perez AV. The case for genetic monitoring of mice and rats used in biomedical research. Mamm Genome. 2013;24(3–4):89–94.
150. Didion JP, Buus RJ, Naghashfar Z, Threadgill DW, Morse HC 3rd, de Villena FP. SNP array profiling of mouse cell lines identifies their strains of origin and reveals cross-contamination and widespread aneuploidy. BMC Genomics. 2014;15:847.
151. Linder CC. The influence of genetic background on spontaneous and genetically engineered mouse models of complex diseases. Lab Anim (NY). 2001;30(5):34–9.
152. Doetschman T. Influence of genetic background on genetically engineered mouse phenotypes. Methods Mol Biol. 2009;530:423–33.
153. Hummel KP, Coleman DL, Lane PW. The influence of genetic background on expression of mutations at the diabetes locus in the mouse. I. C57BL-KsJ and C57BL-6J strains. Biochem Genet. 1972;7(1):1–13.
154. Dietrich WF, Lander ES, Smith JS, Moser AR, Gould KA, Luongo C, et al. Genetic identification of Mom-1, a major modifier locus affecting Min-induced intestinal neoplasia in the mouse. Cell. 1993;75(4):631–9.
155. Threadgill DW, Dlugosz AA, Hansen LA, Tennenbaum T, Lichti U, Yee D, et al. Targeted disruption of mouse EGF receptor: effect of genetic background on mutant phenotype. Science. 1995;269(5221):230–4.
156. Kuperwasser C, Hurlbut GD, Kittrell FS, Dickinson ES, Laucirica R, Medina D, et al. Development of spontaneous mammary tumors in BALB/c p53 heterozygous mice. A model for Li-Fraumeni syndrome. Am J Pathol. 2000;157(6):2151–9.
157. Freeman D, Lesche R, Kertesz N, Wang S, Li G, Gao J, et al. Genetic background controls tumor development in PTEN-deficient mice. Cancer Res. 2006;66(13):6492–6.
158. Calyjur PC, Almeida Cde F, Ayub-Guerrieri D, Ribeiro AF Jr, Fernandes Sde A, Ishiba R, et al. The mdx mutation in the 129/Sv background results in a milder phenotype: transcriptome comparative analysis searching for the protective factors. PLoS One. 2016;11(3):e0150748.
159. Asamoto M, Hokaiwado N, Cho YM, Shirai T. Effects of genetic background on prostate and taste bud carcinogenesis due to SV40 T antigen expression under probasin gene promoter control. Carcinogenesis. 2002;23(3):463–7.
160. Dang R, Torigoe D, Suzuki S, Kikkawa Y, Moritoh K, Sasaki N, et al. Genetic background strongly modifies the severity of symptoms of Hirschsprung disease, but not hearing loss in rats carrying Ednrb(sl) mutations. PLoS One. 2011;6(9):e24086.
161. Vanden Berghe T, Hulpiau P, Martens L, Vandenbroucke RE, Van Wonterghem E, Perry SW, et al. Passenger mutations confound interpretation of all genetically modified congenic mice. Immunity. 2015;43(1):200–9.
162. Stevens JC, Banks GT, Festing MF, Fisher EM. Quiet mutations in inbred strains of mice. Trends Mol Med. 2007;13(12):512–9.
163. Specht CG, Schoepfer R. Deletion of the alpha-synuclein locus in a subpopulation of C57BL/6J inbred mice. BMC Neurosci. 2001;2:11.

164. Bourdi M, Davies JS, Pohl LR. Mispairing C57BL/6 substrains of genetically engineered mice and wild-type controls can lead to confounding results as it did in studies of JNK2 in acetaminophen and concanavalin A liver injury. Chem Res Toxicol. 2011;24(6):794–6.
165. Poltorak A, He X, Smirnova I, Liu MY, Van Huffel C, Du X, et al. Defective LPS signaling in C3H/HeJ and C57BL/10ScCr mice: mutations in Tlr4 gene. Science. 1998;282(5396):2085–8.
166. Wakeland E, Morel L, Achey K, Yui M, Longmate J. Speed congenics: a classic technique in the fast lane (relatively speaking). Immunol Today. 1997;18(10):472–7.
167. Markel P, Shu P, Ebeling C, Carlson GA, Nagle DL, Smutko JS, et al. Theoretical and empirical issues for marker-assisted breeding of congenic mouse strains. Nat Genet. 1997;17(3):280–4.
168. Wolfer DP, Crusio WE, Lipp HP. Knockout mice: simple solutions to the problems of genetic background and flanking genes. Trends Neurosci. 2002;25(7):336–40.
169. Chen S, Kadomatsu K, Kondo M, Toyama Y, Toshimori K, Ueno S, et al. Effects of flanking genes on the phenotypes of mice deficient in basigin/CD147. Biochem Biophys Res Commun. 2004;324(1):147–53.
170. Brommage R, Liu J, Hansen GM, Kirkpatrick LL, Potter DG, Sands AT, et al. High-throughput screening of mouse gene knockouts identifies established and novel skeletal phenotypes. Bone Res. 2014;2:14034.
171. Brown SDM, Holmes CC, Mallon AM, Meehan TF, Smedley D, Wells S. High-throughput mouse phenomics for characterizing mammalian gene function. Nat Rev Genet. 2018;19(6):357–70.
172. Mallon AM, Blake A, Hancock JM. EuroPhenome and EMPReSS: online mouse phenotyping resource. Nucleic Acids Res. 2008;36(Database issue):D715–8.
173. de Angelis MH, Nicholson G, Selloum M, White J, Morgan H, Ramirez-Solis R, et al. Analysis of mammalian gene function through broad-based phenotypic screens across a consortium of mouse clinics. Nat Genet. 2015;47(9):969–78.
174. Paigen K, Eppig JT. A mouse phenome project. Mamm Genome. 2000;11(9):715–7.
175. Brown SD, Moore MW. The International Mouse Phenotyping Consortium: past and future perspectives on mouse phenotyping. Mamm Genome. 2012;23(9–10):632–40.
176. Koscielny G, Yaikhom G, Iyer V, Meehan TF, Morgan H, Atienza-Herrero J, et al. The International Mouse Phenotyping Consortium Web Portal, a unified point of access for knockout mice and related phenotyping data. Nucleic Acids Res. 2014;42(Database issue):D802–9.
177. Bradley A, Anastassiadis K, Ayadi A, Battey JF, Bell C, Birling MC, et al. The mammalian gene function resource: the International Knockout Mouse Consortium. Mamm Genome. 2012;23(9–10):580–6.
178. Skarnes WC, Rosen B, West AP, Koutsourakis M, Bushell W, Iyer V, et al. A conditional knockout resource for the genome-wide study of mouse gene function. Nature. 2011;474(7351):337–42.
179. Meehan TF, Conte N, West DB, Jacobsen JO, Mason J, Warren J, et al. Disease model discovery from 3,328 gene knockouts by The International Mouse Phenotyping Consortium. Nat Genet. 2017;49(8):1231–8.

Animal and Environmental Factors That Influence Reproducibility

José M. Sánchez-Morgado, Aurora Brønstad, and Kathleen Pritchett-Corning

Abstract

In this chapter we address factors that may bias experiments and impact results unless they are controlled for. This apply for factors in the environment that the animal interacts with to assure optimal homeostasis or to fulfil basic needs. It also includes intrinsic properties of the animal themselves that should be taken into consideration when designing studies and applying results from animal research.

Keywords

Therioepistemology · Environment · Sex · Circadian rhythm · Hormones · Reproduction · Enrichment · Diet · Water · Noise · Vibration · Temperature · Humidity

J. M. Sánchez-Morgado (✉)
Comparative Medicine, Trinity College Dublin, The University of Dublin, Dublin, Ireland
e-mail: Jose.Sanchez-Morgado@tcd.ie

A. Brønstad
Department of Clinical Medicine, University of Bergen, Bergen, Norway
e-mail: Aurora.Bronstad@uib.no

K. Pritchett-Corning
Faculty of Arts and Sciences, Harvard University, Cambridge, MA, USA
e-mail: pritchettcorning@fas.harvard.edu

Department of Comparative Medicine, University of Washington, Seattle, WA, USA
e-mail: pritchettcorning@fas.harvard.edu

1 Introduction

Animals used in research must cope with the environment we provide them, and their homeostatic system must adjust to changes in this environment to maintain optimal physiology. Changes in this environment cause the animal to adapt to new conditions by physiologic accommodation. This response may affect experimental outcomes, be a confounding variable or a source of variation. In order to obtain reliable, meaningful results, an attempt should be made to understand and account for all known biological, environmental and social factors when conducting experiments involving animals. This may mean changing experimental designs to maximise variation [1] or listing a wide variety of environmental and animal information in supplemental materials [2]. This chapter will focus on biological and environmental factors that affect animal physiology and thereby also output of experiments. These are also factors useful to assess in comparing studies and addressing questions of non-reproducibility.

In chapter "Rodent Genetics", the authors of that chapter address the genetics of rodents and how this can have an impact on the reproducibility

© Springer Nature Switzerland AG 2021
J. M. Sánchez Morgado, A. Brønstad (eds.), *Experimental Design and Reproducibility in Preclinical Animal Studies*, Laboratory Animal Science and Medicine 1,
https://doi.org/10.1007/978-3-030-66147-2_3

of animal experiments. Even though we will not consider genetics in this chapter, the factors we will discuss here are dependent and related to the genome of the animal. What is more, there is also an interdependence between the genome, the microbiome (addressed in chapter "Microbiology and Microbiome") and the other factors described in this chapter [3–6]. We cannot separate them, and they need to be treated together as potential causes of variability leading to irreproducible animal research if not taken into account in the experimental design (see also Part II in this book dealing with statistics and experimental design).

1.1 Therioepistemology

In 2017, Garner and collaborators introduced the term *therioepistemology* to describe the study of how knowledge is gained from animal research. They coined the word from the study of the theory of knowledge and the mechanisms by which rational inference is formed, known as *epistemology*, and the prefix *therio*, of animals [2]. They proposed six questions to help address the problem of those factors in animal research that we cannot control but should acknowledge instead of ignoring them [2]:

1. What features of model biology are ignored? Physiological, anatomical and behavioural particularities of the animal model will differ from humans; nevertheless, they are consistently ignored. We have dealt with some in this chapter but also in chapters "Rodent Genetics" and "Microbiology and Microbiome" of this book.
2. What features of human biology are ignored? Sometimes it is not the characteristics of the animal model that are ignored but the human condition in itself; thus, we try to replicate human pathologies using genetically modified mice that can only replicate partially a molecular pathway or mimic a specific aspect of a much broader human pathology.
3. What features of the measures are ignored? Part of this problem is how to deal with type I errors, which is consistently ignored throughout the animal research literature. The reader can find more on this question on chapters "Statistical Tests and Sample Size Calculations", "Design of Experiments" and "Scholarly Publishing and Scientific Reproducibility", dealing with statistics and experimental design.
4. What features of background methodology and husbandry are ignored? This relates to the well-known justification of the historical standardisation, i.e. if a model works, why change the conditions, even though there could potentially be refinements and improvements made? The answer will be that if a model stops working under different experimental backgrounds, it lacks external validity, and, thus, it will not translate to humans.
5. What animal well-being issues are ignored? Preclinical research should be treated exactly the same as clinical research, i.e. the animal should be seen as a patient, not as a reagent. The reader is also referred to chapter "Systematic Reviews" in this book.
6. What principles of experimental design and statistics are ignored? In general, preclinical research lacks proper experimental design and statistics. The reader is referred to chapters "Statistical Tests and Sample Size Calculations", "Design of Experiments" and "Scholarly Publishing and Scientific Reproducibility" for more on this.

1.2 Standardisation of the Environment

It has been shown that environmental standardisation will increase test sensitivity, which is the proportion of correctly identified data, and reduce the variation in the obtained data, but, as Richter et al. [1] questioned, will these lead to an increase in reproducibility? The answer is no, as they found in a set of experiments with 18 standardised replicated cohorts and 18 heterogenised replicated cohorts. Through heterogenisation, they better understood the systematic variation of the experimental conditions. Environmental standardisation resulted in poorer reproducibility and introduced a systematic source of false-positive results above that expected by chance alone. This work was criticised because the conclusions were based on a retrospective analysis. The authors went on to do a prospective study and also found that standardised experiments increased test sensitivity at the expense of external validity, i.e. the applicability of a result to other conditions, populations or species [7]. For this study, they used 3 behavioural tests on 256 female mice from 2 different strains, C57BL/6 and BALB/c, within 4 standardised and 4 heterogenised cohorts taking 36 different behavioural measures. They confirmed their previous findings [1] and that even simple forms of heterogenisation may guarantee robust results across experiments [7]. This is something that Michael Festing had already proposed, in terms of the genome, 30 years earlier. In 1980, he published his first proposition to change the way toxicology was carried out in outbred stocks by using instead several inbreds of F1 hybrid strains in a factorial experiment design [8].

2 The Animal Sex

Sex is an important variable to consider, not only for the obvious reason that several physiological processes are different between sexes but also because in a majority of manuscripts either the sex of the animals is not reported or only one sex is used. This is a major source of reduced external validity of those studies. When sex is reported, it is readily apparent there is a generalised male bias across preclinical research disciplines, and this has been criticised for several years. In 2011, Beery et al. [9] reported male bias in eight out of ten fields analysed, including pharmacology, endocrinology, animal behaviour, behavioural physiology, neuroscience, general biology, zoology and physiology. They also found a female skew in the fields of reproduction and immunology, although in this last field less than 40% of manuscripts reported the sex of the animals used [9]. The reasons for omitting one sex, mainly females, in preclinical studies have been poorly justified, consisting of citation of confounding hormonal variations during the oestrus cycle [10, 11], a reduction in statistical power by the introduction of a second sex [10] and historical reasons [11]. This exclusion of one sex in preclinical research and the consequent inadequate analysis has also been cited as a reason for the lack of reproducibility in preclinical research [11]. On the 25th of January 2016, the National Institutes of Health (NIH) implemented the requirement to consider sex as a biological variable within their grant submissions [12]. Nevertheless, some researchers have protested this policy, arguing that to adequately design experiments using both sexes will be more expensive and space-intensive [13] and will result in unnecessary duplication and slow the progress due to more workload [14]. If we, as scientists, are truly serious about moving forwards from a lack of reproducibility, these arguments are both specious and detrimental. Clearly, both sexes need to be included in scientific endeavours, and using just one sex based on those arguments will hinder not only reproducibility but also translational research. As Cara Tannenbaum et al. [15] clearly expressed, "researchers and peer reviewers are being asked to thoughtfully consider whether a single-sex study is justified when research results are to be applied to both sexes". She proposed a set of questions for peer reviewers to consider that we have included here (Table 1).

Physiological processes which are different between sexes include pain and its control, which clearly affects not just pain research but any research which will cause some degree of pain that must be relieved or it will otherwise interfere with the aim of the study. In 2011, Robert E. Sorge, then working in the laboratory of Jeffrey S. Mogil, made a seminal discovery in pain research, namely, that the afferent pain pathway is different in female and male mice [16]. Whereas in male mice, microglia have a major role in pain sensitivity, they realised by working in both sexes that in female mice T cells, instead of microglia, are the preferred afferent pathway. What is more, they discovered that testosterone is the switch that allows the use of microglia instead of T cells by using castrated males and intact females [17]. Since then other discoveries have been made to explain, for example, the attenuated response to morphine observed in females [18]. Thus, unless

Table 1 Question reviewers should consider when evaluating sex as a biological variable (SABV) taken with permission from Ref. [15]

1	Clarity of the research question
2	Clarity of rationale for the research approach and methodology
3	Appropriateness of the research design
4	Appropriateness of the research methods
5	Feasibility of the research approach
6	Anticipation of difficulties that may be encountered in the research and plans for management
7	Quality and appropriateness of SABV
8	Justification for a single-sex study
9	Evidence that the research question incorporates SABV
10	Potential for the research to add value to the current state of knowledge on a given topic that has potential to, but has not yet fully elucidated the impact of sex on biological mechanisms, pathophysiology or translational science
11	Impact of research incorporating SABV
12	Potential for a significant contribution to the improvement of women and men's health, the health of boys and girls or the health of gender-diverse persons
13	Appropriateness and adequacy of the proposed plan for knowledge dissemination and exchange

laboratories were using both sexes, preclinical research on pain would reach very different outcomes depending on the sex of animals used. Memory research is another field of neuroscience that has been shown to be biased because of the use of only male animals [19]. It has been demonstrated that females show a more prominent basal amygdala activation compared with hippocampus activation in males during memory retrieval [20]. In cardiovascular research, we now know that the ability of ventricular myocytes to contract declines with age in male rodents more than in female rodents [21]. There are also well-documented differences in haematology and biochemical analytes between sexes of the same species and even the same strain [22].

2.1 Circadian Rhythm

Circadian rhythm has a significant impact in animal physiology [23, 24]. Circadian rhythms are generated by solar time, with photons impacting the cells in the retina, which in turn send electric signals to the suprachiasmatic nucleus (SCN) within the hypothalamus through the retino-hypothalamic tract. These electric signals will cause SCN neurons spontaneously firing. Signals from the SCN will travel then to the hypothalamus, cortex, brain stem and the different circadian clocks around the body [25]. The retinal evoked firing in the SCN will only persist for the duration of the light pulse [25]. This is the mechanistic reason for the physiological changes evoked by light of enough intensity during the night part of the cycle, which have been documented to occur after a light pulse of less than a second.

Adaption to seasonal changes is an important quality for survival and reproduction, and this quality is deeply conserved in animals even after many generations in captivity. Light, and change in daylight, is an important regulator of the reproduction cycle of many species, and disturbances in light cycle may be responsible for drops in reproductive performance [26]. Standardised light regimes are commonly used to control circadian rhythm variations. Attention should also be paid to indirect light coming through inspection windows, light leakage around doors and daylight in adjacent corridors [27]. Furthermore, attention must be paid to light exposure when animals are brought from animal holding rooms to specially equipped laboratories (imaging, telemetry, behavioural suites, etc.). Laboratories built for humans are usually equipped with windows to allow daylight in and also with a higher light intensity than the one found in the animal holding rooms. The European Guidelines for the Accommodation and Care of Animals Used for Experimental and Other Scientific Purposes (ETS 123) [28] defines standards for light/dark cycle in rodent facilities as typically 12 hours of dark and 12 hours of light, but also other light regimes with longer or shorter day periods are used depending on the species [29]. Artificial induction of seasonal change has been accomplished by modulation of light/dark cycles to expedite or delay developmental stages and reproduction performance [30].

Rodents are nocturnal animals and normally sleep during the daytime. Received wisdom states that frequent sleep disturbance during daytime due to daily routines in the animal facility may cause stress and sleep deprivation in the animals, although this may not be true [31]. Even though efforts have been made to standardise light/dark cycles in duration, few labs keep their animals on reverse day/night cycles, and most experiments are still performed during daytime (since humans trend to be diurnal) [32]. The observation of clinical signs and animal welfare assessments is difficult to perform during daylight hours as animals do not express normal night-time activity levels when they rest. ETS 123 therefore recommends some observation of animals under frequencies of red light undetectable to the rodents, as this is not perceived as bright daylight by rodents [33]. However, this has recently been challenged in an article by Niklaus and collaborators [34] where they claimed that rats are sensitive to light wavelengths longer than 620 nm, reaching opposite results to previous work by De Farias Rocha and collaborators [35], by using a different experimental setup. The question, thus, remains certainly open, but more work needs to be done to support one or the other.

Animal facilities have, more and more, automated means of controlling light/dark periods and light intensity within the room. Thus, we rely on systems such as building management systems software to keep the room environment within the regulatory limits. These systems sometimes fail, and unless there are strong processes in place, there may be a gap of hours or days before the staff working in the facility realise there is a problem. One of the more common failures is constant light exposure due to a failure to start the dark cycle. Mice will increase body weight and become insulin resistant with constant light exposure [36]. A similar effect has been observed in rats, with constant light reducing glucose-stimulated insulin secretion due to a disruption in the pancreatic beta cell circadian clock [37] and accelerating the development of diabetes in transgenic rats for human islet amyloid polypeptide [38].

2.2 Light and the Laboratory Mouse

Light quality (referring here to the spectral composition of light), and its influence in the circadian regulation, is not generally considered by current regulations [28, 39]. However, this can be an important source of variability between different laboratories, especially those working with certain mouse strains or with rats. Thus, most animal facilities do not pay due attention to this important factor, apart from controlling the intensity to avoid rodent light retinopathy and to establish a constant light/dark cycle throughout the year [40]. Research has found that the more light in the 465–485 nm wavelength, which is the blue colour of the visible light spectrum, the better the animal health and welfare compared to cool white fluorescent (CWF) light [41]. Melatonin has been shown to be six- to sevenfold higher in rodents under this blue-appearing wavelength than with CWF lighting [41, 42]. There is now consensus on how to quantify and report light stimuli in experimental studies [43, 44], which should be used to harmonise reporting and thus improve the reproducibility of experimental work between laboratories [41].

2.3 Age and Developmental Stage of the Animal

Studies using animals often use animals at one age, or body weight group, so the external validity of such studies is limited to that age or body weight. This can be critical when other researchers try to reproduce the experiments, especially when the publication does not provide any details of the age or life stage of the animals used. Not only that, but when interpreting the results, the difference found in the data might be the consequence of a normal age-related maturity process taking place in the particular age range chosen for the study like puberty or the beginning of feeding in fish larvae.

The Jackson Laboratory conducted a study with 31 different inbred strains and published data on median lifespans and circulating IGF1 levels at 6, 12 and 18 months for the first cohort of 32 females and 32 males of each strain [45]. They documented that males from C57BL/6 J or 129S1/SvImJ lived twice as long as males from FVB/NJ. These are just three of the inbred strains in which genetically modified mice have been produced worldwide and are used in most, if not all, of the studies using genetically modified mice. Thus, studies using animals in these different backgrounds, but the same genetic modification should take into account the differences in lifespan, which may account for maturation or aging processes that may affect the experimental data.

There are also many examples in the recent literature on how different organs and tissues will mature, and thus change, with age. For example, the developing spleen is an active haematopoietic centre from approximately day 15 of gestation until several weeks after birth in mice, rather than a secondary lymphoid organ as in the adult [46]. In humans, the experimental evidence is that the haematopoietic stem cells (HSCs) naturally migrate back and forth from the bone marrow periodically [47]. In vertebrates, the origins of the haematopoietic tissue are non-singular, with a shifting source and localisation over time. In total, the haematopoietic system is composed of HSCs, multiple terminally differentiated lineages and multiple intermediate committed progenitors [48]. In mice, the haematology goes through various stages as the animal ages. Thus, erythrocyte morphology in the young mouse is quite variable, and there is also a larger count of reticulocytes than in the adult mouse. Leukocytes, on the other hand, have a low count at birth to only reach adult numbers by 6–7 weeks of age. Depending on the mouse strain used, some haematological changes associated with age will be more pronounced. Another aging change in the haematology of mice is a reduction in the haematocrit due to a plasma expansion, which occurs with age and is often misinterpreted as anaemia [49, 50]. Table 2 shows normal haematological reference intervals for different inbred strains at 9 weeks of age [51]. These age-related changes have also been shown to occur in 26 biochemical analytes [22]. In 2008, Mazzaccara et al. [22] examined three mouse strains, C57BL/6 J, 129SV/Ev and C3H/HeJ, and showed that most of the biochemical analytes analysed differed according to age. They also evaluated five haematology parameters of which red blood cell counts, haemoglobin, haematocrit and platelet counts increased with the animal's age only in C57BL/6 J mice [22] (for an excellent review on mouse haematology, we refer the reader to *The Mouse in Biomedical Research, Volume III: Normative Biology, Husbandry and Models*) [52].

Aging is another variable affecting studies using animal models. If the age of mice used in the study is not documented, results may be irreproducible. The mouse cochlea, for example, continues to mature during the first 2 weeks of life [53], and some strains of mice carry alleles causing age-related hearing loss [54, 55]. In the central nervous system, it has also been shown that pain modulation changes with age in rats from a facilitation of spinal pain transmission before day 21 of age to both facilitation and inhibition after 28 days of age [56–58]. Also, the heart changes with age and activity. There is epicardial fat deposition and aortic valve calcifications in older guinea pigs and rats [21]. There is also evidence for atrial hypertrophy and dilation in older rodents, and left ventricular wall thickness increases with age in older rats and mice [21]. There is also strong evidence that the heart's responsiveness to β-adrenergic stimulation declines with age in animals [21]. In aged zebrafish, myocyte hypertrophy, increased ventricular density and fibrosis, valvular lesions and reductions in coronary vasculature have been described [59] (for an excellent review on age-associated changes in zebrafish, see Stoyek MR and collaborators review [59]).

2.4 Hormones and Reproduction

Reproductive performance and animal activity are very much influenced by circadian rhythm, and the reader is advised to read the Circadian Rhythm section for more information.

The mammalian nose contains the main olfactory epithelium, the septal organ of

Table 2 Empirical haematological reference intervals for different inbred strains at 9 weeks of age. We have run Kolmogorov-Smirnov test with Bonferroni correction for the multiple testing. Results are separately shown for both sexes; there is only one entry using data for both sexes when differences between the sexes were not significant [51]

129S2/SvPasCrlf	WBC (10^9/l)	RBC (10^{12}/l)	HGB (g/dl)	HCT (PCV) (%)	MCV (fl)	MCH (pg)	MCHC (g/dl)	RDW (%)	PLT (10^9/l)	MPV (fl)	NEUT (%)	LYMPH (%)	MONO (%)	EO (%)	BASO (%)	NEUT # (10^9/l)	LYMPH # (10^9/l)	MONO # (10^9/l)	EO # (10^9/l)	BASO # (10^9/l)
Mean	12.83	11.23	18.37	53.57	47.64	16.36	34.66	7.98	562.28	10.07	4.63	93.65	0.65	0.80	0.28	0.59	12.02	0.08	0.09	0.03
Low (2.5%)	5.95	9.11	14.83	43.78	47.00	15.90	33.20	7.10	368.85	9.40	3.00	88.65	0.30	0.20	0.10	0.18	5.27	0.02	0.04	0.00
High (97.5%)	19.45	12.62	20.66	59.88	49.00	16.90	43.30	10.06	676.30	12.81	8.07	95.65	1.05	2.21	0.71	0.98	18.62	0.18	0.21	0.10
N	100	100	100	100	100	100	200	100	100	200	100	100	100	100	200	200	100	200	100	200
Mean	10.42	10.66	17.69	51.00	47.77	16.65		8.72	478.60		5.88	91.95	0.77	1.13			9.55		0.12	
Low (2.5%)	4.94	6.44	11.82	28.04	39.48	16.00		7.35	264.95		1.30	87.40	0.30	0.10			4.49		0.01	
High (97.5%)	15.86	11.99	19.71	57.27	49.00	18.25		11.03	701.35		9.65	97.07	1.40	2.36			14.55		0.23	
N	100	100	100	100	100	100		100	100		100	100	100	100			100		100	
129/SvJEv-Gpi 1c	WBC (10^9/l)	RBC (10^{12}/l)	HGB (g/dl)	HCT (PCV) (%)	MCV (fl)	MCH (pg)	MCHC (g/dl)	RDW (%)	PLT (10^9/l)	MPV (fl)	NEUT (%)	LYMPH (%)	MONO (%)	EO (%)	BASO (%)	NEUT # (10^9/l)	LYMPH # (10^9/l)	MONO # (10^9/l)	EO # (10^9/l)	BASO # (10^9/l)
Mean	11.40	10.89	17.85	51.94	47.70	16.40	34.43	8.20	553.00	9.96	5.32	92.97	0.67	0.78	0.26	0.59	10.60	0.08	0.08	0.03
Low (2.5%)	6.60	8.83	14.61	41.54	46.00	15.65	33.21	7.10	388.55	9.40	3.10	89.05	0.25	0.20	0.10	0.32	5.84	0.02	0.02	0.00
High (97.5%)	16.60	12.11	19.55	57.25	49.00	17.05	35.25	9.85	677.80	10.60	8.34	95.60	1.30	1.90	0.90	0.96	15.62	0.16	0.22	0.11
N	182	182	182	182	182	182	182	182	82	182	182	182	182	182	182	182	182	182	82	182
Mean									467.08										0.10	
Low (2.5%)									332.95										0.04	
High (97.5%)									594.00										0.18	
N									100										100	
CD-1	WBC (10^9/l)	RBC (10^{12}/l)	HGB (g/dl)	HCT (PCV) (%)	MCV (fl)	MCH (pg)	MCHC (g/dl)	RDW (%)	PLT (10^9/l)	MPV (fl)	NEUT (%)	LYMPH (%)	MONO (%)	EO (%)	BASO (%)	NEUT # (10^9/l)	LYMPH # (10^9/l)	MONO # (10^9/l)	EO # (10^9/l)	BASO # (10^9/l)
Mean	8.47	9.93	16.40	47.92	47.27	16.35	34.28	8.98	1151.72	10.98	8.79	87.92	1.23	1.47	0.27	0.87	8.12	0.10	0.14	0.02
Low (2.5%)	4.25	8.73	14.40	38.64	40.48	14.95	32.70	7.00	683.30	10.20	2.74	76.94	0.50	0.20	0.10	0.15	3.40	0.03	0.02	0.00

(Continued)

Table 2 Continued

129S2/SvPasCrlf	WBC $(10^9/l)$	RBC $(10^{12}/l)$	HGB (g/dl)	HCT (PCV) (%)	MCV (fl)	MCH (pg)	MCHC (g/dl)	RDW (%)	PLT $(10^9/l)$	MPV (fl)	NEUT (%)	LYMPH (%)	MONO (%)	EO (%)	BASO (%)	NEUT # $(10^9/l)$	LYMPH # $(10^9/l)$	MONO # $(10^9/l)$	EO # $(10^9/l)$	BASO # $(10^9/l)$
High (97.5%)	14.20	11.29	18.45	54.55	51.00	17.81	42.31	11.85	1493.15	12.60	18.32	94.61	2.45	5.40	0.70	2.02	13.41	0.24	0.45	0.06
N	220	220	220	220	100	100	220	220	100	220	220	220	220	100	220	100	100	220	220	220
Mean					49.12	16.65			1018.70					2.05		0.62	6.93			
Low (2.5%)					46.98	15.50			541.80					0.30		0.38	3.73			
High (97.5%)					52.00	17.70			1342.00					6.62		1.12	11.87			
N					120	120			120					120		120	120			
C57BL/6JOlaHsd	WBC $(10^9/l)$	RBC $(10^{12}/l)$	HGB (g/dl)	HCT (PCV) (%)	MCV (fl)	MCH (pg)	MCHC (g/dl)	RDW (%)	PLT $(10^9/l)$	MPV (fl)	NEUT (%)	LYMPH (%)	MONO (%)	EO (%)	BASO (%)	NEUT # $(10^9/l)$	LYMPH # $(10^9/l)$	MONO # $(10^9/l)$	EO # $(10^9/l)$	BASO # $(10^9/l)$
Mean	9.58	10.75	16.31	50.04	46.64	15.07	32.40	8.77	1114.30	11.82	8.97	88.63	1.42	0.70	0.27	0.85	8.50	0.14	0.06	0.03
Low (2.5%)	5.19	9.07	13.89	42.39	45.00	14.60	31.55	7.20	803.45	10.60	4.90	79.40	0.60	0.20	0.10	0.40	4.57	0.04	0.02	0.00
High (97.5%)	15.71	11.94	17.90	55.41	49.00	15.70	33.81	11.21	1365.75	16.20	17.70	93.41	2.80	1.91	0.70	1.84	13.71	0.28	0.20	0.08
N	200	200	200	200	200	100	100	200	100	100	200	200	200	200	200	200	200	200	200	200
Mean						15.29	32.77		975.96	11.42										
Low (2.5%)						14.70	31.84		507.50	10.39										
High (97.5%)						16.05	33.81		1343.15	17.22										
N						100	100		100	100										
C57BL/6J	WBC $(10^9/l)$	RBC $(10^{12}/l)$	HGB (g/dl)	HCT (PCV) (%)	MCV (fl)	MCH (pg)	MCHC (g/dl)	RDW (%)	PLT $(10^9/l)$	MPV (fl)	NEUT (%)	LYMPH (%)	MONO (%)	EO (%)	BASO (%)	NEUT # $(10^9/l)$	LYMPH # $(10^9/l)$	MONO # $(10^9/l)$	EO # $(10^9/l)$	BASO # $(10^9/l)$
Mean	9.04	11.01	16.52	51.49	46.77	15.11	32.33	9.05	1073.49	12.21	11.29	86.13	1.64	0.75	0.19	1.01	7.80	0.14	0.06	0.02
Low (2.5%)	5.24	9.81	14.66	46.54	45.00	14.70	31.41	7.50	648.00	10.20	5.15	67.78	0.57	0.20	0.10	0.38	4.25	0.04	0.02	0.00
High (97.5%)	15.40	11.96	17.90	56.06	48.55	15.63	33.10	10.90	1324.60	16.71	28.04	92.90	3.36	1.53	0.40	2.55	13.56	0.31	0.17	0.04
N	109	219	109	219	219	109	109	219	109	219	109	109	109	109	219	109	109	219	219	219
Mean	11.15		17.02			15.35	32.81		901.24		6.81	91.30	1.12	0.58		0.74	10.21			
Low (2.5%)	5.79		15.20			14.80	31.95		652.15		4.05	86.05	0.50	0.10		0.39	5.17			
High (97.5%)	16.97		18.43			15.73	33.50		1053.10		10.86	94.63	2.03	2.08		1.23	15.71			
N	110		110			110	110		110		110	110	110	110		110	110			

Masera, the vomeronasal organ (VNO) and the Grueneberg ganglion; all are related to olfactory functions including social communications. The major player in social communication through olfactory signals is the VNO, which collects information from the environment through the nose and vomeronasal duct, feeding the vomeronasal sensory neurons (VSNs) with chemicals taken up by the approximately 300 different vomeronasal receptors. The VSN axon passes through the ethmoid cribriform plate to access the accessory olfactory bulb, and from here reaches the amygdala and the hypothalamus [60]. The main olfactory system is also involved in eliciting behaviour from olfactory cues, together with the accessory olfactory system, and they both will interact at different levels in the CNS: olfactory bulbs, amygdala and hypothalamus [60]. The VNO conveys information about pheromones, which are anonymous signals, not being used to identify individuals; predators, the kairomones of Wyatt [61]; prey; and individual identity and may also identify pathogenic states in mice [60]. These olfactory cues in mice are very strongly shaped by a specific set of polymorphic communication proteins that has evolved to provide a distinctive signal of identity: the major urinary proteins (MUPs) [62]. These MUPs are a group of 18–20 kDa lipocalins involved in mouse chemical signalling, synthesised, in their majority, in the liver for excretion in the urine [63]. These MUPs are encoded by a cluster of 21 major urinary protein (MUP) genes on mouse chromosome 4 [62] and released at a high concentration in mouse urine. These genes are rearranged and expressed in a combinatorial form, particularly to each individual in a non-inbred population, and also discriminated through a set of vomeronasal sensory neurons using a combinatorial coding strategy [62]. These proteins are known to bind and slowly release volatile pheromones [63]. Some are involved in male aggression and attraction to females, like MUP20 [60]. There are also 38 exocrine gland-secreting peptide (ESP) genes; some of their translated products are involved in stopping male sexual behaviour (ESP22), and some in starting female lordosis (ESP1) [60].

Urine marking plays an important role in communication between female mice as well [64]. Some of the odours will have signalling effects, i.e. these odours will change the behaviour of other mice, whereas others will have primer effects, i.e. these odours will change the physiology of other mice. This primer effect is the cause of well-known reproductive effects in mice. Female mouse urine is known to contain pheromones and inhibit the reproductive physiology of other females under conditions linked to competition for reproductive opportunities, such as overcrowding. This is known as the Lee-Boot effect, which is a prolongation of the oestrus cycle in group-housed females [65, 66]. The key compound causing the Lee-Boot effect is 2,5-dimethylpyrazine [67], and its excretion is at its peak during metestrus. This compound has also been found to have a negative effect on male mice by depressing the maturation of reproductive organs and the level of immunocompetence [68]. If females are exposed to male urine pheromones, there is an induction of oestrus, a shortening of the oestrous cycle, and oestrus synchronisation of female mice; together this constellation of effects is known as the Whitten effect [69, 70]. Pregnancy failure, known as the Bruce effect [71, 72], is a phenomenon where pregnant rodents terminate their pregnancy after being exposed to the scent of an unfamiliar male. This occurs when female mice in early pregnancy are exposed to odour from an unfamiliar male at the same time as twice daily surges in their prolactin levels. This is stimulated by differences in low-molecular-weight urinary components that include MHC peptides or by differences in the amount of exocrine gland-secreting peptide 1 in male tear fluids, compared to the remembered stud male [62]. The unfamiliar male scent will trigger an increase of dopamine in the hypothalamus and a decrease of prolactin secretion from the anterior pituitary gland resulting in a subsequent decrease in progesterone, which is essential to maintain pregnancy, and the female returns to oestrus within a week [68]. Another primer effect is the accelerated onset of puberty in females exposed to male odours during their prepubertal period, also known as the Vandenbergh effect [73]. In this case, there has been found a correlation between the exposure to male odours and an activation of the posteroventral medial amygdala, posterodorsal medial amygdala, the anterior cortical nucleus of the amygdala, the medial preoptic area and the ventromedial nucleus, showing that these areas are differentially sensitive to intact male odours [74]. In both the Whitten and the Vandenbergh effects, several compounds have been potentially found to have an effect. These compounds have all a strong affinity to MUPs in male mice [75]. Male mouse odours have also a primer effect in male mice. The odour of dominant male mice suppresses sperm motility in subordinates [76].

The reader is directed to Sachiko Koyama's excellent review for more information about the effects of primer marking in mice [68].

2.5 Handling

In 2010, Jane Hurst and Rebecca West published the results of a study that has had a profound impact in the husbandry of laboratory mice [77]. Briefly, they showed that picking up mice using tunnels or the open hand led to a voluntary approach from the animals, low anxiety and acceptance of physical restraint [77]. They also showed that picking them up by the tail induced aversion and high anxiety [77]. In a series of later publications, Jane Hurst and Kelly Gouveia demonstrated that mice do not even have to be familiar with the tunnel, although previous familiarisation helped in an outbred stock, for the anxiety levels to be reduced [78]; that tail handled mice performed poorly in behavioural studies, and this was only slightly improved by prior familiarisation [79]; that mice handled by tunnel explored readily and showed robust responses to test stimuli regardless of prior familiarisation or stimulus location [79]; that very brief handling (just 2 s) was sufficient to familiarise mice with tunnel handling, even when experienced only during cage cleaning [80]; and that experience of repeated immobilisation and subcutaneous injection did not reverse the positive effects of tunnel handling [80]. In spite of all this evidence, there are still laboratories and facilities picking up mice by the base of the tail, some of them even used sterile forceps, as a recent article by Henderson and collaborators [81] has shown. The group sent an online survey worldwide and received 390 complete responses to eight questions addressing the uptake of these non-aversive methods for handling mice. Even though most of the participants were aware of the benefit of using non-aversive handling methods, just 18% of them were using these methods exclusively, with 43% using a combination of non-aversive methods and tail handling and a 35% using only tail handling methods despite all the evidence against this [81]. The authors of this chapter speculate that this failure of uptake is due to concerns about transmission of infectious disease, the resistance of researchers to change that might affect "historical data" and concerns about disruption of established routines.

3 The Environment

3.1 Primary Enclosure (Cage, Pen and Tank)

3.1.1 Size of the Primary Enclosure

The European Union and the United States have defined minimum standards for enclosure dimensions and space allowances for housing research animals in their regulations and guidelines, which are rather similar [28, 39]. These usually define a minimum area (in m^2 or cm^2) per animal of a certain weight and state that all animals should be able to assume normal body postures. For example, the ethological needs of mice include resting, grooming, exploration, gnawing, nesting, hiding and social interaction, so at a minimum, consideration should be given to cage designs which allow performance of these behaviours. Both sets of regulations established a "one-size-fits-all" paradigm that does not necessarily correspond to the wide range of different breeds, stocks or strains used in the laboratory. What is more, there were no studies to sustain these arbitrary standards at the time of their publication.

Even though mice are highly motivated to work for incremental space, there are no biological markers that will clearly indicate a negative effect with reduced space allocation. Attention should be paid to qualitative space, where animals can display the full behavioural repertoire, rather than to quantitative space, simply assigning a minimum area per animal [82].

The three-dimensional design of the primary enclosure is less well defined, though it has been shown that opportunity to use three-dimensional space is important for the development of the brain [83]. For many species, using both horizontal and vertical spaces provided is a natural behaviour. Implementation of "enrichment" programmes may meet some of the demands, but it is important that animals' natural needs and behaviour are the focus of enrichment programmes and that any enrichment is consistently applied.

3.1.2 Enrichment of the Primary Enclosure

Enrichment of the barren cage environment to meet animals' basic needs is now the default way to house research animals [28, 84] and is also regarded as refinement of animal research with the expectation to continuously refine enriched housing conditions based on updated information. Research animals are typically housed under conditions very different from their natural habitat and with limited opportunities to express normal behaviours. Such conditions impose constraints on behaviour and brain development and result in altered brain functions [85]. It has been shown that 2½-week-old rat pups already have a rudimentary map of space [86]. Histological examination of the brains of animals exposed to either a complex ("enriched") environment compared to unenriched controls has revealed experience-induced morphological plasticity in the brain through life [83]. André and collaborators [87] checked 164 physiological parameters under three different conditions: no environmental enrichment, nesting and nesting and shelter. They found that nesting material and shelters may be used to improve animal welfare without impairment of experimental outcome or loss of comparability to previous data collected under barren housing conditions. These results and conclusions contrast with the ones obtained by Macri and collaborators in 2013 [88], where they claim that some effects of the synthetic compound JWH-018, a potent cannabinoid receptor agonist [89], are environmentally mediated. However, this article has many experimental design flaws potentially leading to bias, i.e. experimental groups differed in their conditions, the authors do not report randomisation or blinding, there is no indication of sample size calculations and they report the mean and standard error of the mean instead of the mean and the confidence interval [90]. Keeping animals without the ability to support their basic behavioural needs leads to suffering and distress that may as well be a confounding factor in experimental work. Animals may respond individually with either stereotypic behaviour, aggression, depression, self-mutilation or other maladaptive behaviour and their response cannot be standardised. It is important that responsible bodies (AWB, IACUC, AWERB or equal) develop and update enrichment programmes that take both animal welfare and scientific considerations into account.

3.1.3 Animal Position in the Room

The position of the cage in the rack and the rack within the room may affect a study as light and worker motion is not equally distributed in the room, and this may affect animal behaviour and results [91–93]. Light intensity will vary significantly between the top shelf, usually more brightly lit, and the cages on the bottom row, which are typically much dimmer. We know that mice find brightly lit, elevated spaces aversive, and this may influence results [94, 95]. In addition, the order of cage handling may bias results, e.g. all cages of one group are placed on the top row and always treated or measured early in the day, while those in a different group are placed at the bottom and are treated at the end. To assure proper randomisation in a study, cage position in the rack should also be randomised [96, 97], and in addition rotation of cage position in the rack during a study is recommended to avoid induction of systematic failure because of cage position.

3.2 Diet

Laboratory animals are fed a wide variety of diets, differing between laboratories and commercial companies. These diets, referred to as standard or regular diets, are made with natural ingredients such as soybean meal, alfalfa, fish meal and animal by-products, have variable nutritional content between batches and contain biologically active components such as phytoestrogens and toxic heavy metals such as arsenic [98, 99]. Diet ingredients cover the minimum requirements for the species and life stage and can be manufactured in various ways [100]. It is important that the chosen diet does not negatively influence the experiments, for example, by containing antinutrients or hormone-mimicking or blocking substances. Also, ingredients should be free of any chemicals, toxins, heavy metals or microbes, and documentation should be available from the producer on the quality analyses performed on different batches. The origin of dietary ingredients, processing and storing will impact the quality of the food and thereby the animal and the experiments. We know, for example, that the total isoflavones of soybeans vary within variety, locations and, over time, even when grown in the same location [101]. To avoid uncontrolled variation in models, the same batch of diet should be used throughout a study, and if it is a long-term study, the diet should be one lot (or mixed at the beginning of the study) and should be frozen and thawed for each feeding. Diet past its expiration date should never be used. Not only is degradation of the nutritional value of the diet a concern, but mould or bacterial overgrowth might also occur. The diet should be stored according to manufacturer's recommendations, and a pest control programme should be in place to avoid compromise of diet by infectious agents carried by pests.

The composition of the major nutritional ingredients, carbohydrates, fat and proteins may have significant impact on animal studies. Prebiotic properties of dietary fermentable oligo-, di-, mono-saccharides and polyols (FODMAPs) are known to have a profound influence on the microbiota [102]. Fatty acids play an important role in inflammatory cascades and oxidative stress, and the source of fatty acids in the diet has immunomodulating effects [103]. Antioxidants are added to the food to avoid nutritional degradation and to avoid rancidity of the diet. The level of fatty acids in a diet influences the need for antioxidants, and fatty diet in general has shorter lifetime and must be stored under more strict conditions. The source of the protein may also impact nutritional content. In general, animal protein sources supply essential amino acids; however a combination of plant protein sources can also supply all essential amino acids. In 2005, Mattson et al. [104] demonstrated that the source of protein and fat in a diet affected the mean arterial pressure in salt-sensitive rats. Food sources, fatty acid and amino acid composition, and interaction with genetic predisposition to develop certain diseases, is an important field of research to better understand mechanism of metabolic diseases like diabetes [105].

For some animal models, food must be sterilised to be sure it is free of infectious agents. Heat sterilising via autoclave is one option. However, autoclaving has a detrimental effect on nutritional content, and only diets formulated to withstand this loss of nutrients should be used if autoclaving is necessary. Also, though autoclaving kills vegetative microbes and spores, it does not necessarily degrade or inactivate heat-stable bacteria toxins or products [106], so the same strict quality requirements for dietary sources still apply. Irradiation, usually via large-scale cobalt 60 gamma rays or electronic beam (E-beam) sources, can be used as an alternative to sterilise the diet when the risk of microbial contamination is an issue. Irradiation has a less negative impact on nutritional value [107].

Ad libitum feeding is the most common feeding regime in rodents; however as opportunities for activity in the rodent cage are low, there is a risk of overfeeding and obesity with subsequent welfare issues and obesity-related complications [108]. Food restriction should therefore be considered for long-term studies [109].

3.2.1 Phytoestrogens

Human clinical and nutritional interest in phytoestrogens during the last decade of the twentieth century led to publications illustrating that natural phytoestrogens present in commercial rodent diets could interfere with some research [110–113]. This is particularly true of steroid research due to the nature of these molecules. Coumestrol is the major phytoestrogen in alfalfa, which is a component of some commercial rodent diets. This phytoestrogen, which binds to the oestrogen receptor (ER), has been shown to alter the reproductive development of rats [110–112]. Isoflavone phytoestrogens, which are present in soy, are structurally similar to 17β-oestradiol and, thus, may bind to oestrogen receptors and have both oestrogenic and antiestrogenic activities [114], leading to induced alterations of normal physiological processes that may interfere with the research question being addressed. Alfalfa and soya are the major natural ingredients responsible for the isoflavone content of the current rodent diets. However, some laboratories have recently found no evidence of a soya-based diet influencing the results of behavioural, reproductive or welfare parameters in C57BL/6NCrl mice [115]. This group also found less despair behaviour in the forced swim test in the soy-free group and sexually dimorphic cognitive behaviour with the soy-containing standard diet [115]. Nevertheless, we know that the phytoestrogens present in the diet can influence oestrogenic studies, toxicology programs and carcinogenic studies [110–113, 116]. We also know that the total isoflavone content in soya varies with the variety and the location where it is grown [101, 117].

Rodent feed manufacturers offer not only phytoestrogen-free diets but also grain-based diets, free of any animal origin protein. This movement, towards an animal protein-free rodent diet, had its origins in the public health crisis related to "mad cow" disease, bovine spongiform encephalopathy (BSE), which was linked to a fatal brain disease in humans called variant Creutzfeldt-Jakob disease (vCJD) in the 1990s [118, 119]. Fishmeal has also been linked with confounding results in chemical toxicity and carcinogenicity studies conducted for the National Toxicology Program (NTP) due to nitrosamines and heavy metal content [120].

For carnivorous species, replacement of animal origin ingredients by plant-based ingredients can cause pathological conditions like soybean-induced enteritis in Atlantic salmon [121, 122].

A cautionary tale on how diet can affect experimental outcomes is illustrated by the Dahl salt-sensitive inbred rat (SS/Jr). In 2016, Margaret Zimmerman and Sarah Lindsey raised awareness over recurrent inconsistencies of the SS/Jr [123–125]. Jane Reckelhoff's group found inconsistencies when testing the same strain from the same vendor (SS/JrHsd) but with different diets in different years [124, 126]. In 2010, the SS/JrHsd rats were given purified AIN-76A diet (American Institute of Nutrition formulated purified diet) [127, 128], which used refined ingredients (casein, DL-methionine, sucrose, corn starch, corn oil, cellulose, mineral mix AIN-76 (170915), vitamin mix AIN-76A (40077), choline bitartrate and ethoxyquin and antioxidant) and does not contain alfalfa, whereas, in 2016, SS/JrHsd rats were given Teklad 7034, a fixed formula diet with a different nutrient composition that does not used refined ingredients and contains alfalfa and soybean, two known sources of phytoestrogens. Thus, as illustrated by the Dalmasso and collaborators, the differences between a purified diet and a natural ingredient diet may have accounted for the variability seen in the model. Or, as pointed out by Zimmerman and Lindsey, through a revision of their own experiments with the model, other uncontrolled factors may have accounted for these differences. In any case, this shows how a well-characterised model that has worked consistently over decades can start producing inconsistent data, which may lead to wrong conclusions and thus lead scientists on equivocal pathways.

The diet provided to experimental animals can also affect the microbiota, but for that, we refer the reader to chapter "Microbiology and Microbiome" on microbiology and microbiome.

3.3 Water

As long as a diet of natural ingredients is used, normal municipality drinking water from the tap may be suitable for research animals.

However, for immunocompromised animals or in studies where strict dietary control is crucial, other sources may be better, and for fish, water treatment is necessary. Autoclaving water will kill microbes and reduce the risk of water-born infections in immunocompromised animals. However, autoclaving does not take away chemical substances or heat-stable toxins. Chlorification or acidification is also used to reduce microbiological growth in the drinking water. However, this can impact the taste of the water and water consumption. Depending on the filter technology, mechanical filtration takes out organic material, and charcoal filtration may take out smell, taste and some chemical substances. In reverse osmosis (RO) treatments of water, a partially permeable membrane is used to remove ions, unwanted molecules and larger particles from the raw water source. Regardless of the source, water should be regularly monitored at the facility level for contaminants, both organic and inorganic [129].

Water is usually provided ad libitum in water bottle or in a centralised watering system. If animals are offered fruit, gels or other water-containing diet in addition to kibble or pellets, this might influence their overall drinking water intake. If test substances are provided per os in the drinking water, it might be necessary to control the water intake to be sure animals get the exact amount of test substance.

3.4 Noise and Vibration

The animal facility acoustic environment was mostly ignored by managers, regulators, scientists, architects, engineers and designers in the past. As recent research has shown, personnel involved with animal facilities recognised that control of environmental factors, such as noise, in animal facilities is important to ensure consistent responses to experimental procedures [130]. It is also well known that construction noise (range 70–90 dBA) affects different reproductive parameters in mice [131]. In Europe, the Commission Recommendation of 18 June 2007 on guidelines for the accommodation and care of animals used for experimental and other scientific purposes (2007/526/EC), under "The Environment and Its Control" section, in its point 2.5 recognises that "noise can be a disturbing factor for animals" and gives vague recommendations on what should be an ideal acoustic environment and what should be avoided, both in terms of actual noise and design of the facilities [28]. By contrast, noise and vibration are dealt with by the *Guide for the Care and Use of Laboratory Animals* extensively in Chapter 3, "Environment, Housing and Management", for terrestrial and aquatic animals, and in Chapter 5, "Physical Plant" [39]. Measurements are routinely taken to monitor ventilation, temperature, humidity and lighting and adequate ranges given for them. However, the acoustic environment is often given relatively little consideration mainly due to the difficulty in consistent noise measurements, the differences in audible frequencies to different species and the unknown limits where there is an effect on the normal physiology of animals.

Some groups advocate for a more detailed definitions of what is a safe acoustic environment for animals in research. The first question we need to address is: what is sound? Sound, in physics terms, is a vibration that propagates through a transmission medium, like air or water, as a pressure wave that is audible. At the reception point, i.e. the ears in humans and other vertebrates, pressure and time are the two elements that will describe every sound we hear. We will see when we read about noise that most of the research refers to sound pressure level. Sound pressure will be the deviation from the atmospheric pressure caused by a sound wave. Sound pressure level is the ratio of the absolute sound pressure and a reference level, usually the threshold of hearing, or the lowest intensity of sound that can be heard by most people. The decibel (dB) is commonly used as the unit for sound pressure level, being the ratio of sound pressure on a logarithmic scale.

Different cardiovascular parameters have already been shown to be affected by noise; environmental noise causes a number of changes in laboratory animals: increase of blood pressure in cats, rats, rhesus monkeys and macaque monkeys [132–137]; increase in heart rate in desert mule deer and rats [138]; increase in vasoconstriction in rats [139–141]; increase in respiratory rates and adrenocorticotropin hormone in cats [142]; hypertension [143, 144]; cardiac hypertrophy [144]; changes in electrolyte metabolism [145]; reduced body weight [146–148]; increased adrenal weight [144]; altered tumour resistance and immune response [149]; slower wound healing [148]; changes in oestrous cycles, increased weight of uterus and ovaries, spontaneous lactation, decreased fertility and termination of pregnancy [150]; and embryonic abnormalities [144]. Mice stressed by sound during pregnancy also produce offspring with poor learning ability [151]. Some researchers in contrast have found that noise induces no change in blood pressure in the rat [152]. Noise has also been associated with a change in sleeping patterns in humans [153]. Sanchez-Morgado and collaborators have also studied the effects of construction noise on different biochemical parameters, heart rate and arterial blood pressure in mice and found that there is an increase in systolic and diastolic blood pressure; in the pulse in males more than in females; in cholesterol, triglycerides and LDL in males; and that males are more affected by noise than females [154]. Researchers working with mice in noisy environments should be aware of variations that could mask valid experimental results.

Water is an excellent medium for transfer of acoustic energy without major attenuation. For aquatic animals the perception of "sound" is not limited to "hearing" by ears, but also – depending on the species – involves the lateral line and the gas bladder, making "hearing" more complex involving near-field and far-field signals. The ability to discriminate sounds of interest from background noise also varies between species so that fish classified as auditory specialists are of greater risk of suffering from hearing loss than auditory generalists [155].

Vibration is the periodic back-and-forth motion of the particles of an elastic body or medium, commonly resulting when almost any physical system is displaced from its equilibrium condition and allowed to respond to the forces that tend to restore equilibrium. Thus, sound is generated by vibrating structures, and sound can also cause vibration of structures. We can see that sound and vibration are intimately related. Nevertheless, contrary to sound, we have little data on vibration and its effects on laboratory animals [156].

The reader is referred to other more in-depth reviews on the hearing of laboratory animals like the one published in 2005 by John Turner et al. [157].

3.5 Temperature

The thermoneutral zone (TNZ) is defined as the range of ambient temperature at which temperature regulation is achieved only by control of sensible heat loss, i.e. without regulatory changes in metabolic heat production (rate of transformation of chemical energy into heat in an organism) or evaporative heat loss. The TNZ will therefore be different when insulation, posture and basal metabolic rate (BMR) vary. In mice, the thermoneutral zone is approximately between 29.6 °C and 30.5 °C, although this varies with the strain, age, sex and activity level. The preferred temperature – which can be defined as the temperature where animals will choose to stay when a range of temperatures is given as a choice – varies in mice depending on behaviour, strain, time of the day, age and sex [158–162]. Generally, it has been found that the 26 °C to 29 °C range is preferred for sleep by both sexes in all mouse strains [160]. Rodents adjust to changes in temperature by adjusting metabolism, so temperature control is extremely important as it has a major impact on experimental results [163]. The European Guidelines for the Accommodation and Care of Animals Used for Experimental and other Scientific Purposes defines standard temperatures for animal housing in Europe [28]. These ranges are measured at the room level and are typically lower than those preferred by the animals. Nevertheless, these temperature ranges are a compromise between the animals' needs and what employees can tolerate as their working environment. Thus, there is a thermal stress associated with the current recommended temperature ranges [28, 39] for many animals. Fischer and collaborators [164] have found that mouse metabolism more closely resembles human metabolism at the thermoneutral zone. This is something important to consider for scientists working in human metabolism and using the mouse as a model. As they established, "at any temperature below thermoneutrality, mice metabolism exceeds the human equivalent: Mice under standard conditions display energy expenditure 3.1 times basal metabolism", whereas "humans usually display average metabolic rates of about 1.6 times basal metabolic rate" [164].

The term thermoneutral zone does not apply to ectotherms [165]. For poikilothermic animals the temperature will have an intrinsic impact on growth, development and behaviour.

3.6 Humidity

Recommendations for humidity levels of rodent housing rooms can be found in the European Guidelines for the Accommodation and Care of Animals Used for Experimental and Other Scientific Purposes [28]. Values for rodents are in general higher than office areas so humidification of the ventilated air is usually necessary. Fluctuation of humidity is stressful for the animals and should therefore be kept within a defined range. Too low relative humidity has been discussed as a cause of the condition "ringtail" in rodents [166], respiratory issue and reproductive problems (pup eating). Too high humidity may cause hygienic problems with microbial growth. Different housing systems can affect the humidity depending on the ventilation range and quality of the ventilated air.

4 Final Word

In any animal research effort, many factors may come into play. Control and standardisation of all variables are impossible on either the scientist or the animal side. Uncontrolled variables will have an influence on the final data, and the acknowledgement of this fact can open new avenues of inquiry or aid other scientists in answering their questions. It is, therefore, important to provide all the information we have in our published manuscripts so others can, at least, try to reproduce our conditions when attempting to reproduce results or explain conflicting results in their facility. Ideally, scientists would only publish robust data with external validity, but we understand this is an incremental goal that requires many small steps and changes to the scientific endeavour. After reading this chapter, we hope scientists will be more aware of how the environment and the animal may affect their research outcome. If the reader stops to think carefully about their next experiment and these influences, we will have attained our goal in writing this chapter. There are other chapters within this book that will help both seasoned researchers and early-career scientists tackle different issues related to animal-based research. Therefore, we encourage the reader to peruse those chapters and obtain a much better overview of these factors.

References

1. Richter SH, Garner JP, Würbel H. Environmental standardization: cure or cause of poor reproducibility in animal experiments? Nat Methods. 2009;6:257–61. https://doi.org/10.1038/nmeth.1312.
2. Garner JP, Gaskill BN, Weber EM, et al. Introducing therioepistemology: the study of how knowledge is gained from animal research. Lab Anim (NY). 2017;46:103–13. 2017/03/23. https://doi.org/10.1038/laban.1224.
3. Bubier JA, Philip VM, Quince C, et al. A microbe associated with sleep revealed by a novel systems genetic analysis of the microbiome in collaborative cross mice. Genetics. 2020;214:719–33. 2020/01/04. https://doi.org/10.1534/genetics.119.303013.
4. Deloris Alexander A, Orcutt RP, Henry JC, et al. Quantitative PCR assays for mouse enteric flora reveal strain-dependent differences in composition that are influenced by the microenvironment. Mamm Genome. 2006;17:1093–104. 2006/11/09. https://doi.org/10.1007/s00335-006-0063-1.
5. Goodrich JK, Waters JL, Poole AC, et al. Human genetics shape the gut microbiome. Cell. 2014;159:789–99. 2014/11/25. https://doi.org/10.1016/j.cell.2014.09.053.
6. Jacobs JP, Braun J. Immune and genetic gardening of the intestinal microbiome. FEBS Lett.

2014;588:4102–11. 2014/03/13. https://doi.org/10.1016/j.febslet.2014.02.052.
7. Richter SH, Garner JP, Auer C, et al. Systematic variation improves reproducibility of animal experiments. Nat Methods. 2010;7:167–8. https://doi.org/10.1038/nmeth0310-167.
8. Festing MF. The choice of animals in toxicological screening: inbred strains and the factorial design of experiment. Acta Zool Pathol Antverp. 1980;117–31. 1980/10/01.
9. Beery AK, Zucker I. Sex bias in neuroscience and biomedical research. Neurosci Biobehav Rev. 2011;35:565–72. https://doi.org/10.1016/j.neubiorev.2010.07.002.
10. Beery AK. Inclusion of females does not increase variability in rodent research studies this review comes from a themed issue on sex and gender. Curr Opin Behav Sci. 2018;23:143–9. https://doi.org/10.1016/j.cobeha.2018.06.016.
11. Clayton JA, Collins FS. Policy: NIH to balance sex in cell and animal studies. Nature. 2014;509:282–3. https://doi.org/10.1038/509282a.
12. NOT-OD-15-102. Consideration of sex as a biological variable in NIH-funded research. 2015.
13. Richardson SS, Reiches M, Shattuck-Heidorn H, et al. Opinion: focus on preclinical sex differences will not address women's and men's health disparities. Proc Natl Acad Sci. 2015;112:13419–20. https://doi.org/10.1073/PNAS.1516958112.
14. Klein SL, Schiebinger L, Stefanick ML, et al. Opinion: sex inclusion in basic research drives discovery. Proc Natl Acad Sci U S A. 2015;112:5257–8. https://doi.org/10.1073/pnas.1502843112.
15. Tannenbaum C, Schwarz JM, Clayton JA, et al. Evaluating sex as a biological variable in preclinical research: the devil in the details. Biol Sex Differ. 2016;7:13. https://doi.org/10.1186/s13293-016-0066-x.
16. Sorge RE, LaCroix-Fralish ML, Tuttle AH, et al. Spinal cord toll-like receptor 4 mediates inflammatory and neuropathic hypersensitivity in male but not female mice. J Neurosci Off J Soc Neurosci. 2011;31:15450–4. https://doi.org/10.1523/JNEUROSCI.3859-11.2011.
17. Sorge RE, Mapplebeck JCS, Rosen S, et al. Different immune cells mediate mechanical pain hypersensitivity in male and female mice. Nat Neurosci. 2015;18:1081–3. https://doi.org/10.1038/nn.4053.
18. Doyle HH, Eidson LN, Sinkiewicz DM, et al. Sex differences in microglia activity within the periaqueductal gray of the rat: a potential mechanism driving the dimorphic effects of morphine. J Neurosci Off J Soc Neurosci. 2017;37:3202–14. https://doi.org/10.1523/JNEUROSCI.2906-16.2017.
19. Tronson NC. Focus on females: a less biased approach for studying strategies and mechanisms of memory this review comes from a themed issue on sex and gender ScienceDirect. Curr Opin Behav Sci. 2018;23:92–7. https://doi.org/10.1016/j.cobeha.2018.04.005.
20. Keiser AA, Turnbull LM, Darian MA, et al. Sex differences in context fear generalization and recruitment of Hippocampus and amygdala during retrieval. Neuropsychopharmacology. 2017;42:397–407. https://doi.org/10.1038/npp.2016.174.
21. Keller KM, Howlett SE. Sex differences in the biology and pathology of the aging heart. Can J Cardiol. 2016;32:1065–73. https://doi.org/10.1016/J.CJCA.2016.03.017.
22. Mazzaccara C, Labruna G, Cito G, et al. Age-related reference intervals of the Main biochemical and hematological parameters in C57BL/6J, 129SV/EV and C3H/HeJ mouse strains. PLoS One. 2008;3:e3772. https://doi.org/10.1371/journal.pone.0003772.
23. Berson DM, Dunn FA, Takao M. Phototransduction by retinal ganglion cells that set the circadian clock. Science. 2002;295:1070–3. 2002/02/09. https://doi.org/10.1126/science.1067262.
24. Hanifin JP, Brainard GC. Photoreception for circadian, neuroendocrine, and neurobehavioral regulation. J Physiol Anthropol. 2007;26:87–94. 2007/04/17. https://doi.org/10.2114/jpa2.26.87.
25. Hastings MH, Maywood ES, Brancaccio M. Generation of circadian rhythms in the suprachiasmatic nucleus. Nat Rev Neurosci. 2018;19:453–69. https://doi.org/10.1038/s41583-018-0026-z.
26. Furudate S, Takahashi A, Takagi M, et al. Delayed persistent estrus induced by continuous lighting after inadequate acclimation in rats. Exp Anim. 2005;54:93–5. 2005/02/24. https://doi.org/10.1538/expanim.54.93.
27. Bedrosian TA, Vaughn CA, Galan A, et al. Nocturnal light exposure impairs affective responses in a wavelength-dependent manner. J Neurosci. 2013;33:13081–7. 2013/08/09. https://doi.org/10.1523/JNEUROSCI.5734-12.2013.
28. European C. Commission recommendation of 18 June 2007 on guidelines for the accommodation and care of animals used for experimental and other scientific purposes (2007/526/EC). 2007. Brussels.
29. Joyner CP, Myrick LC, Crossland JP, et al. Deer mice as laboratory animals. ILAR J. 1998;39:322–30. 2001/06/15. https://doi.org/10.1093/ilar.39.4.322.
30. Banerjee S, Chaturvedi CM. Testicular atrophy and reproductive quiescence in photorefractory and scotosensitive quail: involvement of hypothalamic deep brain photoreceptors and GnRH-GnIH system. J Photochem Photobiol B. 2017;175:254–68. 2017/09/20. https://doi.org/10.1016/j.jphotobiol.2017.09.005.
31. Robinson-Junker A, O'Hara B, Durkes A, et al. Sleeping through anything: the effects of unpredictable disruptions on mouse sleep, healing, and affect. PLoS One. 2019;14:e0210620. 2019/02/01. https://doi.org/10.1371/journal.pone.0210620.
32. Hawkins P, Golledge HDR. The 9 to 5 rodent – time for change? Scientific and animal welfare implications of circadian and light effects on laboratory mice and rats. J Neurosci Meth-

ods. 2018;300:20–5. 2017/05/16. https://doi.org/10.1016/j.jneumeth.2017.05.014.

33. European Parliament and Council of Europe. Council directive 86/609/EEC of 24 November 1986 on the approximation of laws, regulations and administrative provisions of the Member States regarding the protection of animals used for experimental and other scientific purposes. Strasbourg: Official Journal of the European Communities, 1986, p. 28.
34. Niklaus S, Albertini S, Schnitzer TK, et al. Challenging a myth and misconception: red-light vision in rats. Animals (Basel). 2020;10. 2020/03/07. https://doi.org/10.3390/ani10030422.
35. Rocha FA, Gomes BD, Silveira LC, et al. Spectral sensitivity measured with electroretinogram using a constant response method. PLoS One. 2016;11:e0147318. 2016/01/23. https://doi.org/10.1371/journal.pone.0147318.
36. Coomans CP, van den Berg SA, Lucassen EA, et al. The suprachiasmatic nucleus controls circadian energy metabolism and hepatic insulin sensitivity. Diabetes. 2013;62:1102–8. 2013/01/01. https://doi.org/10.2337/db12-0507.
37. Qian J, Block GD, Colwell CS, et al. Consequences of exposure to light at night on the pancreatic islet circadian clock and function in rats. Diabetes. 2013;62:3469–78. https://doi.org/10.2337/db12-1543.
38. Gale JE, Cox HI, Qian J, et al. Disruption of circadian rhythms accelerates development of diabetes through pancreatic beta-cell loss and dysfunction. J Biol Rhythms. 2011;26:423–33. 2011/09/17. https://doi.org/10.1177/0748730411416341.
39. The National Research C. Guide for the care and use of laboratory animals. Washington, DC: National Academies Press; 2011. p. 246.
40. Peirson SN, Brown LA, Pothecary CA, et al. Light and the laboratory mouse. J Neurosci Methods. 2018;300:26–36. 2017/04/18. https://doi.org/10.1016/j.jneumeth.2017.04.007.
41. Dauchy RT, Blask DE, Hoffman AE, et al. Influence of daytime LED light exposure on circadian regulatory dynamics of metabolism and physiology in mice. Com Med. 2019;69:350–73. https://doi.org/10.30802/AALAS-CM-19-000001.
42. Dauchy RT, Wren-Dail MA, Hoffman AE, et al. Effects of daytime exposure to light from blue-enriched light-emitting diodes on the nighttime melatonin amplitude and circadian regulation of rodent metabolism and physiology. Comp Med. 2016;66:373–83. 2016/10/26
43. Lucas RJ, Brainard GC, Berson DM, et al. Report on the first international workshop on circadian and neurophysiological photometry, 2013. The Commission Internationale de l'Eclairage; 2015.
44. Lucas RJ, Peirson SN, Berson DM, et al. Measuring and using light in the melanopsin age. Trends Neurosci. 2014;37:1–9. 2013/11/25. https://doi.org/10.1016/j.tins.2013.10.004.
45. Yuan R, Tsaih S-W, Petkova SB, et al. Aging in inbred strains of mice: study design and interim report on median lifespans and circulating IGF1 levels. Aging Cell. 2009;8:277–87. https://doi.org/10.1111/j.1474-9726.2009.00478.x.
46. Holladay SD, Blaylock BL. The mouse as a model for developmental immunotoxicology. Hum Exp Toxicol. 2002;21:525–31. https://doi.org/10.1191/0960327102ht292oa.
47. Rieger MA, Schroeder T. Hematopoiesis. Cold Spring Harb Perspect Biol. 2012;4. https://doi.org/10.1101/CSHPERSPECT.A008250.
48. Schmitt CE, Lizama CO, Zovein AC. From transplantation to transgenics: mouse models of developmental hematopoiesis. Exp Hematol. 2014;42:707–16. https://doi.org/10.1016/J.EXPHEM.2014.06.008.
49. Loeffler M, Pantel K. A mathematical model of erythropoiesis suggests an altered plasma volume control as cause for anemia in aged mice. Exp Gerontol. 1990;25:483–95.
50. Boggs DR, Patrene KD. Hematopoiesis and aging III: Anemia and a blunted erythropoietic response to hemorrhage in aged mice. Am J Hematol. 1985;19:327–38. https://doi.org/10.1002/ajh.2830190403.
51. Sorzano COS, Sánchez-Morgado JM. Normal haematological reference intervals for different inbred strains at 9 weeks of age. Dublin: Trinity College Dublin; 2020.
52. Fox JG. The mouse in biomedical research. Volume III, Normative biology, husbandry and models. 2nd ed. Amsterdam/Boston: Elsevier; 2007.
53. Walters BJ, Zuo J. Postnatal development, maturation and aging in the mouse cochlea and their effects on hair cell regeneration. Hear Res. 2013;297:68–83. https://doi.org/10.1016/j.heares.2012.11.009.
54. Johnson KR, Zheng QY, Erway LC. A major gene affecting age-related hearing loss is common to at least ten inbred strains of mice. Genomics. 2000;70:171–80. 2000/12/09. https://doi.org/10.1006/geno.2000.6377.
55. Kane KL, Longo-Guess CM, Gagnon LH, et al. Genetic background effects on age-related hearing loss associated with Cdh23 variants in mice. Hear Res. 2012;283:80–8. 2011/12/06. https://doi.org/10.1016/j.heares.2011.11.007.
56. Hathway GJ, Koch S, Low L, et al. The changing balance of brainstem-spinal cord modulation of pain processing over the first weeks of rat postnatal life. J Physiol. 2009;587:2927–35. https://doi.org/10.1113/jphysiol.2008.168013.
57. Kwok CHT, Devonshire IM, Imraish A, et al. Age-dependent plasticity in endocannabinoid modulation of pain processing through postnatal development. Pain. 2017;158:2222–32. https://doi.org/10.1097/j.pain.0000000000001027.
58. Schwaller F, Kanellopoulos AH, Fitzgerald M. The developmental emergence of differential brainstem

serotonergic control of the sensory spinal cord. Sci Rep. 2017;7. https://doi.org/10.1038/S41598-017-02509-2.
59. Stoyek MR, Rog-Zielinska EA, Quinn TA. Age-associated changes in electrical function of the zebrafish heart. Prog Biophys Mol Biol. 2018;138:91–104. https://doi.org/10.1016/j.pbiomolbio.2018.07.014.
60. Mohrhardt J, Nagel M, Fleck D, et al. Signal detection and coding in the accessory olfactory system. Chem Senses. 2018;43:667–95. https://doi.org/10.1093/chemse/bjy061.
61. Wyatt TD. Pheromones. Curr Biol. 2017;27:R739–43. https://doi.org/10.1016/j.cub.2017.06.039.
62. Roberts SA, Prescott MC, Davidson AJ, et al. Individual odour signatures that mice learn are shaped by involatile major urinary proteins (MUPs). BMC Biol. 2018;16:48. 2018/04/29. https://doi.org/10.1186/s12915-018-0512-9.
63. Nodari F, Hsu F-F, Fu X, et al. Sulfated steroids as natural ligands of mouse pheromone-sensing neurons. J Neurosci. 2008;28:6407–18. https://doi.org/10.1523/jneurosci.1425-08.2008.
64. Stockley P, Bottell L, Hurst JL. Wake up and smell the conflict: odour signals in female competition. Philos Trans R Soc Lond B Biol Sci. 2013;368:20130082. 2013/10/30. https://doi.org/10.1098/rstb.2013.0082.
65. Van Der Lee S, Boot LM. Spontaneous pseudopregnancy in mice. II. Acta Physiol Pharmacol Neerl. 1956;5:213–5. 1956/12/01
66. Van Der Lee S, Boot LM. Spontaneous pseudopregnancy in mice. Acta Physiol Pharmacol Neerl. 1955;4:442–4. 1955/11/01
67. Ma W, Miao Z, Novotny MV. Role of the adrenal gland and adrenal-mediated chemosignals in suppression of estrus in the house mouse: the lee-boot effect revisited. Biol Reprod. 1998;59:1317–20. 1998/11/26. https://doi.org/10.1095/biolreprod59.6.1317.
68. Koyama S. Primer effects by conspecific odors in house mice: a new perspective in the study of primer effects on reproductive activities. Horm Behav. 2004;46:303–10. https://doi.org/10.1016/j.yhbeh.2004.03.002.
69. Whitten WK. Modification of the oestrous cycle of the mouse by external stimuli associated with the male. J Endocrinol. 1956;13:399–404. 1956/07/01. https://doi.org/10.1677/joe.0.0130399.
70. Whitten WK. Modification of the oestrous cycle of the mouse by external stimuli associated with the male; changes in the oestrous cycle determined by vaginal smears. J Endocrinol. 1958;17:307–13. 1958/09/01. https://doi.org/10.1677/joe.0.0170307.
71. Bruce HM. An exteroceptive block to pregnancy in the mouse. Nature. 1959;184:105. 1959/07/11. https://doi.org/10.1038/184105a0.
72. Parkes AS, Bruce HM. Olfactory stimuli in mammalian reproduction. Science. 1961;134:1049–54. 1961/10/13. https://doi.org/10.1126/science.134.3485.1049.
73. Vandenbergh JG. Male odor accelerates female sexual maturation in mice. Endocrinology. 1969;84:658–60. 1969/03/01. https://doi.org/10.1210/endo-84-3-658.
74. Szymanski LA, Keller M. Activation of the olfactory system in response to male odors in female prepubertal mice. Behav Brain Res. 2014;271:30–8. https://doi.org/10.1016/j.bbr.2014.05.051.
75. Bacchini A, Gaetani E, Cavaggioni A. Pheromone binding proteins of the mouse, *Mus musculus*. Experientia. 1992;48:419–21. 1992/04/15. https://doi.org/10.1007/bf01923448.
76. Koyama S, Kamimura S. Effects of vomeronasal organ removal on the sperm motility in male mice. Zoolog Sci. 2003;20:1355–8. 2003/11/19. https://doi.org/10.2108/zsj.20.1355.
77. Hurst JL, West RS. Taming anxiety in laboratory mice. Nat Methods. 2010;7:825–6. 2010/09/14. https://doi.org/10.1038/nmeth.1500.
78. Gouveia K, Hurst JL. Reducing mouse anxiety during handling: effect of experience with handling tunnels. PLoS One. 2013;8:e66401. 2013/07/11. https://doi.org/10.1371/journal.pone.0066401.
79. Gouveia K, Hurst JL. Optimising reliability of mouse performance in behavioural testing: the major role of non-aversive handling. Sci Rep. 2017;7:44999. 2017/03/23. https://doi.org/10.1038/srep44999.
80. Gouveia K, Hurst JL. Improving the practicality of using non-aversive handling methods to reduce background stress and anxiety in laboratory mice. Sci Rep. 2019;9:20305. https://doi.org/10.1038/s41598-019-56860-7.
81. Henderson LJ, Smulders TV, Roughan JV. Identifying obstacles preventing the uptake of tunnel handling methods for laboratory mice: An international thematic survey. PLoS One. 2020;15:e0231454. 2020/04/15. https://doi.org/10.1371/journal.pone.0231454.
82. Whittaker AL, Howarth GS, Hickman DL. Effects of space allocation and housing density on measures of wellbeing in laboratory mice: a review. Lab Anim. 2012;46:3–13. https://doi.org/10.1258/la.2011.011049.
83. Markham JA, Greenough WT. Experience-driven brain plasticity: beyond the synapse. Neuron Glia Biol. 2004;1:351–63. 2006/08/22. https://doi.org/10.1017/s1740925x05000219.
84. European Parliament and Council of Europe. Directive 2010/63/EU of the European Parliament and of the Council of 22 September 2010 on the protection of animals used for scientific purposes. Strasbourg: Official Journal of the European Union; 2010.
85. Wurbel H. Ideal homes? Housing effects on rodent brain and behaviour. Trends Neurosci. 2001;24:207–11. 2001/03/16. https://doi.org/10.1016/s0166-2236(00)01718-5.

86. Langston RF, Ainge JA, Couey JJ, et al. Development of the spatial representation system in the rat. Science. 2010;328:1576–80. 2010/06/19. https://doi.org/10.1126/science.1188210.
87. André V, Gau C, Scheideler A, et al. Laboratory mouse housing conditions can be improved using common environmental enrichment without compromising data. PLoS Biol. 2018;16:e2005019. https://doi.org/10.1371/journal.pbio.2005019.
88. Macri S, Ceci C, Altabella L, et al. The Directive 2010/63/EU on animal experimentation may skew the conclusions of pharmacological and behavioural studies. Sci Rep. 2013;3:2380. 2013/08/09. https://doi.org/10.1038/srep02380.
89. Atwood BK, Huffman J, Straiker A, et al. JWH018, a common constituent of 'Spice' herbal blends, is a potent and efficacious cannabinoid CB receptor agonist. Br J Pharmacol. 2010;160:585–93. 2010/01/27. https://doi.org/10.1111/j.1476-5381.2009.00582.x.
90. Motulsky H. Intuitive biostatistics. A nonmathematical guide to statistical thinking. 4th ed. New York: Oxford University Press; 2018. p. 568.
91. Gaskill BN, Garner JP. Stressed out: providing laboratory animals with behavioral control to reduce the physiological effects of stress. Lab Anim (NY). 2017;46:142–5. 2017/03/23. https://doi.org/10.1038/laban.1218.
92. Greenman DL, Bryant P, Kodell RL, et al. Relationship of mouse body weight and food consumption/wastage to cage shelf level. Lab Anim Sci. 1983;33:555–8. 1983/12/01
93. Greenman DL, Kodell RL, Sheldon WG. Association between cage shelf level and spontaneous and induced neoplasms in mice. J Natl Cancer Inst. 1984;73:107–13. 1984/07/01
94. Ader DN, Johnson SB, Huang SW, et al. Group size, cage shelf level, and emotionality in non-obese diabetic mice: impact on onset and incidence of IDDM. Psychosom Med. 1991;53:313–21. 1991/05/01. https://doi.org/10.1097/00006842-199105000-00005.
95. Okva K, Nevalainen T, Pokk P. The effect of cage shelf on the behaviour of male C57BL/6 and BALB/c mice in the elevated plus maze test. Lab Anim. 2013;47:220–2. 2013/06/14. https://doi.org/10.1177/0023677213489280.
96. Young SS. Are there local room effects on hepatic tumors in male mice? An examination of the NTP eugenol study. Fundam Appl Toxicol. 1987;8:1–4. 1987/01/01
97. Young SS. A blind reanalysis of a random subset of NCI bioassay studies: agreement between rats and mice. Fundam Appl Toxicol. 1989;12:232–41. 1989/02/01
98. Kozul CD, Nomikos AP, Hampton TH, et al. Laboratory diet profoundly alters gene expression and confounds genomic analysis in mouse liver and lung. Chem Biol Interact. 2008;173:129–40. https://doi.org/10.1016/J.CBI.2008.02.008.
99. Brown NM, Setchell KDR. Animal models impacted by phytoestrogens in commercial chow: implications for pathways influenced by hormones. Lab Investig. 2001;81:735–47. https://doi.org/10.1038/labinvest.3780282.
100. Carter RL, Lipman NS. Feed and bedding. In: Weichbrod RH, Thompson GAH, et al., editors. Management of animal care and use programs in research, education, and testing. Boca Raton: CRC Press; 2018. p. 639–54.
101. Eldridge AC. Determination of isoflavones in soybean flours, protein concentrates, and isolates. J Agric Food Chem. 1982;30:353–5. https://doi.org/10.1021/jf00110a035.
102. Tuck CJ, Caminero A, Jimenez Vargas NN, et al. The impact of dietary fermentable carbohydrates on a postinflammatory model of irritable bowel syndrome. Neurogastroenterol Motil. 2019;31:e13675. 2019/07/11. https://doi.org/10.1111/nmo.13675.
103. Li M, van Esch B, Wagenaar GTM, et al. Pro- and anti-inflammatory effects of short chain fatty acids on immune and endothelial cells. Eur J Pharmacol. 2018;831:52–9. 2018/05/12. https://doi.org/10.1016/j.ejphar.2018.05.003.
104. Mattson DL, Meister CJ, Marcelle ML. Dietary protein source determines the degree of hypertension and renal disease in the Dahl salt-sensitive rat. Hypertension. 2005;45:736–41. https://doi.org/10.1161/01.HYP.0000153318.74544.cc.
105. Svard J, Rost TH, Sommervoll CEN, et al. Absence of the proteoglycan decorin reduces glucose tolerance in overfed male mice. Sci Rep. 2019;9:4614. 2019/03/16. https://doi.org/10.1038/s41598-018-37501-x.
106. Hrncir T, Stepankova R, Kozakova H, et al. Gut microbiota and lipopolysaccharide content of the diet influence development of regulatory T cells: studies in germ-free mice. BMC Immunol. 2008;9:65. 2008/11/08. https://doi.org/10.1186/1471-2172-9-65.
107. Caulfield CD, Cassidy JP, Kelly JP. Effects of gamma irradiation and pasteurization on the nutritive composition of commercially available animal diets. J Am Assoc Lab Anim Sci. 2008;47:61–6. 2008/12/04
108. Martin B, Ji S, Maudsley S, et al. "Control" laboratory rodents are metabolically morbid: why it matters. Proc Natl Acad Sci U S A. 2010;107:6127–33. https://doi.org/10.1073/pnas.0912955107.
109. Hubert MF, Laroque P, Gillet JP, et al. The effects of diet, ad Libitum feeding, and moderate and severe dietary restriction on body weight, survival, clinical pathology parameters, and cause of death in control Sprague-Dawley rats. Toxicol Sci. 2000;58:195–207. 2000/10/29. https://doi.org/10.1093/toxsci/58.1.195.
110. Whitten PL, Lewis C, Russell E, et al. Potential adverse effects of phytoestrogens. J Nutr. 1995;125:771S–6S. https://doi.org/10.1093/jn/125.3_suppl.771s.

111. Whitten PL, Russell E, Naftolin F. Effects of a normal, human-concentration, phytoestrogen diet on rat uterine growth. Steroids. 1992;57:98–106. https://doi.org/10.1016/0039-128X(92)90066-I.
112. Whitten PL, Naftolin F. Effects of a phytoestrogen diet on estrogen-dependent reproductive processes in immature female rats. Steroids. 1992;57:56–61. https://doi.org/10.1016/0039-128X(92)90029-9.
113. Ashby J, Tinwell H, Soames A, et al. Induction of hyperplasia and increased DNA content in the uterus of immature rats exposed to coumestrol. Environ Health Perspect. 1999;107:819–22. https://doi.org/10.1289/ehp.99107819.
114. Dixon RA. Phytoestrogens. Annu Rev Plant Biol. 2004;55:225–61. https://doi.org/10.1146/annurev.arplant.55.031903.141729.
115. Mallien AS, Soukup ST, Pfeiffer N, et al. Effects of soy in laboratory rodent diets on the basal, affective, and cognitive behavior of C57BL/6 mice. J Am Assoc Lab Anim Sci. 2019;58:532–41. https://doi.org/10.30802/AALAS-JAALAS-18-000129.
116. Thigpen JE, Setchell KD, Goelz MF, et al. The phytoestrogen content of rodent diets. Environ Health Perspect. 1999;107:A182–3. https://doi.org/10.1289/ehp.107-1566530.
117. Eldridge AC, Kwolek WF. Soybean isoflavones: effect of environment and variety on composition. J Agric Food Chem. 1983;31:394–6. https://doi.org/10.1021/jf00116a052.
118. Collinge J, Sidle KCL, Meads J, et al. Molecular analysis of prion strain variation and the aetiology of 'new variant' CJD. Nature. 1996;383:685–90. https://doi.org/10.1038/383685a0.
119. Will RG, Ironside JW, Zeidler M, et al. A new variant of Creutzfeldt-Jakob disease in the UK. Lancet. 1996;347:921–5. https://doi.org/10.1016/S0140-6736(96)91412-9.
120. Rao GN, Knapka JJ. Contaminant and nutrient concentrations of natural ingredient rat and mouse diet used in chemical toxicology studies. Fundam Appl Toxicol. 1987;9:329–38. https://doi.org/10.1016/0272-0590(87)90055-8.
121. Knudsen D, Jutfelt F, Sundh H, et al. Dietary soya saponins increase gut permeability and play a key role in the onset of soyabean-induced enteritis in Atlantic salmon (*Salmo salar* L.). Br J Nutr. 2008;100:120–9. 2008/01/03. https://doi.org/10.1017/S0007114507886338.
122. Refstie S, Korsøen ØJ, Storebakken T, et al. Differing nutritional responses to dietary soybean meal in rainbow trout (*Oncorhynchus mykiss*) and Atlantic salmon (*Salmo salar*). Aquaculture. 2000;190:49–63. https://doi.org/10.1016/S0044-8486(00)00382-3.
123. Zimmerman MA, Lindsey SH. Inconsistent blood pressure phenotype in female Dahl salt-sensitive rats. Am J Physiol Renal Physiol. 2016;311:F1391–2. https://doi.org/10.1152/ajprenal.00454.2016.
124. Dalmasso C, Maranon R, Patil C, et al. 20-HETE and CYP4A2 ω-hydroxylase contribute to the elevated blood pressure in hyperandrogenemic female rats. Am J Physiol Renal Physiol. 2016;311:F71–7. https://doi.org/10.1152/ajprenal.00458.2015.
125. Gillis EE, Williams JM, Garrett MR, et al. The Dahl salt-sensitive rat is a spontaneous model of superimposed preeclampsia. Am J Phys Regul Integr Comp Phys. 2015;309:R62–70. https://doi.org/10.1152/ajpregu.00377.2014.
126. Sartori-Valinotti JC, Venegas-Pont MR, LaMarca BB, et al. Rosiglitazone reduces blood pressure in female Dahl salt-sensitive rats. Steroids. 2010;75:794–9. https://doi.org/10.1016/J.STEROIDS.2009.10.010.
127. Report of the American Institute of Nutrition Ad Hoc Committee on Standards for Nutritional Studies. J Nutr. 1977;107:1340–8. https://doi.org/10.1093/jn/107.7.1340.
128. Bieri JG. Second report of the ad hoc committee on standards for nutritional studies. J Nutr. 1980;110:1726. https://doi.org/10.1093/jn/110.8.1726.
129. Allen ED, Czarra EF, De Tolla L. Water quality and water delivery systems. In: Weichbrod RH, GAH T, Norton JN, editors. Management of animal care and use programs in research, education, and testing. Boca Raton: CRC Press; 2018. p. 655–73.
130. Baldwin AL, Schwartz GE, Hopp DH. Are investigators aware of environmental noise in animal facilities and that this noise may affect experimental data? J Am Assoc Lab Anim Sci. 2007;46:45–51. 2007/01/06
131. Rasmussen S, Glickman G, Norinsky R, et al. Construction noise decreases reproductive efficiency in mice. J Am Assoc Lab Anim Sci. 2009;48:363–70. 2009/08/06
132. Hudak WJ, Buckley JP. Production of hypertensive rats by experimental stress. J Pharm Sci. 1961;50:263–4. https://doi.org/10.1002/JPS.2600500321.
133. Buckley JP, Smookler HH. Cardiovascular and biochemical effects of chronic intermittent neurogenic stimulation. In: Welch BL, Welch AS, editors. Physiological effects of noise: based upon papers presented at an international symposium on the extra-auditory physiological effects of audible sound, held in Boston, Massachusetts, December 28–30, 1969, in conjunction with the annual meeting of the American Association for the Advancement of Science. Boston: Springer; 1970. p. 75–84.
134. Ising HHUM. Endocrine and cardiovascular effects of noise. Rockville: American Speech, Language, and Hearing Association; 1980.
135. Peterson EA, Augenstein JS, Tanis DC, et al. Noise raises blood pressure without impairing auditory sensitivity. Science. 1981;211:1450–2. 1981/03/27. https://doi.org/10.1126/science.7466404.
136. Peterson EA, Augenstein JS, Hazelton CL, et al. Some cardiovascular effects of noise. J Aud Res. 1984;24:35–62. 1984/01/01

137. Peterson EA, Haselton CL, Augenstein JS. Daily noise duration influences cardiovascular responses. J Aud Res. 1984;24:69–86. 1984/04/01
138. Weisenberger ME, Krausman PR, Wallace MC, et al. Effects of simulated jet aircraft noise on heart rate and behavior of desert ungulates. J Wildl Manag. 1996;60(1):52–61.
139. Borg E. Peripheral vasoconstriction in the rat in response to sound. III. Dependence of pause characteristics in continuous noise. Acta Otolaryngol. 1978;86:155–9. 1978/09/01. https://doi.org/10.3109/00016487809124732.
140. Borg E. Peripheral vasoconstriction in the rat in response to sound. II. Dependence on rate of change of sound level. Acta Otolaryngol. 1978;85:332–5. 1978/05/01. https://doi.org/10.3109/00016487809121460.
141. Borg E. Peripheral vasoconstriction in the rat in response to sound. I. Dependence on stimulus duration. Acta Otolaryngol. 1978;85:153–7. 1978/03/01. https://doi.org/10.3109/00016487809111921.
142. Kristensen MP, Rector DM, Poe GR, et al. Activity changes of the cat paraventricular hypothalamus during stressor exposure. Neuroreport. 2004;15:43–8. 2004/04/27. https://doi.org/10.1097/00001756-200401190-00010.
143. Rosecrans JA, Watzman N, Buckley JP. The production of hypertension in male albino rats subjected to experimental stress. Biochem Pharmacol. 1966;15:1707–18. https://doi.org/10.1016/0006-2952(66)90078-5.
144. Geber WF. Cardiovascular and teratogenic effects of chronic intermittent noise stress. In: Welch BL, Welch AS, editors. Physiological effects of noise: based upon papers presented at an international symposium on the extra-auditory physiological effects of audible sound, held in Boston, Massachusetts, December 28–30, 1969, in conjunction with the annual meeting of the American Association for the Advancement of Science. Boston: Springer; 1970. p. 85–90.
145. Lockett MF. Effects of sound on endocrine function and electrolyte excretion. In: Welch BL, Welch AS, editors. Physiological effects of noise: based upon papers presented at an international symposium on the extra-auditory physiological effects of audible sound, held in Boston, Massachusetts, December 28–30, 1969, in conjunction with the annual meeting of the American Association for the Advancement of Science. Boston: Springer; 1970. p. 21–41.
146. Am S, As W, Bradshaw M, et al. Endocrine changes due to auditory stress. Acta Endocrinol. 1959;31. https://doi.org/10.1530/ACTA.0.XXXI0405
147. Fink GB, Iturrian WB. Influence of age, auditory conditioning, and environmental noise on sound-induced seizures and seizure threshold in mice. In: Welch BL, Welch AS, editors. Physiological effects of noise: based upon papers presented at an international symposium on the extra-auditory physiological effects of audible sound, held in Boston, Massachusetts, December 28–30, 1969, in conjunction with the annual meeting of the American Association for the Advancement of Science. Boston: Springer; 1970. p. 211–26.
148. Wysocki AB. The effect of intermittent noise exposure on wound healing. Adv Wound Care J Prev Heal. 1996;9:35–9.
149. Jensen MM, Rasmussen AF. Audiogenic stress and susceptibility to infection. In: Welch BL, Welch AS, editors. Physiological effects of noise: based upon papers presented at an international symposium on the extra-auditory physiological effects of audible sound, held in Boston, Massachusetts, December 28–30, 1969, in conjunction with the annual meeting of the American Association for the Advancement of Science. Boston: Springer US; 1970. p. 7–19.
150. Zondek B, Wolstenholme GE, O'Connor M. Effects of external stimuli on reproduction. In honour of Professor B. Zondek. London: Churchill; 1967. p. 4–19.
151. Barlow SM. Teratogenic effects of restraint, cold and audiogenic stress in mice and rats. London: University of London; 1972.
152. Borg E, Moller AR. Noise and blood pressure: effect of lifelong exposure in the rat. Acta Physiol Scand. 1978;103:340–2. 1978/07/01. https://doi.org/10.1111/j.1748-1716.1978.tb06223.x.
153. Snyder-Halpern R. The effect of critical care unit noise on patient sleep cycles. Ccq. 1985;7:41–51. 1985/02/09
154. Gutierrez Llaneza S, López Romero P, García Camacho M, et al. Effects of construction noise on mouse cardiovascular parameters: arterial blood pressure. In: FELASA meeting Helsinki, Finland, June 14–17, 2010
155. Jobling M. Fish in aquaculture environments. In: Huntingford F, Jobling M, Kadri S, editors. Aquaculture and behavior. Ames: Blackwell Publishing Ltd.; 2012. p. 36–64.
156. Reynolds RP, Li Y, Garner A, et al. Vibration in mice: a review of comparative effects and use in translational research. Anim Mod Exp Med. 2018;1:116–24. https://doi.org/10.1002/ame2.12024.
157. Turner JG, Parrish JL, Hughes LF, et al. Hearing in laboratory animals: strain differences and nonauditory effects of noise. Comp Med. 2005;55:12–23.
158. Ogilvie DM, Stinson RH. The effect of age on temperature selection by laboratory mice (*mus musculus*). Can J Zool. 1966;44:511–7. https://doi.org/10.1139/z66-055.
159. Eedy JW, Ogilvie DM. The effect of age on the thermal preference of white mice (*Mus musculus*) and gerbils (*Meriones unguiculatus*). Can J Zool. 1970;48:1303–6. https://doi.org/10.1139/z70-221.
160. Gaskill BN, Gordon CJ, Pajor EA, et al. Heat or insulation: behavioral titration of mouse preference for warmth or access to a nest. PLoS

One. 2012;7:e32799. https://doi.org/10.1371/journal.pone.0032799.

161. Gaskill BN, Rohr SA, Pajor EA, et al. Working with what you've got: changes in thermal preference and behavior in mice with or without nesting material. J Therm Biol. 2011;36:193–9. https://doi.org/10.1016/j.jtherbio.2011.02.004.
162. Gaskill BN, Rohr SA, Pajor EA, et al. Some like it hot: mouse temperature preferences in laboratory housing. Appl Anim Behav Sci. 2009;116:279–85. https://doi.org/10.1016/j.applanim.2008.10.002.
163. Baumans V. The laboratory mouse. In: Hubrecht RC, Kirkwood J, editors. The UFAW handbook on the care and management of laboratory and other research animals. Oxford: Wiley; 2010. p. 276–310.
164. Fischer AW, Cannon B, Nedergaard J. Optimal housing temperatures for mice to mimic the thermal environment of humans: an experimental study. Mol Metab. 2018;7:161–70. 2017/11/11. https://doi.org/10.1016/j.molmet.2017.10.009.
165. IUPS Thermal Commission. Glossary of terms for thermal physiology. Third ed. Revised by The Commission for Thermal Physiology of the International Union of Physiological Sciences. Jap J Physiol. 2001;51:245–80.
166. Crippa L, Gobbi A, Ceruti RM, et al. Ringtail in suckling Munich Wistar Fromter rats: a histopathologic study. Comp Med. 2000;50:536–9. 2000/12/01

Microbiology and Microbiome

Axel Kornerup Hansen

Abstract

A mammal harbours a vast number of microorganisms in the form of bacteria, viruses, protozoans, parasites, fungi and archaea, which is known as the microbiota. The animal host contains approximately 20,000 genes, while the microbiota contains more than 1 million genes. Therefore, many of the competences of a laboratory animal have arisen from the microbiota rather than the mammal genome. As there is substantial variation in composition between animals, animal units and commercial production sites and little information available on this, it is a challenge for experimental design, reproducibility and translatability of animal experiments. Some of the microorganisms are pathogens, i.e. they can induce spontaneous clinical disease in the animals, while others are commensals, i.e. their presence is latent. Traditionally, pathogens have been eradicated from so-called specific pathogen-free breeding colonies of research rodents to decrease mortality, disease incidence, inter-individual parameter variation and other forms of research interference. However, today it can also be argued that animals which have never been infected with pathogens have an under-stimulated immune system and, therefore, may be less translational compared to humans. Many of the commensals have been shown to be important for the induction of animal models, and variation in microbiota composition is responsible for a substantial part of the inter-individual variation in responses of many models and for different outcomes in different facilities. It is still a good principle that rodents for research only are bought from colonies bred behind a specific pathogen protecting barrier and that they are subjected to current health monitoring, which should be documented. However, it can also for individual studies be necessary to include a characterization of the microbiota, which has been made possible by modern sequencing techniques, which over the last decade have become more efficient and cheaper. Characterization can be done on a colony level, but eventually it can also be done on all animals in a specific study, which will allow the incorporation of the information in the data evaluation. It may also be important to ensure that specific bacteria needed for a proper model expression are present in the animals to be used. Before progressing from preclinical animal studies to clinical human studies, it might be considered

A. K. Hansen (✉)
Department of Veterinary and Animal Sciences, Faculty of Health and Medical Sciences, University of Copenhagen, Frederiksberg C, Denmark
e-mail: akh@sund.ku.dk

© Springer Nature Switzerland AG 2021

J. M. Sánchez Morgado, A. Brønstad (eds.), *Experimental Design and Reproducibility in Preclinical Animal Studies*, Laboratory Animal Science and Medicine 1,
https://doi.org/10.1007/978-3-030-66147-2_4

wise to supplement the studies in SPF animals with animals infected with pathogens.

Keywords

Microbiota · Microbiome · Microbiology · Specific pathogen-free organisms · Animal experimentation · Germ-free · Laboratory animal science

1 Introduction to Laboratory Animal Microbiology

Most animals host a huge number, approximately 10^{14}, of microorganisms [1] (Fact Box 1, Table 1). Traditionally, the reason for showing interest in specific infectious microorganisms in veterinary medicine has been their *pathogenicity* (Fact Box 2), and such infections may have a major impact on the expression of animal models, and thereby the reproducibility, and in an infected colony, animals may be at different stages of infection, which will increase inter-individual variation. The microbiome, based upon all the symbionts, which can be divided into thousands of species of microorganisms, is a massive collection of functional genes: actually more than 1 million genes compared to the little more than 20,000 genes of its mammal host. All the bacteria have their own viruses, so-called phages, which further increase the biodiversity in an animal. In addition, the mammal gut will normally house enteric protozoans, and the skin surface will in addition to bacteria also harbour various fungi. Mammals will also normally house a number of latent viruses, but it is unclear to which extent this also is the case for commercially reared laboratory rodents, as routine screening for a limited number of viruses (Table 2) mostly does not reveal the presence of any of these. The animal and its microbiota may be called a *superorganism*. Two experiments conducted with exactly the same strain of animals may in principle have been done on very distinct superorganisms, if the animals origin from two different units with different microbiotas, and, therefore, the one study may not reproduce the other.

Fact Box 1: Terms Used Within Laboratory Animal Microbiology

Symbionts
Microorganisms colonizing an animal.

Pathogens
Microorganisms capable of causing a disease in an animal defined by *Koch's third postulate* as a microorganism causing a specific disease when introduced into a healthy organism.

Commensals
Microorganisms capable of colonizing in animals, however without being able to cause a disease.

Mutualists
Microorganisms colonizing in animals so that both parties benefit from the symbiosis.

Microbiota
The complex community of all microorganisms colonizing an animal.

Microbiome
The collection of genes in the microbiota.

Microflora (or just flora)
A more popular term used for the microbiota. It indicates that microorganisms are plants, which is not the case.

Table 1 The *microbiota* of animals consists of zoologically different domains or kingdoms of organisms. Some of these are built from eukaryotic cells like the animal itself. This is the case for one-cell protozoans, such as *Tritrichomonas*, or one-cell fungi, such as *Candida*, and for multicell parasites, i.e. endoparasites, such as the large intestine helminth, *Syphacia*, or the ectoparasitic mite, *Myobia musculi*. Others, like all the bacteria and eventually archaea on the surfaces of the animal, are prokaryotic organisms. Some are not even cells, but rather complicated structures of organic chemistry, i.e. viruses, such as *mouse hepatitis virus*, or phages, that is, the viruses of bacteria

	Taxon	Kingdom
Biota	*Procaryota*	*Bacteria*
		Archaea
	Eucaryota	*Protozoa*
		Fungi
		Animalia
Non-biota	*Virus*	

Rearing with a fully defined microbiota or even germ-free is called *gnotobiotechnology* (Fact Box 2), which is now a common practice in a range of laboratories all over the world. While the germ-free rodents are not subject to inter-individual variation caused by bacteria, they have a lot of so-called germ-free associated characteristics [2], and therefore they are not very translatable for humans. However, also SPF animals have a microbiota diversity that low and a microbiota composition that different from feral mice that they do not express all natural characteristics of a mammal [3].

Fact Box 2: Developments Within Rodent Microbiology [4–17]

1890 – 1900 – 1910 – 1920 – 1930 – 1940 – 1950 – 1960 – 1970 – 2010

The first experiences with germ-free animals

It becomes clear that animals can live without germs for extended periods[4].

The first descriptions of hazardous infections in rodents

The first infections fatal to laboratory animals, such as *Bordetella bronchiseptica*[5] and *Clostridium piliforme*[6] are described.

Gnotobiotic animals

The first animals either fully germ-free or with only specifically defined bacteria, i.e. *gnotobiotic* animals, are reared in isolators[7, 8].

SPF-animals

The first reported use of caesarian section to produce so-called *specific pathogen-free* (SPF) breeding animals for the upstart of new colonies housed in a protected unit, i.e. a *barrier*[9] (Figure 1), mainly to get rid of zoonotic and fatal infections.

The Schaedler Flora

Some of the more dominant bacteria in conventional and SPF mice[10] are selected as *The Schaedler Flora* and used for association with ex-germ-free mice to normalize their enlarged cecum and abnormal intestinal histology[11].

Description of additional rodent pathogens

New agents, such as *Citrobacter rodentium*[12], are described as causative agents of problematic disease outbreaks, and eliminated from the breeding colonies, as well. As the more severe pathogens are eliminated, new ones with a more discrete impact on the research models, such as several different virus infections, are eliminated.

The Altered Schaedler Flora

The *Schaedler* flora is revised and becomes known as *The altered Schaedler Flora* (ASF)[13] (Table 9.3).

Considering the commensal microbiota

A concern is raised that some commensals are important for induction of human diseases in animal models[3, 14].

The call for dirty animals

A concern is raised on SPF animals having become that clean that their immune system mostly resembles that of a newborn human[15, 16, 17].

Table 2 Examples of facultative pathogens found in mice. + frequently present, (+) occasionally present and – rarely present in populations of wild, conventionally housed and barrier-bred mice [15, 18 –25, 45, 48 –55],

	Wild and pet shop mice	Conventional laboratory mice	Barrier-bred laboratory mice	Recommended for testing by FELASA
Viruses				
Mouse adenovirus	+	+	–	+
Mouse hepatitis virus	+	+	–	+
Mouse norovirus	+	+	–	+
Mouse parvovirus	+	+	–	+
Mouse rotavirus	+	+		+
Minute virus of mice	+	+	–	+
Theiler's murine encephalomyelitis virus	+	+	–	+
Sendai virus	+	+	–	+
Lymphocytic choriomeningitis virus	+	+	–	+
Polyomavirus	+	+	–	+
Pneumonia virus of mice	+	+	–	+
Reovirus type 3	+	+	–	+
Bacteria				
Streptococcus pneumoniae				+
Mycoplasma spp.	+	+	–	+
Rodentibacter spp.*	+	+	(+)	+
Clostridium piliforme	+	+	–	+
Citrobacter rodentium	?	–	–	+
Corynebacterium kutscheri	?	–	–	+
Salmonella spp.	+	–	–	+
Streptobacillus moniliformis	+	–	–	
Helicobacter spp.	+	+	(+)	+
Parasites				
Syphacia spp.	+	+	–	+
Mites	+	(+)	–	+

*Formerly named Pasteurella pneumotropica

2 Methods to Control the Impact of Microorganisms on Animal Studies

2.1 Barrier-Protected Specific Pathogen-Free Animals

Since Henry Foster, the founder of the Charles River breeding company, produced the first SPF rodents in the late 1950s, rodents for research have been produced by a three-step method. Colony founding breeders are delivered in an aseptic rederivation. Caesarean section, as originally applied by Henry Foster, may even eliminate infections with a potential to pass the placenta, as not every foetus of an infected mother will harbour the infection [26]. Caesarean section has over the last decades gradually been replaced by embryo transfer [27]. For both techniques recipient mothers may have either SPF or germ-free status. After rederivation the animals are given a standardized microbiota. This has for years been the altered Schaedler flora (ASF), i.e. a collection of eight bacterial species [13] (Table 3). As embryos may be stored indefinitely in liquid nitrogen and viability is normally above 90% [28, 29], animals can be rederived not only for hygienic purposes but also for the turn back of genetic drift to a specified basic generation of

Table 3 The altered Schaedler flora used as upstart microbiota for laboratory rodents

Phylum	ASF number	Description
Firmicutes	ASF 356	Closely related to *Clostridium propionicum*
	ASF 360	*Lactobacillus* spp. clustering with *L. acidophilus* and *L. lactis*
	ASF 361	*Lactobacillus* spp.
	ASF 492	*Eubacterium pexicaudatum*
	ASF 500	A novel unnamed genus related to *Bacillaceae* and *Clostridiaceae*
	ASF 502	*Clostridium* cluster XIV
Deferribacteres	ASF 457	*Mucispirillum schaedleri*
Bacteroidetes	ASF 519	*Bacteroides* spp. clustering with *B. forsythus, B. distasonis, B. merdae* and CDC group DF-3

the strain. This is regarded as a way to increase reproducibility, but if the microbiota of the colony is eliminated at each rederivation and only ASF is given back, a new microbiota will be established at each rederivation based on environment and circumstances, and therefore rederivations at current intervals may decrease reproducibility.

To reduce the risk of infections, the rederived animals after a thorough examination are transferred to facilities, in which certain protective measures are implemented, a so-called barrier facility (Fig. 1). Here they are used for the upstart of a breeding colony large enough to deliver the animals needed for projects. A barrier-protected unit should also be applied in the experimental facilities to avoid specific infections in the period, when the animals are used for studies. In most such facilities, a quarantine period of 24–72 h is applied for staff having had contact with either animals from unreliable sources or wild animals, as these may be infected with some of the unwanted pathogens [30, 31]. This is mostly based upon experience and tradition, and as most murine pathogens are species specific, passive transfer of pathogens is more likely prevented by the daily bath and change of clothes and not the length of the quarantine period. Microorganisms, which colonize the human caretakers, will obviously not be eliminated by a quarantine period. If animals come from unsafe sources with an unknown health status, these animals should be handled accordingly. Any facility not being a large commercial breeder should be considered unsafe. The best option for such animals is to rederive the strain or stock for in-house breeding, if the experimental facility has a barrier-protected breeding facility of its own. Second best is to have an isolated unit, where animals of unknown health status are housed. This may be a smaller unit or an isolator, where the delivered animals are housed without any contact to other animals and after a quarantine period of, for example, 4 weeks can be tested and transferred to another animal unit.

Many of the infections eliminated from barrier-protected laboratory rodent colonies are still found in the wild population of rodents, as well as in pets and other unprotected rodents [15, 18–25] (Table 2).

2.2 Health Monitoring

In both breeding colonies and experimental facilities, it is important to document that the protective measures in reality protect the animals and that these are free of infection, as these may spread to a number of studies. Therefore, a number of animals are sampled from the colony at frequent intervals and subjected to a range of tests. This practice is called *health monitoring*, although microbiological monitoring would be a more appropriate term. The *Federation of European Laboratory Animal Science Associations* (FELASA) has issued guidelines for health monitoring of various species: rodents and rabbits under breeding as well as experimental conditions [25] and pigs, dogs and cats [32], primates [33] and ruminants [34]. These recommend the agents to test for (Table 2), the methods to use, the number of animals to test, the frequency of testing and the

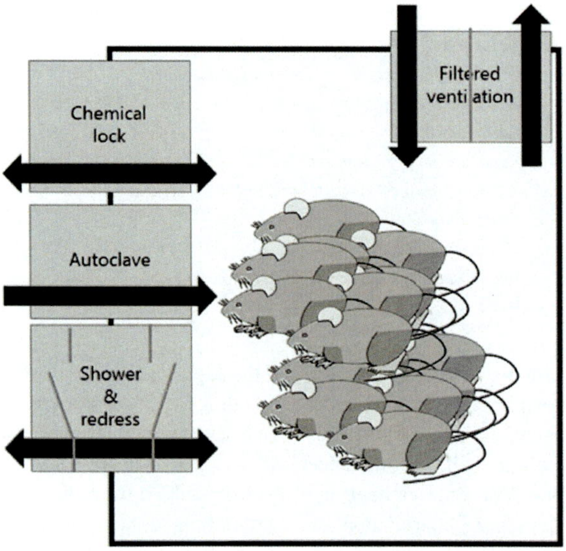

Fig. 1 Barrier-protection. To prevent specific infections in laboratory animals, these must be housed in a barrier-protected facility. Staff enters through a three-room shower, where they undress, shower and redress in clean clothes. Diet and materials can be transferred into the barrier through an autoclave, and in the lock larger equipment can be introduced through a chemical disinfection procedure. Animals can be transferred to the exterior through this lock. The facility is ventilated with filtered air. Staff is normally subject to quarantine if they have had contact with animals of the same species in another facility

format for reporting results. It should be a routine procedure when receiving rodents for research that an up-to-date health report generated in the submitting colony is studied prior to the receipt of the animals. Any commercial vendor will be able to issue such a report, and this should as a minimum adhere to the FELASA guidelines. Also, a large multinational commercial vendor will be able to guarantee that the animals have been bred and housed in barrier-protected facilities. It is, however, still important to take a critical look at any health report received. To obtain a statistically high probability of detecting infections, the sample size should be calculated for each agent tested for based upon the expected prevalence during an infection in a colony and the sensitivity of the assay applied [35], which is normally not done properly in many health reports. For example, it is extremely rare to report infection with lymphocytic choriomeningitis virus (LCMV) in commercially produced laboratory mice [19, 24, 36–38]. It probably is rare, but due to the low prevalence of this virus in infected mouse colonies, a proper sample size would be at least 50 animals, which is seldomly sampled by commercial breeders. In a more thorough investigation done by the US Centers for Disease Control and Prevention in 2014 in one commercial facility, LCMV was isolated from eight mice [39]. Another example is *Clostridium piliforme*, the causative agent of Tyzzer's disease. In some rat colonies, screening is done by histopathology of liver samples. However, as many rat strains do not develop liver changes, and those strains, which do, do it with an extremely low prevalence, such investigations have no statistical validity [40, 41].

2.3 Characterisation of the Microbiota

Microbiota characterization methods are evolving extremely rapidly [42]. Before the millennium a combination of selective and indicative

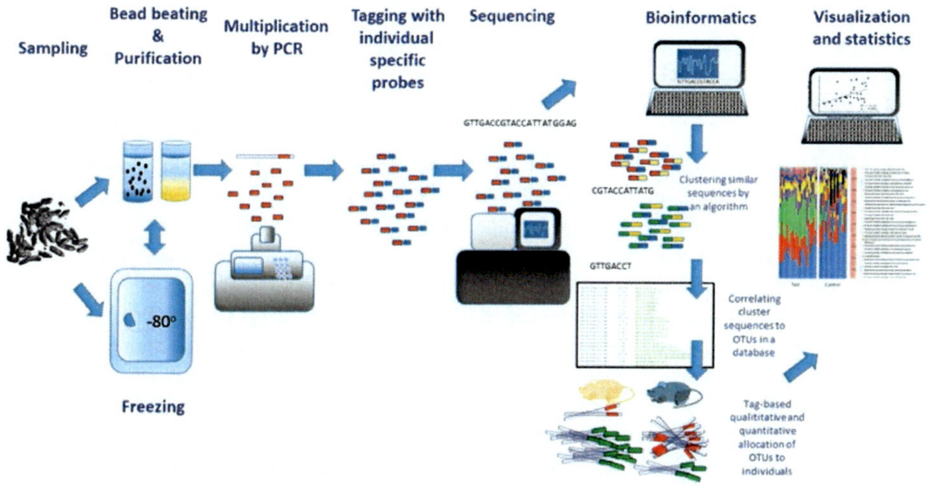

Fig. 2 The procedure of amplicon sequencing The samples are bead beaten and purified to obtain pure bacterial DNA. The DNA strings are multiplied by PCR and tagged with a sequence code specific for the animal of origin. The DNA strings are sequenced in a high-throughput sequencer, and an algorithm is used to cluster the sequences of similar coding. The sequences of the clusters are used to find the correlating operational taxonomic units (OTUs) in a database, and based upon the tags, the identification can be allocated qualitatively and quantitatively to the individual animals. The results can be visualized in various ways (Fig. 3), and statistics can be used to illustrate the probability of the identifications and compare findings between groups of animals

cultivation media was applied [43–45]. However, such cultivations identify less than 20% of the microbiota members, as most of the microbes are uncultivable by traditional methods. In the beginning of the twenty-first century, methods such as gas-liquid chromatography of bacterial cellular fatty acids [46] and some PCR-based gel electrophoresis methods [47] were applied, which effectively identified differences between groups of mice, however without identification or quantification of individual bacteria. For a short period combinations of multiple qPCRs [48] were used to give a qualitative and quantitative picture of the microbiota composition, which, however, needed all target bacteria to be predefined, and therefore species not included were not detected. Since the first high-throughput sequencing platform, the 454 GS20 pyrosequencing platform (454 Life Sciences, Branford, USA) which marketed a primary tool has been amplicon sequencing, i.e. sequencing of a short region of the bacterial DNA with a subsequent probability-based identification of the bacterium (Fig. 2). Due to the development of equipment and lowering of costs, metagenomics sequencing is now increasingly used, i.e. the entire genome is sequenced directly on the sampled DNA, and therefore the outcome is not only bacterial identification but also a full description of the capacity of this bacterium, as all of its genes are identified.

First, it is important to consider, where to sample from, as animals will cluster differently from different sites, such as faeces or caecum [49], and some sites, such as the ileum with all its lymphatic tissue, may be more important for immune stimulation than other sites. Many bacteria are linked to the mucosa, so including enteric surface in the sampling may be important. It is difficult to give general and precise directions for each specific model investigated, so the sampling site and methodology should for the sake of reproducibility be carefully described and reported [49]. Samples can be stored for months in liquid nitrogen or at −80 °C. Next, microbial DNA needs to be purified from the samples. Commercial kits, e.g. the Stool Kit (Qiagen, Valencia, USA) or the PowerSoil Kit (MoBio Laboratories, Carlsbad, USA), are widely used [50], but in-house solutions, e.g. phenol/chloroform extraction-based methods, may also be applied. Complete lysis of microbial cells is essential, and therefore bead beating is often used for mechanical cell disruption [51].

Amplicon sequencing starts by a PCR-based amplification of a target gene. For bacteria the 16S rRNA gene is the most common target, while either the 18S or the 26S rRNA (D1 region) genes are usually preferred for fungal identification. The principle is that primers should bind to some conserved regions of the gene, while the amplification will produce DNA sequences also based upon the variable regions of the gene, i.e. the regions used to differ the one organism from another. A range of 'universal' prokaryotic primer sets targeting different regions of the 16S rRNA gene are available including the V1, V1–V3, V3, V4 and V6–V8 regions, but although termed 'universal', the choice of primers influences which species will be detected or not [52]. Also, most universal primers only detect species with an abundance >1% of the total population. This can be improved by selecting more species-specific primers [53], if there is a specific need to look for specific species.

The DNA strings are tagged with an identification sequence unique for each sample/mice and sequenced using a high-throughput bench-top sequencer [54]. These have become far more cost-effective since 2005, because they can do far more reads in one run and they can read far more base pairs on each DNA string. The first sequencers could deliver around 1 million reads, while the present sequencers can deliver more than 1 billion reads. While the read length of the first sequencers, such as the 454 GS20 pyrosequencing platform, was less than 500 bases, the present machines, such as the MinION (Oxford Nanopore, Oxford, UK), make ultra-long read lengths possible, i.e. hundreds of kb. Therefore, such sequencers can now also be applied for metagenomic sequencing, i.e. instead of only reading one target gene, several genes can be read.

To transform sequence data into usable knowledge on microbe and gene identities, these must subsequently be subjected to bioinformatic analysis to identify single bacteria to a phylum, genus or even species level depending on how informative the gene region chosen is. In very long reads functional genes may also be identified. Clustering algorithms such as UPARSE [55] have been developed, which can group similar reads into clusters, which in combination with a database, e.g. the 16S rRNA databases Green Genes (http://greengenes.secondgenome.com/) or Silva (https://www.arb-silva.de/), can be identified as individual organisms, termed operational taxonomic units (OTUs) [56]. Identification is normalized to the lowest number of reads obtained, for example, if the normalization is done at 1200 reads per sample, sequences with longer reads are interpreted several times based upon several random selections of 1200 reads. Even for amplicon sequencing, the PICRUSt (Phylogenetic Investigation of Communities by Reconstruction of Unobserved States) (http://picrust.github.io/picrust/) tool offers the possibility to predict the functional composition of a microbiota on the basis of the targeted gene data [57]. However, as far as only target genes are sequenced, both identification and prediction of functional capability will be probability based, and different approaches can lead to different results. There are tools, such as BLAST (https://blast.ncbi.nlm.nih.gov/Blast.cgi), which can be used to achieve a statistical significance of a database match. Identification is obtained both as a qualitative identification, i.e. which species have been identified, and as a quantitative identification, i.e. how abundant is each species.

The OTU community can be described by alpha and beta diversity. Alpha diversity describes the diversity inside each individual animal. The qualitative OTU count is termed the 'species richness', i.e. how many different OTUs could simply be counted in each sample. The quantitative expression of alpha diversity is termed 'species richness' or 'the Shannon index', i.e. do OTUs appear with equal abundances or are some dominant in relation to others. Beta diversity describes how different the microbial composition is between the individual samples. 'Bray-Curtis dissimilarity' describes the quantitative differences between two samples on a 0–1 scale, in which 0 means that both samples share the same species at exactly the same abundances, while 1 means that both samples have completely different species abundances. In the same way, 'Jaccard distance' describes the qualitative distance between two samples on a 0–1 scale. UniFrac is based upon sequence distances, i.e. based upon the fraction of branch length that is shared between two samples or unique to one or the other sample. An unweighted UniFrac is purely based on sequence distances, while in a weighted UniFrac, branch lengths are weighted by relative abundances, i.e. it includes both sequence and abundance information [58].

Data can be presented in a table presenting the individual OTUs and the abundances of each in two or several groups of animals using parametric or non-parametric descriptions, or the abundances of the phylua, genera or species can be presented as a bar plot (Fig. 3a) or a heat map (Fig. 3b) for each individual animal. The abundance of each OTU can be compared between groups by ordinary parametric and non-parametric quantitative statistics. In addition to presenting the p-values of such tests, one should also correct for multiple comparisons by false discovery rate (FDR), which will result in a row of similar q-values. It is important to present both p- and q-values, but to make solid conclusions based upon p-values, strong hypotheses should be available on each OTU, e.g. as it is the case when oligosaccharides are tested in mice, because it is well known that if efficient, they will have a strong impact on *Bifidobacterium* spp. [59]. Also, the G-test of independence can be used to determine whether a given OTU is more or less likely to be associated with one of the groups, and analysis of similarity (ANOSIM) can be used for testing for differences between groups of mice on the UniFrac distance matrices.

Visually, UniFrac differences can be used to present a cluster analysis (Fig. 3c), i.e. a phylogenetic tree on how different the individuals are. Data can be further presented as a simple dissimilarity matrix which can be visualized graphically by multidimensional scaling such as principal coordinate analysis (PCoA) (Fig. 3d) [60]. Quantitative expressions, such as the principal coordinates as an expression on the entire variation in gut microbiota composition or the individual abundances of each OTU, can be correlated to quantitative research parameters by Spearman's correlation (Fig. 3e). This will reveal a correlation coefficient expressing how much of the variation in the research parameter, which is determined by the gut microbiota composition or the abundance of the individual OTU, as well as a p-value as an indication on whether this correlation is significant.

Several platforms have been developed for analysing rRNA gene-targeted amplicon sequences, which include tools for the steps from initial identification to a descriptive presentation of the data. Very commonly used is the QIIME (http://qiime.org/, Quantitative Insights Into Microbial Ecology) platform [61], but analytical techniques are constantly improved.

3 The Impact of Microorganisms on Inter-individual Variation and Model Expression

3.1 The Impact of the Microbiota

There seems to be no doubt that the microbiota plays an important role in mediating or preventing chronic inflammatory and metabolic diseases in humans and animals [62–64], and this is relevant to address in animal research to achieve higher reproducibility and translationability [14].

The typical rodent gut microbiota contains bacteria of the phyla *Actinobacteria*, *Tenericutes*, *Firmicutes*, *Bacteroidetes*, *Verrucomicrobia* and *Proteobacteria* and in contrast to humans also one species from *Deferribacteres*, because it has been given to them with the ASF [54] (Table 3). On the phylum level, laboratory rodents are quite similar, but at the family, genus and species level, there is a huge variation between colonies and breeders both in relation to bacteria [65] and to the phages [66] of these bacteria, and they differ substantially from humans [54]. Inside the colony the beta diversity is typically approximately 40% for an outbred stock and 30% for an inbred strain

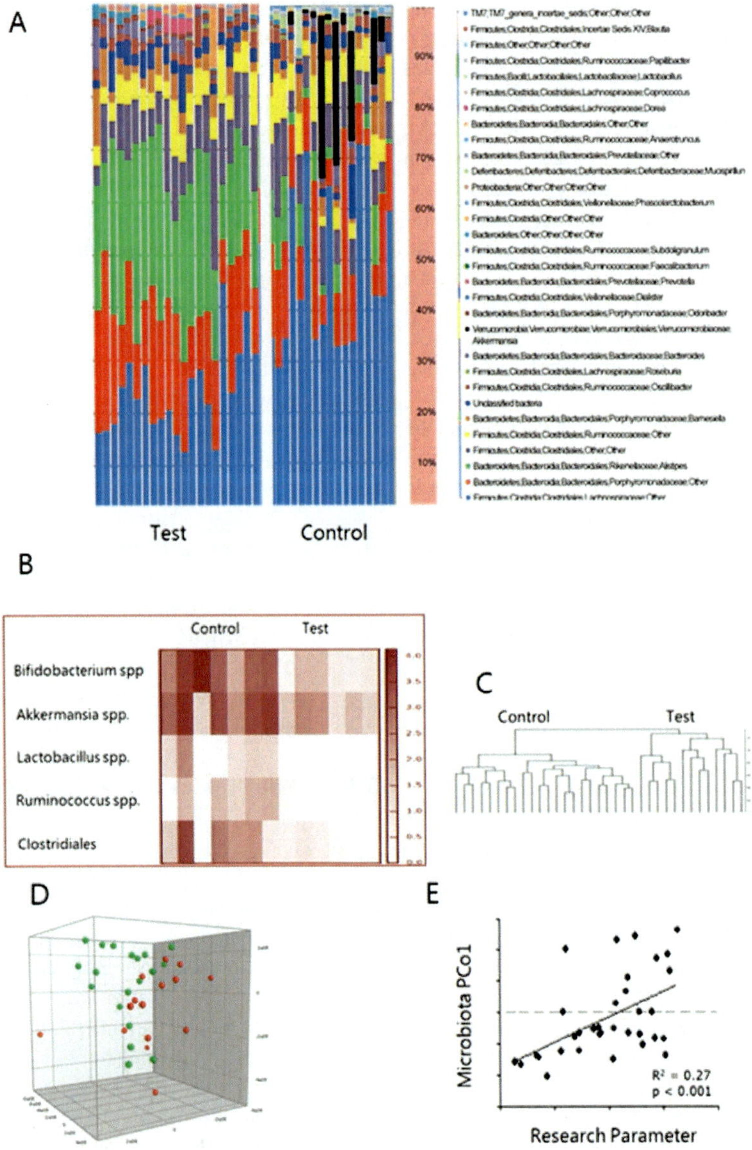

Fig. 3 Visualization of microbiota characterization. Results of a microbiota characterization may be shown on a phylum, genus or species level. In a bar plot (**a**), these different groups are shown as bars, in which each colour represents one of these groups and the size of the bar correlates to the abundance. In a heat map (**b**), the colour intensity correlates to the abundance. A phylogenetic clustering tree (**c**) may be used to show how different the individual animals are from one another. A principal coordinate analysis (PCoA, based upon dissimilarities) or a principal component analysis (PCA, based upon similarities) may also be used to calculate a series of dissimilarity/similarity scales between the animals called principal coordinates (PCo) or principal components (PC), respectively. These can be put into a two- or three-dimensional graph (**d**), which will visualize the differences between the animals, and in which animals of different groups can be given different colours. The quantitative values of PCos and PCs can be correlated to the quantitative values monitored for a research parameter in each animal to show the correlation coefficient (R^2) and the p-value (**e**)

[65], but this difference between inbred and outbred is probably more related to differences in breeding systems than to genetics [47]. There is a substantial cage effect [67]. Between different colonies at different commercial vendors, there are substantial differences in microbiota composition, richness and diversity [68]. Therefore, much of the inter-individual variation observed in various rodent models has its origin in variation in the microbiota of the animals [69]. Studies should always be planned, so that one experimental group is not just housed all in the same cage. It should be noted that mice from not only different breeders but even from different rooms at the same breeder may respond differently and that such a difference may even be larger than the experimental factor itself [70]. To increase reproducibility such information, i.e. which breeder, which room and that mice in the same group were housed in more than one cage, should at least be collected and reported. In the upper part of the gut, e.g. in the ileum with its huge accumulation of lymphatic tissue [71–77], the microbiota is normally not very diverse, i.e. the species mostly belong to the two phyla *Bacteroidetes* and *Firmicutes*, and there can be huge inter-individual differences [73]. The gut microbiota becomes gradually much more diverse during the passage through the large intestine, and the highest diversity is found in faeces [71–78]. Individuals clustering in the upper part of the gut may differ essentially in the lower part of the gut, in which other individuals may cluster [49, 77]. A low microbiota diversity in man as well as in the mouse is indicative of an increased risk of developing inflammatory disease [79, 80]. The microbiotas in the respiratory system, on the skin and in the reproductive tracts are not as complex as the gut microbiota, but these may also be important for disease protection or induction [81, 82]. Both in humans [83] and rodents [43], *Actinobacteria* and *Proteobacteria* are readily isolated from the vagina, and at least in humans, *Firmicutes* dominates the vaginal microbiota [83]. The skin microbiota of laboratory mice, which normally is less diverse than what is known from humans [84], differs among the specific sites of the body surface [84], and it may exhibit a substantial inter-individual variation [85]. The members of the microbiota of a barrier-bred rodent colony are apart from those, which are ASF derived, most likely of human or dietary origin [86, 87], while very little if any of it originates from the natural habitat of mice. For example, *Staphylococcus aureus* is common in laboratory mice, but extremely uncommon in wild mice [88]. In fact, the microbiota of wild mice differs substantially from the microbiota of barrier-bred laboratory mice [89]. Compared to either feral or conventional mice, barrier-bred laboratory mice seem to harbour a less complex microbiota, less *Bacteroides,* less *Paraprevotella* and *Lactobacillus* spp. but more *Clostridia* spp. [75, 88, 90].

Sole differences in microbiota composition are responsible for marked differences in phenotypic expression. In a range of animal models [14], there is a strong correlation between microbiota composition and the expression of key parameters, e.g. within type 1 diabetes [45, 77, 91], type 2 diabetes [69, 92, 93], colon cancer [94–96], atopic dermatitis [51, 97], inflammatory bowel disease (IBD) [62, 98], depression [99] and schizophrenia [100]. The microbiota significantly influences the inter-individual variation [69, 101] through the host immune system as well as through the host metabolism and frequently through both. Differences in metabolites as a result of microbiota differences between animals of the same strain maintained in different rooms may lead to different drug response phenotypes [101]. Even after inoculation with the ASF, mice still have a metabolism most comparable with germ-free mice, and to develop their metabolism further, they need a more complex microbiota [3]. Furthermore, for neuro-psychiatric models, the cross-talk between the gut bacteria, the immune system and the brain through the vagal nerves and the hypothalamus-pituitary axis, known as the *gut-brain axis*, has an essential impact on the models, because animals with different microbiotas send different cytokine signals from their macrophages to the brain [102]. For example, the behavioural phenotypes of NIH Swiss mice and BALB/c mice may be swabbed by microbiota transfer, which leads to the conclusion that behaviour to a certain extent is more determined by the microbiota than by host genetics [103].

Table 4 Examples of commensal bacterial species, which as latently appearing in the rodent gut microbiota, may have an impact on models for human disease

Phylum	Species	Importance
Firmicutes	*Candidatus Savagella* (segmented filamentous bacteria (SFBs)) [105–109]	A pro-inflammatory bacterium with in inductive impact on inflammatory bowel disease in adoptive transfer SCID mice or rheumatoid arthritis in K/BxN mice but also with a protective impact on type 1 diabetes in NOD mice and bacterial enterocolitis, e.g. caused by *Citrobacter rodentium* and *Salmonella*
	Enterococcus faecalis [110, 111]	May increase severity of inflammatory bowel disease in IL-10 knockout mice
	Faecalibacterium prausnitzii [112–116]	The most common bacterial species in the human gut with an anti-inflammatory impact on inflammatory bowel disease in both men and mice
	Lactobacillus spp. [59, 117, 118],	Anti-inflammatory bacteria, which also have been shown to decrease stress-induced corticosterone and anxiety- and depression-related behaviour
Actinobacteria	*Bifidobacterium* spp. [59, 119–123]	Anti-inflammatory bacteria with a protective impact on allergy in germ-free mice, inflammatory bowel disease in IL-10 knockout mice and myocardial infarction in ischemia/reperfusion injury in Dahl/S rats
Bacteroidetes	*Bacteroides vulgatus* [124]	A pro-inflammatory bacterium with an inductive effect on inflammatory bowel disease
	Bacteroides fragilis [125–128]	A pro-inflammatory bacterium with an inductive effect on inflammatory bowel disease, colon cancer and a protective effect on *Helicobacter hepaticus*-induced colitis and autism in the maternal immune activation mouse model
	Prevotella spp. [69, 71, 94, 129]	Bacteria with both pro- and anti-inflammatory capabilities, e.g. increasing glucose intolerance in leptin-deficient obese mice and inflammatory bowel disease in the dextran sodium sulphate model while decreasing colon cancer in the azoxymethane/dextran sodium sulphate model
	Alistipes spp. [130, 131]	Correlated to stress and depression in both mice and men
Proteobacteria	*Escherichia coli* [124]	A pro-inflammatory bacterium with an inductive impact on inflammatory bowel disease in HLA-B27-overexpressing rats
Verrucomicrobia	*Akkermansia muciniphila* [69, 94, 132–137]	An anti-inflammatory bacterium with a protective impact on obesity/type 2 diabetes, type 1 diabetes and inflammatory bowel disease and an inductive effect on allergic asthma, *Salmonella typhimurium* enteritis and colon cancer in the azoxymethane/dextran sodium sulphate model

3.2 The Impact of Specific Commensals

Some specific bacterial species may be regarded as being of crucial importance for certain models (Table 4). Some bacteria can be clearly defined as pro- or anti-inflammatory. However, even if so, they may have both inductive and protective impacts on the models, e.g. because inflammation in early life may increase anti-inflammation later in life or the activation of T-helper cell type 2 may favour the development of diseases related to these, such as atopic dermatitis, while protecting against diseases relating to T-helper cells type1, such as type 1 diabetes [104] or the opposite. In contrast to pathogens, the impact of such bacteria is based as much on their quantitative as on their qualitative presence, and they may work both inductive and protective in relation to disease development. Many of these can only exert their actions in conjunction with other microbiota members or other host and environmental factors. However, it has also been proposed that the impact of single bacteria may be amplified in

SPF mice with a low microbiota diversity and no contact with pathogens [17].

3.3 The Impact of Pathogens

Some pathogens, such as ectromelia virus, are obviously unwanted guests in laboratory animal facilities. However, even the highly pathogenic ectromelia virus, which is a DNA virus causing mousepox, is more fatal in some mice than in others, e.g. DBA, C3H and BALB/c mice are very sensitive, while C57BL/6 mice seem to be relatively resistant and may even carry latent infections [138, 139]. Most other DNA viruses do not induce overt clinical symptoms in rodents, while RNA viruses vary more in their morbidity. The mouse coronavirus, known as *mouse hepatitis virus*, which is the most common virus infection observed to bypass the protective measures in barrier-protected SPF colonies [19, 24], causes diarrhoea in suckling mice [140] and high mortality in immunodeficient mice, such as SCID [141] and nude mice [142]. However, in many mouse colonies, it is asymptomatic. Although mechanisms differ in relation to infections with bacteria and parasites, some of the same concerns may be related to these [143]. Often, a good environment is the most important factor for avoiding the transition of latent infections into clinically overt infections, e.g. lowered air exchange may raise air concentrations of NH_3 [144], which again may induce respiratory disease in rats latently infected with, e.g. *Mycoplasma pulmonis* or even with bacteria with low pathogenicity such as *Staphylococcus xylosus* [145]. Dietary deficiency of vitamins A and E may have the same effect [146]. Viral infections along with a range of specific bacterial infections and parasite infestations are listed on various lists for the definition of SPF status, mostly due to the impact that these may have even as latent infections on a range of organ systems and the parameters related to these. Many of the agents on such lists do not necessarily cause clinically overt infections. Viruses may alter the response of the immune system. In the active phase, i.e. when the virus is present and propagating in the host, it may infect the immune cells themselves [147] and thereby elicit an immune suppressing effect, while when battling the infection, the abundance of immune cells will increase and eventually make the animal less sensitive to other infections [15]. When injecting the parvovirus H1 virus into hamsters, Helene Toolan discovered that they became far more resistant to both spontaneous [148] and induced cancers [149]. Therefore, animals may function differently as models whether they are non-infected, carry an active infection or have recovered from the infection. Additionally, viruses may contaminate biological products, such as cells and serum, sampled from the animals, and with these become spread to other facilities [150]. As not all viruses are equally infective, they may balance at lower prevalence rates, and this may increase inter-individual variation in a colony, when not all animals are under viral impact. DNA viruses, such as parvoviruses, normally cause persisting infections, while RNA viruses, with such exceptions as *lymphocytic choriomeningitis virus,* in immune competent animals are eliminated from the host after a period of infection. However, this may be different in immunodeficient and transgenic animals, and, therefore, viral infections are highly uncontrollable.

3.4 The Need for Pathogenic Stimulation

Exactly the reasons why obligate and facultative pathogens have been eliminated from modern breeding colonies of laboratory rodents may also be used as an argument why they should still be there. It has been claimed that mice reared without the encounter of pathogenic infections do not resemble humans [17]. This may be especially important within studies relating to the immune system [151], which may account for failures of translating results from preclinical research to the clinical phase. For example, within type 1 diabetes research, not a single one of the interventions from a range of successful preclinical intervention studies on the most commonly applied model, the nonobese diabetic (NOD) mouse, has translated into useful therapies in humans [152]. A range of viruses in humans have been indicated as causative for the development of type 1 diabetes [153–165], so even though it is not possible to conclude that the lack of virus infections in the mouse model is the cause of lacking translation, it is clear that a very clean mouse is not very comparable to the human patients. Parts of the immune system of adult laboratory mice to a higher extent resemble the immune system of a newborn rather than an adult human being, in the sense that meeting virus infections in early life would normally generate a cytotoxic T-cell and a T-helper cell response [166]. These cell types often have a very low abundance in SPF mice [15], while the abundance is much higher in pet shop and feral mice, which have been reared exposed to the 'childhood' infections eliminated in laboratory animal facilities [15]. Co-housing such mice with laboratory mice transferred some of these virus infections to the laboratory mice [15]. This caused a high mortality, but in those laboratory mice, surviving it induced the lacking T-cell responses and a blood cell gene expression of a pattern more similar to adult humans [15]. In addition, the infected laboratory mice became more resistant to other infections [15]. In the same way, transferring the clearly differing natural gut microbiome from a population of wild mice closely related to laboratory mice made these recipients exhibit reduced inflammation and increased survival following influenza virus infection and improved resistance against mutagen/inflammation-induced colorectal tumorigenesis [89]. While humans with defects in the *Hoil-1* gene (*Rbck1*) vary in their degree of hyperinflammation and immune deficiency, knockout mice deficient of the *Hoil-1* gene had greater susceptibility to infection with pathogens, such as *Listeria monocytogenes* [167]. However, infection with γ-herpesvirus protected them from this *Listeria* challenge by promoting a hyperinflammatory state similar to humans [167].

4 Measures to Reduce or Control Microbiota Impact

4.1 Early Life Handling and Housing

In early life, when there seems to be a window open during which it is easier to stimulate the formation of regulatory T cells [168], a core microbiota is established, and oral tolerance towards it is established to protect the host against inflammatory disease later in life [169]. It is often difficult precisely to describe the core microbiome [170]. In the respiratory system, the ability for induction of tolerance is easier than in the gut later in life [171]. Approximately 15 days after weaning, the core microbiota of a mouse becomes stable unless subjected to dramatic environmental or dietary impacts [172]. It is, therefore, important in order to avoid later variation in expression of animal models that the breeder is well aware, how the young animals are handled and able to describe this in details, as a range of human diseases modelled in rodents are driven by specific T-cell subsets primed early in life [14]. It is important that the breeder secures a uniform colonisation of the microbiota in the pups, and, therefore, in contrast to experimental facilities, the use of individually ventilated cage (IVC) system may not necessarily be the best option in breeding facilities. It may also be an option to exchange pups between mothers, because cross-fostering makes the offspring cluster with their foster mothers [173], although it may not fully counteract the genetic impact on microbiota composition [174].

4.2 Later Life Handling and Housing

In addition to the core microbiota established in early life, there is a more variable part of the microbiota [175], which may rapidly respond to the environmental impact from, e.g. caging, diet or stressors, which may, therefore, interfere with the model or increase inter-individual variation. Co-housed mice will after some time cluster according to their microbiota [176]. This will not necessarily influence the oral tolerance and other kinds of immune stimulation obtained in the early life [168, 176], but it may be observed that a genetically induced phenotype is changed by co-housing with wild-type mice. For example, caspase-3 knockout mice have a reduced response to induction of colitis with dextran sodium sulphate (DSS), but co-housing with wild-type mice increases the abundance of *Prevotella* spp., which weakens the protective effect of the gene deletion [129]. Co-housing effects have also been observed in mice humanized with microbiota from twins discordant in relation to obesity [177]. Therefore, a phenotypic characterisation of transgenic animals may be most optimal if including both animals co-housed and not co-housed with the wild-type animals. There can be substantial inter-cage variation in rodent colonies [178], and approximately 30% of the gut microbiota variation may be related to caging or cage environment [79]. It is, therefore, important to include a sufficient number of cages in each experimental group, i.e. each group must be housed in at least two cages, and it should be tested if there is a cage factor in the post-experimental data analysis. If groups are not co-housed, it is only possible to test for the cage factor and get an idea of its magnitude within the groups. If possible, it might, therefore, be wise to house test and control animals in the same cages, because it enables the cage to be included as a factor in a post-experiment multifactorial data evaluation. However, due to the co-housing impact on the microbiota, this is not a simple matter, and it must be considered carefully. In addition, there can be several other study elements, which will disfavour co-housing. In experimental facilities, the inter-individual variation has been shown to be lower in IVC systems, and mice housed in open cages compared to IVC housed mice had higher abundances of *Enterobacteriaceae*, *Bacteroides/Prevotella* spp. and *Lactobacillus* spp. and lower abundances of *Bifidobacterium* spp. [179]. Housing mice on grid floors should be avoided, as it induces stress, which will change the gut microbiota [130].

4.3 Feeding Procedures

The gut microbiota is also extremely sensitive to dietary changes and responds to these within few days [180]. The diet manufacturer will typically deliver a fixed composition scheme and do a current batch control according to this. However, this guaranteed composition only includes the large fractions, i.e. digestible carbohydrates, fibres, fats and proteins, as well as some micronutrients such as minerals and vitamins, and eventually some well-defined toxins. Changes in relation to the major fractions will clearly change the microbiota. Dietary fat increases plasma lipopolysaccharide (LPS) levels, which may induce the phenomenon known as *metabolic endotoxemia* [181], which causes specific changes in the gut microbiota with a markedly reduced abundance of, e.g. the anti-inflammatory *Bifidobacterium* spp. and pro-inflammatory *Bacteroides*-related bacteria [182]. Differences in proteins lead to less dramatic microbiota changes, but the phenotype, e.g. growth and fat deposition, is likely to change according to protein type in the diet [183–186]. A diet rich in proteins increases the abundance of *Bacteroides* spp., while a diet rich in carbohydrates increases the abundance of *Prevotella* spp. [187]. High levels of dietary fibres influence the microbial short-chain fatty acid production and their interaction with specific G-protein receptors and may, therefore, alleviate dextran sulphate sodium-induced colitis [188]. It is also important to consider the source of nutrients of different brands. Wheat and barley contain substantial amounts of gluten, which, e.g. is essential for the development of type 1 diabetes in NOD mice [45, 176], while corn does not contain gluten. However, manufacturers of corn-based diets have often added wheat middlings, and, therefore, corn-based diets may not necessarily be gluten-free. Therefore, it is important to consider the diet type carefully for each study, and obviously the use of different brands of diets may lead to differences in study outcomes. However, the use of specific diets can easily be and should be precisely described in manuscripts, and if in-house diets are used, these should be clearly declared in publications and research reports. However, this will not fully elucidate dietary influences on study outcomes, as in natural diets there are batch variations which cannot easily be controlled and described and which have a profound impact on microbiota composition, immune stimulation and metabolism. Very small amounts of trace elements in the diet may influence the microbiota [189]. Even if the processed and sterilized natural diet may not contain live bacteria, it will contain varying amounts of LPS from killed bacteria, which may influence the number of regulatory T cells and alter cytokine levels [190], which are known to be important for a range of animal models [99, 125, 191–193]. Even trace amounts of LPS increases the level of long-term blood glucose (HbA1c%) in the diet-induced obese mouse [194] and if given in early life decreases the gene expressions of *tnfα*, *il10*, *il6*, *ifnγ*, *il1β*, *il2*, *il4* and *foxp3* in NOD mice [194–196]. Various types of saccharides, such as starch, form the structural elements of plants, such as corn, wheat and barley, which are the main components of a rodent diet. Different types of starch may be more or less resistant to small intestine decomposition, and the resistant starch will pass to the large intestine, where it is decomposed to new poly- and oligosaccharides [197]. Oligosaccharides, which also may be contained in the diet before digestion, have a growth-promoting effect on *Bifidobacterium* spp. and other anti-inflammatory bacteria [59, 198]. Other non-starch saccharides, such as β-glycans with a documented reducing impact on plasma cholesterol, glycaemic index and colon cancer and arabinoxylan, with a documented antioxidant effect, are present in plant-based diets and likely to influence animal models [199]. The saccharide composition of the diet will vary according to season, geographical origin and processing and is, therefore, totally uncontrollable [200–202]. Therefore, to avoid uncontrolled variation in the models, e.g. induced by varying amounts and types of saccharides and LPS in the diet, the same batch of diet should be used throughout a study, and if it is a long-term study, the diet should be frozen and thawed for each feeding.

Furthermore, a simple thing such as acidification of drinking water may have a strong impact on the gut microbiota composition, e.g. in relation to the development of type 1 diabetes in NOD mice [203]. Therefore, it should be carefully considered whether this is needed in the facility, and it should be clearly described in publications.

4.4 Securing the Presence of Key Bacteria in the Microbiota

In the same way as classical health monitoring documents the absence of pathogens, it may be necessary prior to a study to test the animals for the presence or absence of specific commensals. The first publications on the impact of *segmented filamentous bacteria (SFB)* (Table 4) on models of IBD came, because a research group observed that the change of vendor caused them problems in inducing their adaptive transfer model in the mice [108, 204]. It turned out that only mice from one of the colonies were colonialized with SFBs, which was then found to induce the T-helper cell type 17, which had not previously been described [108, 204]. In contrast, a later study has shown that the absence of SFBs dramatically lowers the incidence of type 1 diabetes in NOD mouse [107], and in contrast to this, the absence of *Akkermansia muciniphila* increases the incidence of type 1 diabetes in the NOD mouse [134, 205]. Some of these bacteria could be the targets for various anti-inflammatory interventions, as it, for example, has been with *Bifidobacterium* spp. For many years this anti-inflammatory bacterium has been used for production of yoghurts with claimed health beneficial effects [206]. However as humans are not likely to consume an amount of yoghurt comparable to amounts fed in a mouse study, a more modern strategy pursued by the food industry is to feed oligosaccharides to propagate *Bifidobacterium* spp. [59, 207, 208]. Therefore, many major industrial players on the food market have various types of oligosaccharides in their pipelines, and they have a need for documenting the effects in mouse studies, as comprehensive immune system studies including immune cell counts, can be difficult to do in humans. However, several if not most of commercial mouse colonies do not harbour *Bifidobacterium* spp. as well as other bacteria of crucial importance for the induction of other animal models, as well as there can be substantial differences between colonies in their abundances of these important bacteria [68] (Table 4). Unfortunately, the presence or absence of commensals is not given major attention in the quality assurance of large commercial breeders, and, therefore, it may be necessary to organize some prescreening of the colonies, before decisions on which animals to be used are taken.

4.5 Incorporation of Microbiota Characterization in Data Evaluation

The traditional dogma that variation is always non-preferable in animal studies has to a certain extent been challenged by the 'omics' techniques. Today, it is possible within a reasonable budget to characterize the microbiota of each individual animal in an experiment. For example, the starting prize for doing sequencing of one study on an Oxford Nanopore Minion is approximately $1000 in 2019. Sequencing the animals may be clustered according to their UniFrac distances, and the cluster relationship can be used as a factor in a multifactorial data analysis, such as the general linear model. In theory, it might be done before the study, and animals most prone to model induction, intervention response, etc. may be selected for the study, thereby avoiding the use of animals not contributing significantly to study power. However, response time for a full 16S sequencing is in practice too long to allow such an approach, and furthermore still too little is known on which microbiota types are the most favourable for which models.

4.6 Inoculation of Rodents with Well-Defined Microbiotas

It is an attractive approach to set up animals for every study with a microbiota specifically aimed at fulfilling the goals of the specific animal model and study type. As there is still very limited exact knowledge on what would be the most favourable microbiota for which model, this is only possible for a very limited number of models. However, it is quite clear that there is a need for a different regime at rederivation rather than nowadays practice, in which new breeding animals are inoculated with ASF, and the remaining part of microbiota composition is left to chance and environment. Rodent colonies given a more diverse starter microbiota eventually with a guaranteed association with important commensals (Table 4) would improve the model expression in animals from the colony, e.g. in relation to IBD [209]. Also, it has been attempted for decades to 'humanize' rodents through inoculation with a human microbiota to have rodents with a more translational gut function for intervention studies [210] or to transfer certain human phenotypes to rodents for the further study of human diseases [177]. This may lead to establishment of a microbiota in both adult [211] and younger mice [180], but a human gut microbiota fails to stimulate the murine immune system in the same way as a murine microbiota does, and in the number of T cells and intra-epithelial lymphocytes, such 'humanized' mice have an immune function comparable to germ-free mice, which again are mostly comparable with newborn humans [212].

For securing a good starter microbiota after rederivation, the most simple approach is to freeze microbiota from well-functioning colonies with a high success in model induction and use this at rederivation. It is reasonable to assume that this microbiota should be sampled from the caecum in an anaerobic chamber but is unclear to which extent it makes a difference compared to simply sampling in the aerobic environment.

The optimal recipient for a fecal microbiota transplant is a germ-free animal [213] (Fig. 4). It is possible to decontaminate mice with antibiotics, such as ampicillin in the dose 1 g per litre drinking water [214] or 200 mg per kg body weight [213] for at least 7 days, eventually in a cocktail with other antibiotics [215], and to use the decontaminated mice for successful transplantation [214]. In addition or as a supplement, polyethylene glycol (PEG 3350) as one dose of 93 mg may be used to wash out the microbiota [213]. However, colonization is not as good as for germ-free mice [213, 216]. It might be possible by faecal microbiota transfer from mouse to germ-free mice to achieve colonization rates as high as 90% [217], while it is much lower when transplanting from humans to germ-free mice. The most optimal window for inoculation seems to

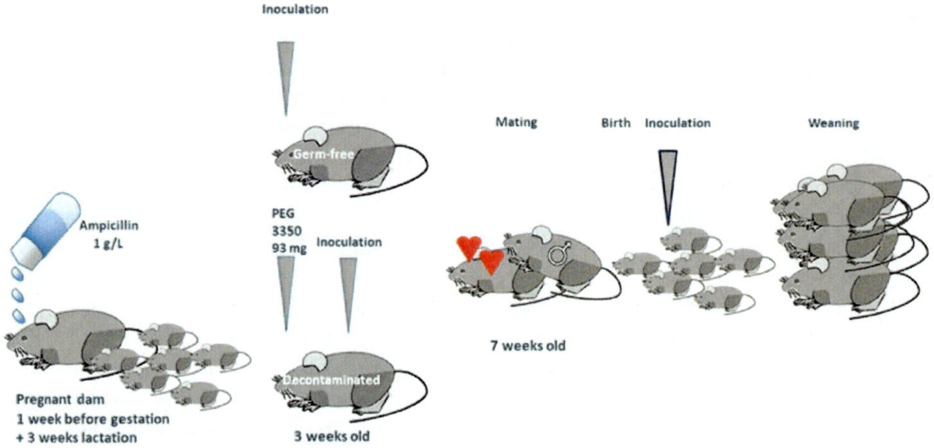

Fig. 4 Faecal microbiota transplantation (FMT). The optimal recipient for FMT is a germ-free animal, but in the lack of such pregnant dams and their litters can be decontaminated with antibiotics and/or polyethylene glycol (PEG 3350). At weaning the mice are inoculated into the oral cavity, by gavage or rectally with the microbiota in a saline suspension. At 7 weeks of age, the inoculated mice are mated, and at weaning the offspring is inoculated again

be around weaning [168], while later inoculation will be subject to a strong environmental impact, as well as it may be more difficult to influence the immune system [168, 213, 218]. As an alternative to the inoculation of a whole batch of mice for a study, it is more useful to inoculate germ-free females, mate these and use their offspring [97, 219]. Both oral and rectal inoculations can be applied, which does not seem to make a difference in mice [217]. Co-housing with animals with the desired microbiota seems to be an applicable tool, but if both animals already have a microbiota, the resulting microbiota will be a mixture, in which the one microbiota composition may dominate the other [220]. After establishment of the microbiota in a few founder animals, a colony with a stable version of the inoculated microbiota can be bred and maintained for several generations in IVC cages [219].

4.7 The Use of Antibiotics

The preferred option for studying the impact of the microbiota on a specific animal model is to induce the model in a germ-free animal [221]. As many models are not available in a germ-free version, the use of antibiotics has been applied in several studies. For example, in rats a schizophrenia-like state can be induced by intraperitoneal injection with phencyclidine (PCP), in a more popular term known as angel dust, twice daily for 7 days [222], which leads to severe memory failure in the animals [223]. However, rats treated with ampicillin from 7 days before model induction until termination are unaffected in their memory [100]. Also, it is possible to induce a temporary state of low microbiota impact by giving antibiotics for shorter periods later in life than just right after birth. For example, in diet-induced obesity in mice, a high-calorie diet is used to induce obesity and a type 2 diabetes-like state characterized by increased HbA1c% and reduced glucose tolerance [224, 225]. Glucose tolerance is improved if the mouse is put on life-long antibiotics [92, 93], but if the mice are treated with antibiotics only prior to weaning or only as adult, it can be shown that antibiotics only affect glucose tolerance in the juvenile animals and only in the acute phase right after treatment, while glucose tolerance in adult mice is unaffected [226]. Ampicillin seems to be essential in cocktails used for this purpose [73, 215]. However, antibiotics do not induce a fully germ-free state no matter which combination is used [215], and ampicillin-treated mice will recover with a microbiota, which is different from the pretreatment microbiota and which contains both members only suppressed by the treatment and members caught from the environment [227]. Furthermore, when using antibiotics for other purposes, such as doxycycline for inducing inducible knockout in recombinase carrying mice, it should be remembered that the antibiotic itself has a strong impact on the immune system due to the inhibition of the microbiota [228].

4.8 The Use of Animals with a Microbiota of Wild Origin

Due to the concern that SPF rodents in their lack of pathogenic stimulation do not reflect humans and that observations in such animals may have a lack of translationability [17, 151], it has been proposed to complement the use of SPF mice with the use of 'dirty' mice, i.e. mice harbouring common pathogens, so that before moving to an expensive clinical trial, therapeutics might be validated in both SPF and dirty mouse models to filter out modalities that are highly sensitive to unique environmental perturbations [17]. It is, however, obvious that if research facilities are to house both SPF and dirty mice with all their viruses, parasites and pathogenic bacteria (Table 2), the first ones must be securely separated from the latter, and it should be considered that many of those pathogens harboured by the dirty mice may not only be persisting as infections in the mice, but they may also survive in the environment for long periods making it difficult to use the facility again for SPF mice without a thorough and expensive decontamination procedure [143].

Dirty mice may be captured in the environment, or they may be purchased from a pet shop [15]. Subsequently they must be housed in a dedicated, underpressure, protected unit [17]. As the dirty mice harbour many of those infections, which were eradicated from rodent colonies of the past, they will also be subject to all those problems, which led to the eradication of the pathogens, i.e. increased mortality, increased variation, risk of zoonoses, decreased animal welfare, etc. [17]. Especially the increased variation may be regarded as a serious problem in an experimental design context. One way to deal with this may be to characterize each individual mouse in an experiment and to incorporate the information on infection status in the data evaluation, during which a multifactorial data evaluation can be used to reveal whether infectious status has an impact on research parameters. It should also be considered that there is no guarantee that exactly those infections harboured by the wild mouse will favour a specific model. Therefore, the dirty mouse model should be regarded more as a supplement rather than as a replacement for the current studies in SPF mice and humans, as reviewed by David Masopust et al. [17]. Furthermore, the use of wild or pet rodents for experimental use is in conflict with the European Union Directive from 2010, which lists that a range of species can only be used for research if produced by licensed breeders or exceptionally allowed by the competent authority [229]. So the use of wild or pet shop rodents needs to be licensed by the competent authority before start. A more pragmatic alternative is to produce the rodents in-house by infecting SPF rodents with a range of pathogens, such as mouse hepatitis virus, murine cytomegalovirus and the intestinal helminth *Heligmosomoides polygyrus* [16]. Such infections has been shown to alter pre- and post-vaccination gene expression, cytokines and antibodies in blood in a direction similar to wild or pet shop mice when mice are vaccinated against yellow fever virus [16].

5 Concluding Remarks

It has become gradually more complicated to consider microbiological aspects, when doing animal experiments. One hundred years ago, no such issues were considered; then 80 years ago, we got the option of working with gnotobiotic animals; then 60 years ago came animals free of specific pathogens; 20 years ago came the discussion on the need to have a well-functioning microbiota for a proper model induction and intervention response; and today it is discussed if we need to have some of the pathogens back to improve model induction and intervention response. The tools for improving animal research by proper microbiota considerations are available today, and as the society and the scientific community have a common interest in improving reproducibility and translationability of animal research while also striving to achieve reduction in animal use and increase power of studies, a scientist should see the increased awareness of microbiological matters as an opportunity to improve research.

References

1. Norman JM, Handley SA, Virgin HW. Kingdom-agnostic metagenomics and the importance of complete characterization of enteric microbial communities. Gastroenterology. 2014;146:1459–69. https://doi.org/10.1053/j.gastro.2014.02.001.
2. Falk PG, Hooper LV, Midtvedt T, et al. Creating and maintaining the gastrointestinal ecosystem: what we know and need to know from gnotobiology. Microbiol Mol Biol Rev. 1998;62:1157.
3. Norin E, Midtvedt T. Intestinal microflora functions in laboratory mice claimed to harbor a "normal" intestinal microflora. Is the SPF concept running out of date? Anaerobe. 2010;16:311–3. https://doi.org/10.1016/j.anaerobe.2009.10.006.
4. Nuttall George HF, Thierfelder H. Thierisches Leben ohne Bakterien im Verdauungskanal. Hoppe Seylers Z Physiol Chem. 1897;23(3):231–5.
5. Smith T. Some bacteriological and environmental factors in the pneumonias of lower animals with special reference to the guinea-pig. J Med Res. 1913;29:291–U227.
6. Tyzzer EE. A fatal disease of the Japanese waltzing mouse caused by a spore-bearing bacillus (Bacillus piliformis N.Sp.). J Med Res. 1917;37:307–38.
7. Glimstedt G. Metabolism of bacteria free animals. I General methods. Skand Arch Physiol. 1936;73:48–62. https://doi.org/10.1111/j.1748-1716.1936.tb01451.x.
8. Reyniers JA, Trexler PC, Ervin RF. Rearing germ-free albino rats. Lobund Rep. 1946:1–84. 1946/11/01.
9. Foster H. Large scale production of rats free of commonly occurring pathogens and parasites. Proc Anim Care Panel. 1958;8:92–100.
10. Schaedler RW, DUBOS R, Costello R. The development of the bacterial flora in the gastrointestinal tract of mice. J Exp Med. 1965;122:59–66.
11. Schaedler RW, DUBS R, Costello R. Association of germfree mice with bacteria isolated from normal mice. J Exp Med. 1965;122:77–82.
12. Barthold SW, Coleman GL, BHATT PN, et al. The etiology of transmissible murine colonic hyperplasia. Lab Anim Sci. 1976;26:889–94.
13. Dewhirst FE, Chien CC, Paster BJ, et al. Phylogeny of the defined murine microbiota: altered Schaedler flora. Appl Environ Microbiol. 1999;65:3287–92.
14. Bleich A, Hansen AK. Time to include the gut microbiota in the hygienic standardisation of laboratory rodents. Comp Immunol Microbiol Infect Dis. 2012;35:81–92. DOI: S0147-9571(11)00125-1 [pii];10.1016/j.cimid.2011.12.006 [doi]
15. Beura LK, Hamilton SE, Bi K, et al. Normalizing the environment recapitulates adult human immune traits in laboratory mice. Nature. 2016;532:512–6. 2016/04/21. https://doi.org/10.1038/nature17655.
16. Reese TA, Bi K, Kambal A, et al. Sequential infection with common pathogens promotes human-like immune gene expression and altered vaccine response. Cell Host Microbe. 2016;19:713–9. Article. https://doi.org/10.1016/j.chom.2016.04.003.
17. Masopust D, Sivula CP, Jameson SC. Of mice, dirty mice, and men: using mice to understand human immunology. J Immunol. 2017;199:383–8. https://doi.org/10.4049/jimmunol.1700453.
18. Dammann P, Hilken G, Hueber B, et al. Infectious microorganisms in mice (Mus musculus) purchased from commercial pet shops in Germany. Lab Anim. 2011;45:271–5. https://doi.org/10.1258/la.2011.010183.
19. Schoondermark-van de Ven EM, Philipse-Bergmann IM, van der Logt JT. Prevalence of naturally occurring viral infections, Mycoplasma pulmonis and Clostridium piliforme in laboratory rodents in Western Europe screened from 2000 to 2003. Lab Anim. 2006;40:137–43. 2006/04/08. https://doi.org/10.1258/002367706776319114.
20. Rodrigues DM, Moreira JCD, Lancellotti M, et al. Murine norovirus infection in Brazilian animal facilities. Exp Anim. 2017;66:115–24. Article
21. Parker SE, Malone S, Bunte RM, et al. Infectious diseases in wild mice (Mus musculus) collected on and around the University of Pennsylvania (Philadelphia) Campus. Comp Med. 2009;59:424–30.
22. Davies RH, Wray C. Mice as carriers of Salmonella enteritidis on persistently infected poultry units. Vet Rec. 1995;137:337–41. 1995/09/30
23. Taylor JD, Stephens CP, Duncan RG, et al. Polyarthritis in wild mice (Mus musculus) caused by Streptobacillus moniliformis. Aust Vet J. 1994;71:143–5. 1994/05/01
24. Pritchett-Corning KR, Cosentino J, Clifford CB. Contemporary prevalence of infectious agents in laboratory mice and rats. Lab Anim. 2009;43:165–73.
25. Mahler Convenor M, Berard M, Feinstein R, et al. FELASA recommendations for the health monitoring of mouse, rat, hamster, guinea pig and rabbit colonies in breeding and experimental units. Lab

Anim. 2014;48:178–92. 2014/02/06. https://doi.org/10.1177/0023677213516312.
26. Hansen AK, Skovgaard-Jensen HJ, Thomsen P, et al. Rederivation of rat colonies seropositive for Bacillus piliformis and the subsequent screening for antibodies [published erratum appears in Lab Anim Sci 1993 Feb; 43(1): 114]. Lab Anim Sci. 1992;42:444–8.
27. Moler TL, Donahue SE, Anderson GB. Simple technique for non-surgical embryo transfer in mice. Lab Anim Sci. 1979;29:353–6. Note
28. El-Gayar M, Gauly M, Holtz W. One-step dilution of open-pulled-straw (OPS)-vitrified mouse blastocysts in sucrose-free medium. Cryobiology. 2008;57:191–4. https://doi.org/10.1016/j.cryobiol.2008.07.012.
29. Jin B, Mochida K, Ogura A, et al. Equilibrium vitrification of mouse embryos. Biol Reprod. 2010;82:444–50. https://doi.org/10.1095/biolreprod.109.077685.
30. Easterbrook JD, Kaplan JB, Glass GE, et al. A survey of rodent-borne pathogens carried by wild-caught Norway rats: a potential threat to laboratory rodent colonies. Lab Anim. 2008;42:92–8.
31. Nakai N, Kawaguchi C, Nawa K, et al. Detection and elimination of contaminating microorganisms in transplantable tumors and cell lines. Exp Anim. 2000;49:309–13.
32. Rehbinder C, Baneux P, Forbes D, et al. FELASA recommendations for the health monitoring of breeding colonies and experimental units of cats, dogs and pigs – report of the Federation of European Laboratory Animal Science Associations (FELASA) Working Group on Animal Health. Lab Anim. 1998;32:1–17.
33. Weber H, Berge E, FInch J, et al. Health monitoring of non-human primate colonies. Recommendations of the Federation of European Laboratory Animal Science Associations (FELASA) Working Group on non-human primate health accepted by the FELASA Board of Management, 21 November 1998. Lab Anim. 1999;33(Suppl 1):S1–18.
34. Rehbinder C, Alenius S, Bures J, et al. FELASA recommendations for the health monitoring of experimental units of calves, sheep and goats Report of the federation of European Laboratory Animal Science Associations (FELASA) Working Group on Animal Health. Lab Anim. 2000;34:329–50.
35. Hansen AK. Statistical aspects of health monitoring of laboratory animal colonies. Scand J Lab Anim Sci. 1993;20:11–4.
36. Hayashimoto N, Morita H, Ishida T, et al. Current microbiological status of laboratory mice and rats in experimental facilities in Japan. Exp Anim. 2013;62:41–8.
37. Manjunath S, Kulkarni PG, Nagavelu K, et al. Sero-prevalence of rodent pathogens in India. PLoS One. 2015;10:e0131706. https://doi.org/10.1371/journal.pone.0131706.
38. McInnes EF, Rasmussen L, Fung P, et al. Prevalence of viral, bacterial and parasitological diseases in rats and mice used in research environments in Australasia over a 5-y period. Lab Anim (NY). 2011;40:341–50. https://doi.org/10.1038/laban1111-341.
39. Knust B, Stroher U, Edison L, et al. Lymphocytic choriomeningitis virus in employees and mice at multipremises feeder-rodent operation, United States, 2012. Emerg Infect Dis. 2014;20:240–7. Article. https://doi.org/10.3201/eid2002.130860.
40. Hansen AK, Andersen HV, Svendsen O. Studies on the diagnosis of Tyzzer's disease in laboratory rat colonies with antibodies against Bacillus piliformis (Clostridium piliforme). Lab Anim Sci. 1994;44:424–9.
41. Hansen AK, Svendsen O, Mollegaard-Hansen KE. Epidemiological studies of Bacillus piliformis infection and Tyzzer's disease in laboratory rats. Z Versuchstierkd. 1990;33:163–9.
42. Hansen AK, Nielsen DS. Molecular biology based methods for microbiota characterization. In: Hansen AK, Nielsen DS, editors. Handbook of laboratory animal bacteriology. 2nd ed. Boca Raton: CRC Press; 2014. p. 93–104.
43. Hansen AK. The aerobic bacterial flora of laboratory rats from a Danish breeding centre. Scand J Lab Anim Sci. 1992;19:59–68.
44. Dahl K, Kirkeby S, d'Apice AJF, et al. The bacterial flora of alpha-gal knock out mice express the alpha-gal epitope comparable to wild type mice. Transpl Immunol. 2005;14:9–16.
45. Hansen AK, Ling F, Kaas A, et al. Diabetes preventive gluten-free diet decreases the number of caecal bacteria in non-obese diabetic mice. Diab Metab Res Rev. 2006;22:220–5.
46. Vaahtovuo J, Erkki E, Paavo T. Comparison of cellular fatty acid profiles of the microbiota in different gut regions of BALB/c and C57BL/6J mice. Antonie Van Leeuwenhoek. 2005;88:67–74.
47. Hufeldt MR, Nielsen DS, Vogensen FK, et al. Family relationship of female breeders reduce the systematic inter-individual variation in the gut microbiota of inbred laboratory mice. Lab Anim. 2010;44:283–9.
48. Bergstrom A, Licht TR, Wilcks A, et al. Introducing GUt low-density array (GULDA): a validated approach for qPCR-based intestinal microbial community analysis. FEMS Microbiol Lett. 2012;337:38–47. https://doi.org/10.1111/1574-6968.12004.
49. Pang W, Vogensen FK, Nielsen DS, et al. Faecal and caecal microbiota profiles of mice do not cluster in the same way. Lab Anim. 2012;46:231–6.
50. Aagaard K, Petrosino J, Keitel W, et al. The human microbiome project strategy for comprehensive sampling of the human microbiome and why it matters. FASEB J. 2013;27:1012–22. https://doi.org/10.1096/fj.12-220806.
51. Lundberg R, Clausen SK, Pang W, et al. Gastrointestinal microbiota and local inflammation during Oxazolone-induced Dermatitis in BALB/cA Mice. Comp Med. 2012;62:371–80.

52. Mao DP, Zhou Q, Chen CY, et al. Coverage evaluation of universal bacterial primers using the metagenomic datasets. BMC Microbiol. 2012;12:66. https://doi.org/10.1186/1471-2180-12-66.
53. Nielsen DS, Moller PL, Rosenfeldt V, et al. Case study of the distribution of mucosa-associated Bifidobacterium species, Lactobacillus species, and other lactic acid bacteria in the human colon. Appl Environ Microbiol. 2003;69:7545–8. https://doi.org/10.1128/Aem.69312.7545-7548.2003.
54. Krych L, Hansen CH, Hansen AK, et al. Quantitatively different, yet qualitatively alike: a meta-analysis of the mouse core gut microbiome with a view towards the human gut microbiome. PLoS One. 2013;8:e62578. 2013/05/10. https://doi.org/10.1371/journal.pone.0062578.
55. Edgar RC. UPARSE: highly accurate OTU sequences from microbial amplicon reads. Nat Meth. 2013;10:996. https://doi.org/10.1038/nmeth.2604.
56. Edgar RC. UPARSE: highly accurate OTU sequences from microbial amplicon reads. Nat Methods. 2013;10:996–8. https://doi.org/10.1038/nmeth.2604.
57. Langille MGI, Zaneveld J, Caporaso JG, et al. Predictive functional profiling of microbial communities using 16S rRNA marker gene sequences. Nat Biotechnol. 2013;31:814. https://doi.org/10.1038/Nbt.2676.
58. Lozupone C, Hamady M, Knight R. UniFrac–an online tool for comparing microbial community diversity in a phylogenetic context. BMC Bioinform. 2006;7:371.
59. Hansen CH, Frokiaer H, Christensen AG, et al. Dietary xylooligosaccharide downregulates IFN-gamma and the low-grade inflammatory cytokine IL-1beta systemically in mice. J Nutr. 2013;143:533–40. 2013/02/22. https://doi.org/10.3945/jn.112.172361.
60. De Angelis M, Piccolo M, Vannini L, et al. Fecal microbiota and metabolome of children with autism and pervasive developmental disorder not otherwise specified. PLoS One. 2013;8:e76993. 2013/10/17. https://doi.org/10.1371/journal.pone.0076993.
61. Caporaso JG, Kuczynski J, Stombaugh J, et al. QIIME allows analysis of high-throughput community sequencing data. Nat Methods. 2010;7:335–6. https://doi.org/10.1038/nmeth.f.303.
62. Bleich A, Mahler M. Environment as a critical factor for the pathogenesis and outcome of gastrointestinal disease: experimental and human inflammatory bowel disease and helicobacter-induced gastritis. Pathobiology. 2005;72:293–307. DOI: PAT2005072006293 [pii];10.1159/000091327 [doi]
63. Itoh K, Narushima S. Intestinal flora of animal models of human diseases as an environmental factor. Curr Issues Intest Microbiol. 2005;6:9–15.
64. Sartor RB. Microbial influences in inflammatory bowel diseases. Gastroenterology. 2008;134:577–94. DOI: S0016-5085(07)02157-9 [pii];10.1053/j.gastro.2007.11.059 [doi]
65. Hufeldt MR, Nielsen DS, Vogensen FK, et al. Variation in the gut microbiota of laboratory mice is related to both genetic and environmental factors. Comp Med. 2010;60:336–42.
66. Rasmussen TS, de Vries L, Kot W, et al. Mouse vendor influence on the bacterial and viral gut composition exceeds the effect of diet. Viruses. 2019;11(5):435. https://doi.org/10.3390/v11050435.
67. Alexander AD, Orcutt RP, Henry JC, et al. Quantitative PCR assays for mouse enteric flora reveal strain-dependent differences in composition that are influenced by the microenvironment. Mamm Genome. 2006;17:1093–104. Article. https://doi.org/10.1007/s00335-006-0063-1.
68. Ericsson AC, Davis JW, Spollen W, et al. Effects of vendor and genetic background on the composition of the fecal microbiota of inbred mice. Plos One. 2015;10:19. Article. https://doi.org/10.1371/journal.pone.0116704.
69. Ellekilde M, Krych L, Hansen CH, et al. Characterization of the gut microbiota in leptin deficient obese mice – correlation to inflammatory and diabetic parameters. Res Vet Sci. 2014;96:241–50. https://doi.org/10.1016/j.rvsc.2014.01.007.
70. Rasmussen TS, de Vries L, Kot W, et al. Mouse vendor influence on the bacterial and viral gut composition exceeds the effect of diet. Viruses. 2019;11:588160. 2019/05/16. https://doi.org/10.3390/v11050435.
71. Scher JU, Sczesnak A, Longman RS, et al. Expansion of intestinal Prevotella copri correlates with enhanced susceptibility to arthritis. eLife. 2013;2:e01202. https://doi.org/10.7554/eLife.01202.
72. Hildebrandt MA, Hoffmann C, Sherrill-Mix SA, et al. High-fat diet determines the composition of the murine gut microbiome independently of obesity. Gastroenterology. 2009;137:1716–24. https://doi.org/10.1053/j.gastro.2009.08.042.
73. Ubeda C, Taur Y, Jenq RR, et al. Vancomycin-resistant Enterococcus domination of intestinal microbiota is enabled by antibiotic treatment in mice and precedes bloodstream invasion in humans. J Clin Invest. 2010;120:4332–41. DOI: 43918 [pii];10.1172/JCI43918 [doi]
74. Antonopoulos DA, Huse SM, Morrison HG, et al. Reproducible community dynamics of the gastrointestinal microbiota following antibiotic perturbation. Infect Immun. 2009;77:2367–75. https://doi.org/10.1128/IAI.01520-08.
75. Wilson KH, Brown RS, Andersen GL, et al. Comparison of fecal biota from specific pathogen free and feral mice. Anaerobe. 2006;12:249–53. DOI: S1075-9964(06)00071-0 [pii];10.1016/j.anaerobe.2006.09.002 [doi]

76. Ley RE, Backhed F, Turnbaugh P, et al. Obesity alters gut microbial ecology. Proc Natl Acad Sci U S A. 2005;102:11070–5.
77. Hansen CH, Krych L, Nielsen DS, et al. Early life treatment with vancomycin propagates Akkermansia muciniphila and reduces diabetes incidence in the NOD mouse. Diabetologia. 2012;55:2285–94. Article. https://doi.org/10.1007/s00125-012-2564-7.
78. Walk ST, Blum AM, Ewing SAS, et al. Alteration of the murine gut microbiota during infection with the parasitic helminth heligmosomoides polygyrus. Inflamm Bowel Dis. 2010;16:1841–9. https://doi.org/10.1002/ibd.21299.
79. Hildebrand F, Nguyen TL, Brinkman B, et al. Inflammation-associated enterotypes, host genotype, cage and inter-individual effects drive gut microbiota variation in common laboratory mice. Genome Biol. 2013;14:R4. 2013/01/26. https://doi.org/10.1186/gb-2013-14-1-r4.
80. Qin J, Li Y, Cai Z, et al. A metagenome-wide association study of gut microbiota in type 2 diabetes. Nature. 2012;490:55–60. https://doi.org/10.1038/nature11450.
81. Gollwitzer ES, Saglani S, Trompette A, et al. Lung microbiota promotes tolerance to allergens in neonates via PD-L1. Nat Med. 2014;20:642–7. https://doi.org/10.1038/nm.3568.
82. Buve A, Jespers V, Crucitti T, et al. The vaginal microbiota and susceptibility to HIV. AIDS. 2014;28:2333–44.
83. The_human_microbiome_project. Structure, function and diversity of the healthy human microbiome. Nature. 2012;486:207–14. https://doi.org/10.1038/nature11234. http://www.nature.com/nature/journal/v486/n7402/abs/nature11234.html#supplementary-information
84. Grice EA, Kong HH, Conlan S, et al. Topographical and temporal diversity of the human skin microbiome. Science. 2009;324:1190–2. https://doi.org/10.1126/science.1171700.
85. Scharschmidt TC, List K, Grice EA, et al. Matriptase-deficient mice exhibit ichthyotic skin with a selective shift in skin microbiota. J Invest Dermatol. 2009;129:2435–42. https://doi.org/10.1038/jid.2009.104.
86. Whyte W, Lidwell OM, Lowbury EJ, et al. Suggested bacteriological standards for air in ultraclean operating rooms. J Hosp Infect. 1983;4:133–9.
87. Zhang CH, Zhang MH, Wang SY, et al. Interactions between gut microbiota, host genetics and diet relevant to development of metabolic syndromes in mice. ISME J. 2010;4:232–41.
88. Hauschild T, Slizewski P, Masiewicz P. Species distribution of staphylococci from small wild mammals. Syst Appl Microbiol. 2010;33:457–60. 2010/10/26. https://doi.org/10.1016/j.syapm.2010.08.007.
89. Rosshart SP, Vassallo BG, Angeletti D, et al. Wild mouse gut microbiota promotes host fitness and improves disease resistance. Cell. 2017;171:1015-1028 e1013. 2017/10/24. https://doi.org/10.1016/j.cell.2017.09.016.
90. Itoh K, Mitsuoka T, Sudo K, et al. Comparison of fecal flora of mice based upon different strains and different housing conditions. Z Versuchstierkd. 1983;25:135–46.
91. Buschard K, Pedersen C, Hansen SV, et al. Antidiabetogenic effect of fusidic acid in diabetes prone Bb rats. Autoimmunity. 1992;14:101–4.
92. Bech-Nielsen GV, Hansen CH, Hufeldt MR, et al. Manipulation of the gut microbiota in C57BL/6 mice changes glucose tolerance without affecting weight development and gut mucosal immunity. Res Vet Sci. 2012;92:501–8.
93. Membrez M, Blancher F, Jaquet M, et al. Gut microbiota modulation with norfloxacin and ampicillin enhances glucose tolerance in mice. FASEB J. 2008;22:2416–26.
94. Zackular JP, Baxter NT, Iverson KD, et al. The gut microbiome modulates colon tumorigenesis. MBio. 2013;4:e00692–13. https://doi.org/10.1128/mBio.00692-13.
95. Klimesova K, Kverka M, Zakostelska Z, et al. Altered gut microbiota promotes colitis-associated cancer in IL-1 receptor-associated kinase M-deficient mice. Inflamm Bowel Dis. 2013;19:1266–77. 2013/04/10. https://doi.org/10.1097/MIB.0b013e318281330a.
96. Ericsson AC, Akter S, Hanson MM, et al. Differential susceptibility to colorectal cancer due to naturally occurring gut microbiota. Oncotarget. 2015;6:33689–704. Article. https://doi.org/10.18632/oncotarget.5604.
97. Zachariassen LF, Krych L, Engkilde K, et al. Sensitivity to oxazolone induced dermatitis is transferable with gut microbiota in mice. Sci Rep. 2017;7:44385. Article. https://doi.org/10.1038/srep44385. http://www.nature.com/articles/srep44385#supplementary-information
98. Sellon RK, Tonkonogy S, Schultz M, et al. Resident enteric bacteria are necessary for development of spontaneous colitis and immune system activation in interleukin-10-deficient mice. Infect Immun. 1998;66:5224–31.
99. Pyndt Jorgensen B, Hansen JT, Krych L, et al. A possible link between food and mood: dietary impact on gut microbiota and behavior in BALB/c mice. PLoS One. 2014;9:e103398. 2014/08/19. https://doi.org/10.1371/journal.pone.0103398.
100. Jorgensen BP, Krych L, Pedersen TB, et al. Investigating the long-term effect of subchronic phencyclidine-treatment on novel object recognition and the association between the gut microbiota and behavior in the animal model of schizophrenia. Physiol Behav. 2015;141:32–9. Article. https://doi.org/10.1016/j.physbeh.2014.12.042.
101. Holmes E, Nicholson J. Variation in gut microbiota strongly influences individual rodent phenotypes.

Toxicol Sci. 2005;87:1–2. Editorial Material. https://doi.org/10.1093/toxsci/kfi259.
102. Quigley EMM. Microbiota-brain-gut axis and neurodegenerative diseases. Curr Neurol Neurosci Rep. 2017;17:9. Review. https://doi.org/10.1007/s11910-017-0802-6.
103. Bercik P, Denou E, Collins J, et al. The intestinal microbiota affect central levels of brain-derived neurotropic factor and behavior in mice. Gastroenterology. 2011;141:599-609.e593. https://doi.org/10.1053/j.gastro.2011.04.052.
104. Engkilde K, Buschard K, Hansen AK, et al. Prevention of diabetes in NOD mice by repeated exposures to a contact allergen inducing a sub-clinical dermatitis. PLoS One. 2010;5:e10591.
105. Stepankova R, Powrie F, Kofronova O, et al. Segmented filamentous bacteria in a defined bacterial cocktail induce intestinal inflammation in SCID mice reconstituted with CD45RB(high) CD4+ T cells. Inflamm Bowel Dis. 2007;13:1202–11.
106. Wu HJ, Ivanov II, Darce J, et al. Gut-residing segmented filamentous bacteria drive autoimmune arthritis via T helper 17 cells. Immunity. 2010;32:815–27. https://doi.org/10.1016/j.immuni.2010.06.001.
107. Kriegel MA, Sefik E, Hill JA, et al. Naturally transmitted segmented filamentous bacteria segregate with diabetes protection in nonobese diabetic mice. Proc Natl Acad Sci USA. 2011;108:11548–53. DOI: 1108924108 [pii];10.1073/pnas.1108924108 [doi]
108. Ivanov II, Atarashi K, Manel N, et al. Induction of intestinal Th17 cells by segmented filamentous bacteria. Cell. 2009;139:485–98. DOI: S0092-8674(09)01248-3 [pii];10.1016/j.cell.2009.09.033 [doi]
109. Garland CD, Lee A, Dickson MR. Segmented filamentous bacteria in the rodent small intestine: their colonization of growing animals and possible role in host resistance toSalmonella. Microb Ecol. 1982;8:181–90.
110. Balish E, Warner T. Enterococcus faecalis induces inflammatory bowel disease in interleukin-10 knockout mice. Am J Pathol. 2002;160:2253–7.
111. Kim SC, Tonkonogy SL, Albright CA, et al. Variable phenotypes of enterocolitis in interleukin 10-deficient mice monoassociated with two different commensal bacteria. Gastroenterology. 2005;128:891–906. DOI: S0016508505001782 [pii]
112. Martin R, Chain F, Miquel S, et al. The commensal bacterium faecalibacterium prausnitzii is protective in DNBS-induced chronic moderate and severe colitis models. Inflamm Bowel Dis. 2014;20:417–30. https://doi.org/10.1097/01.mib.0000440815.76627.64.
113. Rosique RM, Bermudez-Humaran LG, Chain F, et al. Protective and curative effect of faecalibacterium prausnitzii in a chronic DNBS-induced murine colitis. Gastroenterology. 2012;142:S392.
114. Zhang M, Qiu X, Zhang H, et al. Faecalibacterium prausnitzii inhibits interleukin-17 to ameliorate colorectal colitis in rats. PLoS One. 2014;9 https://doi.org/10.1371/journal.pone.0109146.
115. Paturi G, Mandimika T, Butts CA, et al. Influence of dietary blueberry and broccoli on cecal microbiota activity and colon morphology in mdr1a(-/-) mice, a model of inflammatory bowel diseases. Nutrition. 2012;28:324–30. https://doi.org/10.1016/j.nut.2011.07.018.
116. Carlsson AH, Yakymenko O, Olivier I, et al. Faecalibacterium prausnitzii supernatant improves intestinal barrier function in mice DSS colitis. Scand J Gastroenterol. 2013;48:1136–44. https://doi.org/10.3109/00365521.2013.828773.
117. Bravo JA, Forsythe P, Chew MV, et al. Ingestion of Lactobacillus strain regulates emotional behavior and central GABA receptor expression in a mouse via the vagus nerve. Proc Natl Acad Sci USA. 2011;108(38):16050.
118. Schultz M, Veltkamp C, Dieleman LA, et al. Lactobacillus plantarum 299V in the treatment and prevention of spontaneous colitis in interleukin-10-deficient mice. Inflamm Bowel Dis. 2002;8:71–80.
119. Madsen K, Cornish A, Soper P, et al. Probiotic bacteria enhance murine and human intestinal epithelial barrier function. Gastroenterology. 2001;121:580–91. DOI: S0016508501903269 [pii]
120. Madsen KL, Doyle JS, Jewell LD, et al. Lactobacillus species prevents colitis in interleukin 10 gene-deficient mice. Gastroenterology. 1999;116:1107–14. DOI: S0016508599004436 [pii]
121. McCarthy J, O'Mahony L, O'Callaghan L, et al. Double blind, placebo controlled trial of two probiotic strains in interleukin 10 knockout mice and mechanistic link with cytokine balance. Gut. 2003;52:975–80.
122. Schwarzer M, Srutkova D, Schabussova I, et al. Neonatal colonization of germ-free mice with Bifidobacterium longum prevents allergic sensitization to major birch pollen allergen Bet v 1. Vaccine. 2013;31:5405–12. Article. https://doi.org/10.1016/j.vaccine.2013.09.014.
123. Lam V, Su J, Koprowski S, et al. Intestinal microbiota determine severity of myocardial infarction in rats. FASEB J. 2012;26:1727–35. 2012/01/17. https://doi.org/10.1096/fj.11-197921.
124. Rath HC, Wilson KH, Sartor RB. Differential induction of colitis and gastritis in HLA-B27 transgenic rats selectively colonized with Bacteroides vulgatus or Escherichia coli. Infect Immun. 1999;67:2969–74.
125. Nakano V, Gomes DA, Arantes RM, et al. Evaluation of the pathogenicity of the Bacteroides fragilis toxin gene subtypes in gnotobiotic mice. Curr Microbiol. 2006;53:113–7. Article. https://doi.org/10.1007/s00284-005-0321-6.
126. Wu S, Rhee KJ, Albesiano E, et al. A human colonic commensal promotes colon tumorigenesis via acti-

vation of T helper type 17 T cell responses. Nat Med. 2009;15:1016–22. Article. https://doi.org/10.1038/nm.2015.
127. Hsiao EY, McBride SW, Hsien S, et al. Microbiota modulate behavioral and physiological abnormalities associated with neurodevelopmental disorders. Cell. 2013;155:1451–63. 2013/12/10. https://doi.org/10.1016/j.cell.2013.11.024.
128. Mazmanian SK, Round JL, Kasper DL. A microbial symbiosis factor prevents intestinal inflammatory disease. Nature. 2008;453:620–5. https://doi.org/10.1038/nature07008. http://www.nature.com/nature/journal/v453/n7195/suppinfo/nature07008_S1.html
129. Brinkman BM, Becker A, Ayiseh RB, et al. Gut microbiota affects sensitivity to acute DSS-induced colitis independently of host genotype. Inflamm Bowel Dis. 2013;19:2560–7. Research Support, Non-U.S. Gov't. https://doi.org/10.1097/MIB.0b013e3182a8759a.
130. Bangsgaard Bendtsen KM, Krych L, Sørensen DB, et al. Gut microbiota composition is correlated to grid floor induced stress and behavior in the BALB/c mouse. PLoS One. 2012;7:e46231.
131. Naseribafrouei A, Hestad K, Avershina E, et al. Correlation between the human fecal microbiota and depression. Neurogastroenterol Motil. 2014;26:1155–62. Article. https://doi.org/10.1111/nmo.12378.
132. Everard A, Belzer C, Geurts L, et al. Cross-talk between Akkermansia muciniphila and intestinal epithelium controls diet-induced obesity. Proc Natl Acad Sci U S A. 2013;110:9066–71. https://doi.org/10.1073/pnas.1219451110.
133. Marietta EV, Gomez AM, Yeoman C, et al. Low incidence of spontaneous type 1 diabetes in non-obese diabetic mice raised on gluten-free diets is associated with changes in the intestinal microbiome. PLoS One. 2013;8:e78687. Article. https://doi.org/10.1371/journal.pone.0078687.
134. Hanninen A, Toivonen R, Poysti S, et al. Akkermansia muciniphila induces gut microbiota remodelling and controls islet autoimmunity in NOD mice. Gut. 2018;67:1445–53. https://doi.org/10.1136/gutjnl-2017-314508.
135. Russell SL, Gold MJ, Hartmann M, et al. Early life antibiotic-driven changes in microbiota enhance susceptibility to allergic asthma. EMBO Rep. 2012;13:440–7. Article. https://doi.org/10.1038/embor.2012.32.
136. Ganesh BP, Klopfleisch R, Loh G, et al. Commensal Akkermansia muciniphila exacerbates gut inflammation in Salmonella Typhimurium-infected gnotobiotic mice. PLoS One. 2013;8:e74963. Article. https://doi.org/10.1371/journal.pone.0074963.
137. Kang CS, Ban M, Choi EJ, et al. Extracellular vesicles derived from gut microbiota, especially Akkermansia muciniphila, protect the progression of dextran sulfate sodium-induced colitis. PLoS One. 2013;8:e76520. Article. https://doi.org/10.1371/journal.pone.0076520.
138. Bhatt PN, Jacoby RO. Mousepox in inbred mice innately resistant or susceptible to lethal infection with ectromelia virus. III. Experimental transmission of infection and derivation of virus-free progeny from previously infected dams. Lab Anim Sci. 1987;37:23–7.
139. Jacoby RO, BHATT PN. Mousepox in inbred mice innately resistant or susceptible to lethal infection with ectromelia virus. II Pathogenesis. Lab Anim Sci. 1987;37:16–22.
140. Broderson JR, Murphy FA, Hierholzer JC. Lethal enteritis in infant mice caused by mouse hepatitis virus. Lab Anim Sci. 1976;26:824.
141. Percy DH, Barta JR. Spontaneous and experimental infections in scid and scid/beige mice. Lab Anim Sci. 1993;43:127–32.
142. Sebesteny A, Hill AC. Hepatitis and brain lesions due to mouse hepatitis virus accompanied by wasting in nude mice. Lab Anim. 1974;8:317–26.
143. Hansen AK. Health status and health monitoring. In: Hau J, Schapiro SJ, editors. Handbook of laboratory animal science. 3rd ed. Boca Raton: CRC Press; 2010. p. 251–306.
144. Graham JE, Schoeb TR. Mycoplasma pulmonis in rats. J Exo Pet Med. 2011;20:270–6. https://doi.org/10.1053/j.jepm.2011.07.004.
145. Detmer A, Hansen AK, Dieperink H, et al. Xylose-positive staphylococci as a cause of respiratory disease in immunosuppressed rats. Scand J Lab Anim Sci. 1991;18:13–8.
146. Tvedten HW, Whitehai CK, Langham RF. Influence of vitamins-A and E on gnotobiotic and conventionally maintained rats exposed to mycoplasma-pulmonis. J Am Vet Med Assoc. 1973;163:605–12.
147. Oldstone MB. Anatomy of viral persistence. PLoS Pathog. 2009;5:e1000523. 2009/08/04. https://doi.org/10.1371/journal.ppat.1000523.
148. Toolan HW. Lack of Oncogenic Effect of the H-Viruses for Hamsters. Nature. 1967;214:1036. https://doi.org/10.1038/2141036a0.
149. Toolan HW, Rhode SL, Gierthy JF. Inhibition of 7,12-Dimethylbenz(a)anthracene-induced tumors in Syrian hamsters by prior infection with H-1 parvovirus. Cancer Res. 1982;42:2552–5.
150. Nicklas W, Kraft V, Meyer B. Contamination of transplantable tumors, cell lines, and monoclonal antibodies with rodent viruses. Lab Anim Sci. 1993;43:296–300.
151. Tao L, Reese TA. Making mouse models that reflect human immune Responses. Trends Immunol. 2017;38:181–93. 2017/02/06. https://doi.org/10.1016/j.it.2016.12.007.
152. von Herrath M, Nepom GT. Animal models of human type 1 diabetes. Nat Immunol. 2009;10:129–32.
153. Bian X, Wallstrom G, Davis A, et al. Immunoproteomic profiling of antiviral antibodies in new-onset type 1 diabetes using protein arrays. Diabetes. 2016;65:285–96. 2015/10/10. https://doi.org/10.2337/db15-0179.

154. Capua I, Mercalli A, Romero-Tejeda A, et al. Study of 2009 H1N1 pandemic influenza virus as a possible causative agent of diabetes. J Clin Endocrinol Metab. 2018;103:4343–56. 2018/09/12. https://doi.org/10.1210/jc.2018-00862.
155. Fujiya A, Ochiai H, Mizukoshi T, et al. Fulminant type 1 diabetes mellitus associated with a reactivation of Epstein-Barr virus that developed in the course of chemotherapy of multiple myeloma. J Diab Invest. 2010;1:286–9. 2010/12/03. https://doi.org/10.1111/j.2040-1124.2010.00061.x.
156. Gale EA. Congenital rubella: citation virus or viral cause of type 1 diabetes? Diabetologia. 2008;51:1559–66. 2008/07/22. https://doi.org/10.1007/s00125-008-1099-4.
157. Hiltunen M, Hyoty H, Karjalainen J, et al. Serological evaluation of the role of cytomegalovirus in the pathogenesis of IDDM: a prospective study. The Childhood Diabetes in Finland Study Group. Diabetologia. 1995;38:705–10. 1995/06/01
158. Honeyman MC, Coulson BS, Stone NL, et al. Association between rotavirus infection and pancreatic islet autoimmunity in children at risk of developing type 1 diabetes. Diabetes. 2000;49:1319–24. 2000/08/03. https://doi.org/10.2337/diabetes.49.8.1319.
159. Krogvold L, Edwin B, Buanes T, et al. Detection of a low-grade enteroviral infection in the islets of langerhans of living patients newly diagnosed with type 1 diabetes. Diabetes. 2015;64:1682–7. 2014/11/26. https://doi.org/10.2337/db14-1370.
160. Laitinen OH, Honkanen H, Pakkanen O, et al. Coxsackievirus B1 is associated with induction of beta-cell autoimmunity that portends type 1 diabetes. Diabetes. 2014;63:446–55. 2013/08/27. https://doi.org/10.2337/db13-0619.
161. Lindberg B, Ahlfors K, Carlsson A, et al. Previous exposure to measles, mumps, and rubella–but not vaccination during adolescence–correlates to the prevalence of pancreatic and thyroid autoantibodies. Pediatrics. 1999;104:e12. 1999/07/02. https://doi.org/10.1542/peds.104.1.e12.
162. Oikarinen S, Tauriainen S, Hober D, et al. Virus antibody survey in different European populations indicates risk association between coxsackievirus B1 and type 1 diabetes. Diabetes. 2014;63:655–62. 2013/09/07. https://doi.org/10.2337/db13-0620.
163. Pak CY, Eun HM, McArthur RG, et al. Association of cytomegalovirus infection with autoimmune type 1 diabetes. Lancet. 1988;2:1–4. 1988/07/02. https://doi.org/10.1016/s0140-6736(88)92941-8.
164. Sano H, Terasaki J, Tsutsumi C, et al. A case of fulminant type 1 diabetes mellitus after influenza B infection. Diabetes Res Clin Pract. 2008;79:e8-9. 2008/01/08. https://doi.org/10.1016/j.diabres.2007.10.030.
165. Aarnisalo J, Veijola R, Vainionpaa R, et al. Cytomegalovirus infection in early infancy: risk of induction and progression of autoimmunity associated with type 1 diabetes. Diabetologia. 2008;51:769–72. 2008/02/19. https://doi.org/10.1007/s00125-008-0945-8.
166. Williamson JSP, Stohlman SA. Effective clearance of mouse hepatitis-virus from the central-nervous-system requires both CD4+ and CD8+ T-cells. J Virol. 1990;64:4589–92. Note
167. MacDuff DA, Reese TA, Kimmey JM, et al. Phenotypic complementation of genetic immunodeficiency by chronic herpesvirus infection. eLife. 2015;4. https://doi.org/10.7554/eLife.04494.
168. Hansen CHF, Nielsen DS, Kverka M, et al. Patterns of early gut colonization shape future immune responses of the host. Plos One. 2012;7:e34043. https://doi.org/10.1371/journal.pone.0034043. [doi];PONE-D-11-21227 [pii]
169. Weng M, Walker WA. The role of gut microbiota in programming the immune phenotype. J Dev Orig Health Dis. 2013;4:203–14. https://doi.org/10.1017/s2040174412000712.
170. Turnbaugh PJ, Hamady M, Yatsunenko T, et al. A core gut microbiome in obese and lean twins. Nature. 2009;457:480-484U487. https://doi.org/10.1038/nature07540.
171. Unger WWJ, Hauet-Broere F, Jansen W, et al. Early events in peripheral regulatory T cell induction via the nasal mucosa. J Immunol. 2003;171:4592–603. Article
172. Schloss PD, Schubert AM, Zackular JP, et al. Stabilization of the murine gut microbiome following weaning. Gut Microbes. 2012;3:383–93. https://doi.org/10.4161/gmic.21008.
173. Hansen CH, Andersen LS, Krych L, et al. Mode of delivery shapes gut colonization pattern and modulates regulatory immunity in mice. J Immunol. 2014;193:1213–22. 2014/06/22. https://doi.org/10.4049/jimmunol.1400085.
174. Org E, Parks BW, Joo JWJ, et al. Genetic and environmental control of host-gut microbiota interactions. Genome Res. 2015;25:1558–69. Article. https://doi.org/10.1101/gr.194118.115.
175. Shade A, Handelsman J. Beyond the Venn diagram: the hunt for a core microbiome. Environ Microbiol. 2012;14:4–12. https://doi.org/10.1111/j.1462-2920.2011.02585.x.
176. Hansen CH, Krych L, Buschard K, et al. A maternal gluten-free diet reduces inflammation and diabetes incidence in the offspring of NOD mice. Diabetes. 2014;63:2821–32. 2014/04/04. https://doi.org/10.2337/db13-1612.
177. Ridaura VK, Faith JJ, Rey FE, et al. Gut microbiota from twins discordant for obesity modulate metabolism in mice. Science. 2013;341:1241214. Research Support, N.I.H., Extramural; Research Support, Non-U.S. Gov't; Twin Study. https://doi.org/10.1126/science.1241214.
178. Lees H, Swann J, Poucher SM, et al. Age and microenvironment outweigh genetic influence on the

Zucker Rat microbiome. Plos One. 2014;9. Article. https://doi.org/10.1371/journal.pone.0100916.
179. Thoene-Reineke C, Fischer A, Friese C, et al. Composition of intestinal microbiota in immune-deficient mice kept in three different housing conditions. PLoS One. 2014;9:e113406. https://doi.org/10.1371/journal.pone.0113406.
180. Turnbaugh P, Ridaura V, Faith J, et al. The effect of diet on the human gut microbiome: a metagenomic analysis in humanized gnotobiotic mice. Sci Transl Med. 2009;1:6ra14.
181. Cani PD, Delzenne NM. Gut microflora as a target for energy and metabolic homeostasis. Curr Opin Clin Nutr Metab Care. 2007;10:729–34. 2007/12/20. https://doi.org/10.1097/MCO.0b013e3282efdebb.
182. Cani PD, Amar J, Iglesias MA, et al. Metabolic endotoxemia initiates obesity and insulin resistance. Diabetes. 2007;56:1761–72. Article. https://doi.org/10.2337/db06-1491.
183. Tranberg B, Madsen AN, Hansen AK, et al. Whey-reduced weight gain is associated with a temporary growth reduction in young mice fed a high-fat diet. J Nutr Biochem. 2015;26:9–15.
184. Tranberg B, Hellgren LI, Lykkesfeldt J, et al. Whey protein reduces early life weight gain in mice fed a high-fat diet. PLoS One. 2013;8:e71439. https://doi.org/10.1371/journal.pone.0071439.
185. Rune I, Rolin B, Lykkesfeldt J, et al. Long-term Western diet fed apolipoprotein E-deficient rats exhibit only modest early atherosclerotic characteristics. Sci Rep. 2018;8:5416. 2018/04/05. https://doi.org/10.1038/s41598-018-23835-z.
186. Rune I, Rolin B, Larsen C, et al. Modulating the gut microbiota improves glucose tolerance, lipoprotein profile and atherosclerotic plaque development in ApoE-deficient mice. PLoS One. 2016;11:e0146439. 2016/01/23. https://doi.org/10.1371/journal.pone.0146439.
187. Wu GD, Chen J, Hoffmann C, et al. Linking long-term dietary patterns with gut microbial enterotypes. Science. 2011;334:105–8. 2011/09/03. https://doi.org/10.1126/science.1208344.
188. Macia L, Tan J, Vieira AT, et al. Metabolite-sensing receptors GPR43 and GPR109A facilitate dietary fibre-induced gut homeostasis through regulation of the inflammasome. Nat Commun. 2015;6. https://doi.org/10.1038/ncomms7734.
189. Nielsen DS, Krych L, Buschard K, et al. Beyond genetics. Influence of dietary factors and gut microbiota on type 1 diabetes. FEBS Lett. 2014;588:4234–43. 2014/04/22. https://doi.org/10.1016/j.febslet.2014.04.010.
190. Hrncir T, Stepankova R, Kozakova H, et al. Gut microbiota and lipopolysaccharide content of the diet influence development of regulatory T cells: studies in germ-free mice. BMC Immunol. 2008;9. Article https://doi.org/10.1186/1471-2172-9-65.
191. Cani PD, Bibiloni R, Knauf C, et al. Changes in gut microbiota control metabolic endotoxemia-induced inflammation in high-fat diet-induced obesity and diabetes in mice. Diabetes. 2008;57:1470–81.
192. Li W, Dowd SE, Scurlock B, et al. Memory and learning behavior in mice is temporally associated with diet-induced alterations in gut bacteria. Physiol Behav. 2009;96:557–67. https://doi.org/10.1016/j.physbeh.2008.12.004.
193. Jorgensen BP, Hansen JT, Krych L, et al. A possible link between food and mood: dietary impact on gut microbiota and behavior in BALB/c mice. PLoS One. 2014;9:ARTN e103398. https://doi.org/10.1371/journal.pone.0103398.
194. Lindenberg FCB, Ellekilde M, Thorn AC, et al. Dietary LPS traces influences disease expression of the diet-induced obese mouse. Res Vet Sci. 2019;123:195–203. 2019/01/27. https://doi.org/10.1016/j.rvsc.2019.01.005.
195. Kihl P, Krych L, Deng L, et al. Oral LPS dosing induces local immunological changes in the pancreatic lymph nodes in mice. 2019.
196. Lindenberg FCB, Ellekilde M, Thörn AC, et al. Dietary LPS traces influence disease expression of the diet-induced obese mouse. Res Vet Sci. 2019;123:195–203.
197. Perin D, Murano E. Starch polysaccharides in the human diet: effect of the different source and processing on its absorption. Nat Prod Commun. 2017;12:837–53.
198. Cani PD, Possemiers S, Van de Wiele T, et al. Changes in gut microbiota control inflammation in obese mice through a mechanism involving GLP-2-driven improvement of gut permeability. Gut. 2009;58:1091–103.
199. Izydorczyk MS, Dexter JE. Barley β-glucans and arabinoxylans: molecular structure, physicochemical properties, and uses in food products–a review. Food Res Int. 2008;41:850–68. https://doi.org/10.1016/j.foodres.2008.04.001.
200. Durr C, Brunel-Muguet S, Girousse C, et al. Changes in seed composition and germination of wheat (Triticum aestivum) and pea (Pisum sativum) when exposed to high temperatures during grain filling and maturation. Crop Pasture Sci. 2018;69:374–86. https://doi.org/10.1071/cp17397.
201. Johansson DP, Gutierrez JLV, Landberg R, et al. Impact of food processing on rye product properties and their in vitro digestion. Eur J Nutr. 2018;57:1651–66. https://doi.org/10.1007/s00394-017-1450-y.
202. Katyal M, Singh N, Chopra N, et al. Hard, medium-hard and extraordinarily soft wheat varieties: comparison and relationship between various starch properties. Int J Biol Macromol. 2019;123:1143–9. https://doi.org/10.1016/j.ijbiomac.2018.11.192.
203. Sofi MH, Gudi R, Karumuthil-Melethil S, et al. pH of drinking water influences the composition of gut microbiome and Type 1 diabetes incidence. Diabetes. 2014;63:632–44. Article. https://doi.org/10.2337/db13-0981.

204. Ivanov II, Frutos RD, Manel N, et al. Specific microbiota direct the differentiation of IL-17-producing T-Helper cells in the mucosa of the small intestine. Cell Host Microbe. 2008;4:337–49. https://doi.org/10.1016/j.chom.2008.09.009.
205. Hansen CHF, Krych L, Nielsen DS, et al. Early life treatment with vancomycin propagates Akkermansia muciniphila and reduces diabetes incidence in non-obese diabetic (NOD) mice. Diabetologia. 2012;55:2285–94.
206. O'Callaghan A, van Sinderen D. Bifidobacteria and their role as members of the human gut microbiota. Front Microbiol. 2016;7. https://doi.org/10.3389/fmicb.2016.00925.
207. Fernandez J, Redondo-Blanco S, Gutierrez-del-Rio I, et al. Colon microbiota fermentation of dietary prebiotics towards short-chain fatty acids and their roles as anti-inflammatory and antitumour agents: a review. J Funct Foods. 2016;25:511–22. https://doi.org/10.1016/j.jff.2016.06.032.
208. Jain I, Kumar V, Satyanarayana T. Xylooligosaccharides: an economical prebiotic from agroresidues and their health benefits. Indian J Exp Biol. 2015;53:131–42.
209. Hart ML, Ericsson AC, Franklin CL. Differing complex microbiota alter disease severity of the IL-10(-/-) mouse model of inflammatory bowel disease. Front Microbiol. 2017;8:15. Article. https://doi.org/10.3389/fmicb.2077.00792.
210. Respondek F, Gerard P, Bossis M, et al. Short-chain fructo-oligosaccharides modulate intestinal microbiota and metabolic parameters of humanized gnotobiotic diet induced obesity mice. PLoS One. 2013;8. https://doi.org/10.1371/journal.pone.0071026.
211. Goodman A, Kallstrom G, Faith J, et al. Extensive personal human gut microbiota culture collections characterized and manipulated in gnotobiotic mice. Proc Natl Acad Sci USA. 2011;108:6252–7.
212. Chung H, Pamp SJ, Hill JA, et al. Gut immune maturation depends on colonization with a host-specific microbiota. Cell. 2012;149:1578–93.
213. Le Roy T, Debédat J, Marquet F, et al. Comparative evaluation of microbiota engraftment following fecal microbiota transfer in mice models: age, kinetic and microbial status matter. Front Microbiol. 2019;9. https://doi.org/10.3389/fmicb.2018.03289.
214. Ellekilde M, Selfjord E, Larsen CS, et al. Transfer of gut microbiota from lean and obese mice to antibiotic-treated mice. Sci Rep. 2014;4:5922. https://doi.org/10.1038/srep05922.
215. Hansen AK, Krych L, Nielsen DS, et al. A review of applied aspects of dealing with gut microbiota impact on rodent models. ILAR J. 2015;56:250–64. https://doi.org/10.1093/ilar/ilv010.
216. Lundberg R, Toft MF, August B, et al. Antibiotic-treated versus germ-free rodents for microbiota transplantation studies. Gut Microbes. 2016;7:68–74.
217. Lützhøft DV, Sánchez-Alcoholado L, Tougaard P, et al. Gut microbial colonization of C57BL/6NTac mouse colon using faecal transfer was equally effective when comparing rectal inoculation and oral inoculation based on 16S rRNA sequencing. Res Vet Sci. 2019;126:227–32.
218. McCafferty J, Muhlbauer M, Gharaibeh RZ, et al. Stochastic changes over time and not founder effects drive cage effects in microbial community assembly in a mouse model. ISME J. 2013;7:2116–25. Article. https://doi.org/10.1038/ismej.2013.106.
219. Lundberg R, Bahl MI, Licht TR, et al. Microbiota composition of simultaneously colonized mice housed under either a gnotobiotic isolator or individually ventilated cage regime. Sci Rep. 2017;7:42245. Article
220. Caruso R, Ono M, Bunker ME, et al. Dynamic and asymmetric changes of the microbial communities after cohousing in laboratory mice. Cell Rep. 2019;27:3401. Article. https://doi.org/10.1016/j.celrep.2019.05.042.
221. Hansen AK, Hansen CH, Krych L, et al. Impact of the gut microbiota on rodent models of human disease. World J Gastroenterol. 2014;20:17727–36. 2014/12/31. https://doi.org/10.3748/wjg.v20.i47.17727.
222. Jentsch JD, Roth RH. The neuropsychopharmacology of phencyclidine: from NMDA receptor hypofunction to the dopamine hypothesis of schizophrenia. Neuropsychopharmacology. 1999;20:201–25. https://doi.org/10.1016/S0893-133X(98)00060-8.
223. Kesner RP, Dakis M. Phencyclidine disrupts acquisition and retention performance within a spatial continuous recognition memory task. Pharmacol Biochem Behav. 1993;44:419–24. Article. https://doi.org/10.1016/0091-3057(93)90484-b.
224. Sinha YN, Thomas JW, Salocks CB, et al. Prolactin and growth-hormone secretion in diet-induced obesity in mice. Horm Metab Res. 1977;9:277–82. Article. https://doi.org/10.1055/s-0028-1093552.
225. Heydemann A. An overview of murine high fat diet as a model for type 2 diabetes mellitus. J Diabetes Res. 2016;14. Review. https://doi.org/10.1155/2016/2902351.
226. Rune I, Hansen CH, Ellekilde M, et al. Ampicillin-improved glucose tolerance in diet-induced obese C57BL/6NTac mice is age dependent. J Diabetes Res. 2013;2013:319321. https://doi.org/10.1155/2013/319321.
227. Castro-Mejia JL, Jakesevic M, Fabricius NF, et al. Gut microbiota recovery and immune response in ampicillin-treated mice. Res Vet Sci. 2018;118:357–64. 2018/04/14. https://doi.org/10.1016/j.rvsc.2018.03.013.
228. Hansen AK, Malm SA, Metzdorff SB. The cre-inducer doxycycline lowers cytokine and chemokine transcript levels in the gut of mice. J Appl Genet. 2017:1–4.
229. European_Union. Directive 2010/63/EU of The European Parliament and The Council of 22 September 2010 on the Protection of Animals used for Scientific Purposes. 2010.

Effects of Untreated Pain, Anesthesia, and Analgesia in Animal Experimentation

Paulin Jirkof and Heidrun Potschka

1 Introduction

A potential cause of suffering in animal experimentation is pain induced by procedures, diseases, and injuries. Pain is not only nociception, the sensory nervous system's response to (potentially) harmful stimuli, but has been defined as a "subjective, sensory and emotional experience" [1, 2] in humans. It is very likely that pain, as an affective experience, also exists in other vertebrate animals than humans. Therefore, anesthesia and pain treatment become ethical and, in most countries, legal obligations in any animal experiment or related procedures, e.g., breeding or marking procedures, that induce more than mild pain of short duration. Article 14 of the EU Directive 2010/63/EU on the protection of animals used for scientific purposes, for example, states that "member states shall ensure that, unless it is inappropriate, procedures are carried out under general or local anesthesia, and that analgesia or another appropriate method is used to ensure that pain, suffering and distress are kept to a minimum."

Next to these ethical and legal obligations, scientific considerations regarding the implementation of adequate analgesia and anesthesia procedures are important. Anesthesia and analgesia have scientific and methodological implications for the design of experiments and the quality of the resulting data. On the one hand, untreated pain is affecting a magnitude of systems and mechanisms in the body, and on the other hand, anesthesia and analgesia can have significant effects on experimental readout parameters. The use or omission of certain anesthesia and analgesia protocols has therefore the potential to affect scientific results and increase the variability of data. Thus, also the proper reporting of these procedures in scientific publications is of high importance to enable the interpretation of published data. A recent review on reporting practices for anesthesia and analgesia protocols after invasive animal procedures revealed that unfortunately many published studies currently do not report, or do not completely report, the anesthetic and analgetic measures involved [3].

Pain management includes the choice of anesthesia and analgesia agents, their dose, administration method, duration and frequency of treat-

P. Jirkof (✉)
Department Animal Welfare and 3Rs,
University of Zurich, Zurich, Switzerland
e-mail: paulin.jirkof@uzh.ch

H. Potschka
Institute of Pharmacology, Toxicology, and Pharmacy,
Ludwig-Maximilians-University Munich, Munich,
Germany
e-mail: potschka@pharmtox.vetmed.uni-muenchen.de

© Springer Nature Switzerland AG 2021

J. M. Sánchez Morgado, A. Brønstad (eds.), *Experimental Design and Reproducibility in Preclinical Animal Studies*, Laboratory Animal Science and Medicine 1,
https://doi.org/10.1007/978-3-030-66147-2_5

ment, and a pain-monitoring scheme for each individual animal. Untreated pain or inadequately chosen or insufficiently reported anesthesia or analgesia protocols may carry the potential to hamper the reproducibility of animal experiments substantially. Respective protocols are therefore an important part of experimental design, and determining an optimal protocol is mandatory when planning animal experiments. In this chapter, we will highlight some important considerations regarding pain management in animal research.

2 Effects of Untreated Pain

The nociceptive system comprises structures of the peripheral and central nervous system involved in the processing of information generated by activation of nociceptors or by direct damage to the nervous system (Fig. 1).

Noxious stimuli that cause tissue damage can result in an increase of mediators that trigger activation of peripheral nociceptors. The two main types of nociceptors are characterized by either thin myelinated Aδ fibers with fast conduction or unmyelinated C fibers with slow conduction. The fibers are responsible for two different components of pain with Aδ fibers mediating sharp momentary pain and C fibers mediating diffuse and dull pain. The information is then processed via the spinal cord dorsal horn reaching ascending pathways, which project from the spinal cord to the brain. Among others, these pathways comprise the spinothalamic and spinoreticulothalamic tract, which render the thalamic nuclei a key structure in the processing of nociceptive signals. Further projections are directly reaching the amygdala. Nociception is defined as the process of information generation and transmission from the periphery via the spinal cord to subcortical structures including the thalamus.

It is important to note that an activation of the nociceptive system can occur without a perception of pain and that it can trigger responses of the endocrine and vegetative nervous system with all its functional consequences without the perception of pain. Moreover, reflex responses to a noxious stimulus do not necessarily require pain perception, and can occur as a consequence of activation of the peripheral nociceptive system.

The perception of pain requires the processing in higher brain centers including the cerebral cortex resulting in the aversive and unpleasant state of pain. In humans pain has been defined by the International Association for the Study of Pain as "an unpleasant sensory and emotional experience associated with actual or potential tissue damage or described in terms of such damage" [1]. Considering the challenges to assess the emotional or affective state of animals, an adjusted definition

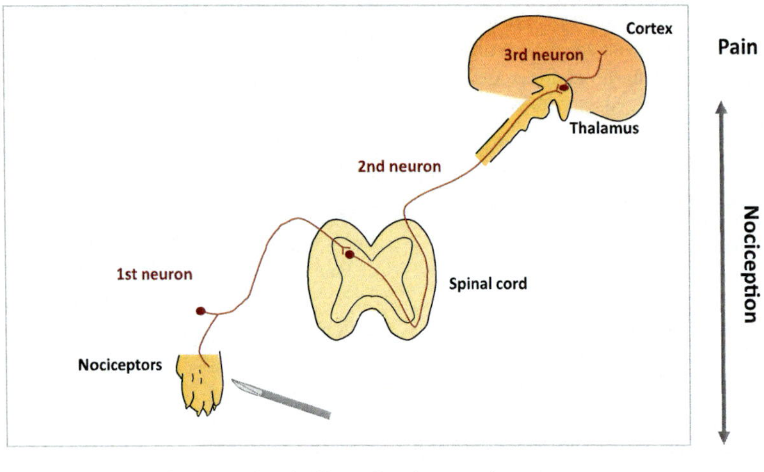

Fig. 1 Nociceptive system and structures involved in nociception vs. pain

has been suggested to describe pain in animals: "Animal pain is an aversive, sensory experience representing awareness by the animal of damage or threat to the integrity of its tissues; (note that there might not be any damage). It changes the animal's physiology and behavior to reduce or avoid the damage, to reduce the likelihood of its recurrence and to promote recovery. Non-functional (non-useful) pain occurs when the intensity or duration of the experience is not appropriate for damage sustained (especially if none exists) and when physiological and behavioral responses are unsuccessful in alleviating it" [4].

Activation of the nociceptive system can trigger processes of peripheral and central sensitization at different levels involving nociceptor activation, transduction in the spinal cord, and changes in the responsiveness of neurons involved in the transmission and processing of nociceptive signals. Sensitization can result in primary and secondary hyperalgesia with an increased sensitivity to noxious stimuli at the site of the injury or in surrounding tissue, in allodynia with an increased sensitivity to non-noxious stimuli, and in chronic and persistent pain states. Thus, every attempt to achieve a prevention or limitation of peripheral and central sensitization processed during an intervention with activation of the nociceptive system is of utmost relevance to limit possible long-term consequences of the procedure.

Pain that is not treated or not sufficiently treated can have many effects. As mentioned above, in the context of painful procedures, it needs to be considered that the mere activation of the nociceptive system can directly cause autonomic nervous system responses. As nerves of the autonomous nervous system innervate almost every organ system, the effects are manifold. Ascending painful impulses lead to hypothalamic activation and increased sympathetic-adrenergic system activity which affect the body's unconscious actions. This activation results, for example, in substantial respiratory and cardiovascular effects, such as changes in blood pressure, heart rate, and heart rate variability. In many species, including laboratory mice [5], the elevation of heart rate and typical changes in heart rate variability can therefore be observed in painful conditions. The same is true for respiratory rate and body temperature, which, like heart rate and heart rate variability, may provide an estimation of the sympathetic and parasympathetic components of autonomic system activity [6, 7].

The activation of the nociceptive system is also accompanied by responses of the hypothalamic pituitary-adrenal axis, which constitutes a major neuroendocrine system. The target organs of these system release catecholamines like adrenaline and noradrenaline or corticosteroids.

Pain, similar to distress, affects the secretion of many hormones, neurotransmitters, and enzymes. For example, untreated pain increases the secretion of catecholamines such as noradrenaline, corticoids, glucagon, adrenocorticotropic hormone (ACTH), and antidiuretic hormone (ADH) and decreases the secretion of thyroxine, insulin, and testosterone in many species [8–10]. Levels of these hormones or their metabolites in blood, serum, urine, feces, milk, or hair can be used to measure the impact of pain in many species.

There is a tight relationship between the immune and the nervous system (for a more detailed discussion, see, e.g., DeMarco (2019)). Untreated pain can affect the immune system, for example, by leading to a reduction of natural killer cells, mixed lymphocyte reactivity, and interleukin-2 as well as the increase of interleukin-10 [11, 12].

As cancer formation and progression are closely linked to immune system functions, it is not surprising that pain is known to increase tumor growth and number of metastases in humans and animals [11, 13]. Increased susceptibility to infection and delayed wound healing are other potential consequences of pain that show the close link of both systems [11].

In humans, unrelieved pain may contribute to psychological distress, sleeplessness or sleep disruption, and impaired rehabilitation. Changes in behavior that might be indicative of negative affective states, i.e., pain, are also observed in animals. Typical changes in rodent behavior include reduced food and water intake and therefore a reduction in body weight, changes in activity, reduced or fragmented sleep, a disturbed circadian rhythm, loss of behavioral diversity, and changes in social behaviors like social grooming, or in nest building or burrowing behavior as well as effects on cognitive function and emotionality [10, 14–18]. These behavioral changes are not only of significance for behavioral research but may also be used for the assessment of animal pain.

3 Effects of Analgetic Substances

The choice of an analgesia protocol for a specific research question is challenging and might best be solved with the help of an expert in veterinary analgesia. The optimal analgesia protocol should relieve pain reliably and lack side effects that might hamper science and animal welfare. In case of surgical or painful procedures, preventive analgesia, defined as pre-, intra-, and postoperative analgesia, must be planned to efficiently cover the temporal development of pain and the estimated intensity.

Analgesia should have a controllable effect on the specific system targeted by the experiment or on experimental procedures. In light of the many aspects that have to be considered, there is no one-size-fits-all analgesia.

Analgetic drugs reduce or suppress pain perception based on an interaction at different levels of the nociceptive system [19]. In earlier times, it was often stated that analgetic treatment may compromise the animal's protection of a wound area or injury site. This rarely applies as most of the analgetic drug regimens can limit and reduce the level of pain, but do not completely block protective responses to an activation of the nociceptive system [20]. While analgetic drugs attenuate the level of dull and throbbing pain, the sharp pain resulting from mechanical pressure to an injured site is still experienced. Thus, while analgesia per definition is the absence of pain, this is rarely achieved, so that animals still protect the surgical area or injury site. Respective caution seems to be only necessary with long-lasting local anesthesia as this can result in a complete control of pain depending on administration site and dose [20].

In view of various mechanisms contributing to peripheral and central sensitization [20–22], any effort should be made to avoid gaps in pain management as these may result in pain states that are more difficult to control. Along this line, preventive concepts should be applied, which are initiated before a painful intervention and are extended into the post-surgical phase. Pre-emptive concepts did not always prove to be very successful in human medicine, a fact that was likely related to gaps in post-surgical pain management [23]. Based on this experience and our current understanding of the mechanisms of sensitization and hyperalgesia development, continuous exposure to therapeutic levels of efficacious analgetic drugs should be guaranteed from the start of a surgical procedure and during the post-surgical phase as long as relevant pain levels are expected following an intervention. It has been reported that the intensity of early post-surgical pain correlates with the risk of chronic persistent post-surgical pain [24].

As further discussed below, efficacious preventive concepts should be based on multimodal regimens with a combination of analgetics that limits the development of hypersensitivity [25, 26].

In order to provide an efficacious pain management, the expected level and type of pain need to be considered to avoid therapeutic failure. Visceral, somatic, and nociceptive pain are characterized by profound differences in the response to specific analgetic drugs [27]. Neuropathic pain resulting from direct injury or damage of the nervous system is in general difficult to control by traditional analgetic drugs [28]. Visceral pain results from activation of nociceptors of internal organs in the thorax, abdomen, or pelvis [29]. In contrast, somatic pain is mediated by activation of nociceptors in the skin, muscles, joints, bones, and connective tissue [27].

In addition, the choice of an analgetic regimen also needs to consider tolerance development, which in case of opioids can occur following prolonged administration but also rapidly even during a short-term drug exposure [30]. The possibility of rapid internalization, which, for instance, has been reported in response to the fentanyl derivative remifentanil [31], needs to be taken into account for a smooth transition of intra-surgical to post-surgical analgesia.

In the following, we report and discuss the main desired and adverse effects of analgetic drugs, which may exert an impact on possible readout parameters in experimental studies. Please note that we can only provide a rough overview with selected specific examples in this book chapter and that during study planning it will be of utmost relevance to carefully check the literature for a description of effects that may be relevant for the specific parameters studied.

In this context, we would also like to refer the reader to more specific reviews focusing on the selection of analgetics and/or anesthetics in specific research areas (e.g., [32, 33]).

3.1 Opioids

Opioid analgetics are opioid receptor agonists that exert their pharmacological effects by binding and activating specific opioid receptors that are widely distributed, mainly in the central but also in the peripheral nervous system and gastrointestinal tract. While some of these synthetic or naturally occurring substances bind to opioid receptors but have little agonist activity like the opioid antagonist naloxone, others are potent analgetics. The pain-relieving effect of opioid analgetics is induced by two mechanisms: inhibitory effects on pain transmission and emotional detachment from pain [34–36].

Given the abundant distribution and distinct receptor characteristics, side effects of opioids are diverse and include constipation, respiratory depression, nausea and urinary retention, as well as sedation, addiction, tolerance, and hyperalgesia [36].

Tolerance is characterized by an acute or progressive lack of response to the drug that can be overcome by increasing the dose [37, 38]. Hyperalgesia is a central sensitization process by which opioids sometimes increase rather than decrease pain [37, 38]. In rodent studies, opioid-induced pain hypersensitivity has been observed after repeated or acute administration and after high as well as low doses of opioids such as morphine, buprenorphine, tramadol, or fentanyl [37, 39–41]. Nevertheless, doubts have been raised regarding the actual significance of opioid-induced hyperalgesia in clinical settings using standard doses of opioids.

A topic of much discussion are the immune modulatory effects of some opioids. Immune modulation refers to stimuli that can alter immune function by affecting the generation, function, and maturation of immune cells by several proposed mechanisms, including action on immunocytes as well as the hypothalamic-pituitary-adrenal (HPA) axis, sympathetic activity, or central immune modulation. Natural killer cell activity, cytokine expression, chemotaxis, or phagocytic activity may be affected [42]. These mechanisms have been characterized in both humans and laboratory animals, and there are differences among opioids. Tramadol seems to have a weak upregulation effect, fentanyl and morphine appear to strongly downregulate the immune system, and buprenorphine causes only weak or no immunosuppression [43, 44].

These effects should be taken into consideration when researchers are interested in immune responses as in many oncological models. Opioids may modulate immune system function, apoptosis, tumor cell invasion, and angiogenesis. All of these play an important role in cancer formation and progression [13]. The effect of opioids on cancer development that was shown in human and animal studies has to be taken into account when planning pain treatment for these models. In mice, for example, tramadol seems to inhibit proliferation, migration, and invasion of breast cancer cells [45], whereas fentanyl inhibits tumor growth and cell invasion in colorectal cancer [46]. For morphine, tumor-enhancing effects after administration of daily morphine, as well as tumor and metastasis suppression, have been observed in mice [47, 48].

The immunosuppressive effects of certain opioids, together with their effects on cardiovascular and respiratory function, have to be carefully considered also in animal models of sepsis as at least in human patients there seems to be a link between the use of certain opioids and sepsis mortality [42].

In addition, it has been recognized that opioid receptors modulate inflammation, and reports are suggestive of both anti-inflammatory and pro-inflammatory effects [35].

Endogenously released opioid peptides, as well as exogenously administered opioids, can have cardioprotective effects [49]. For example, in rodent ischemia reperfusion experiments, reduced infarct size was seen after preconditioning with fentanyl [50].

In humans and animals, chronic opioid use alters endocrine function by inhibiting the hypothalamic-pituitary-gonadal axis and possibly the HPA axis [51]. Negative effects of short-term treatment with common opioids, for example, buprenorphine, on reproductive parameters after embryo transfer are not known in mice [52].

Although the effects listed above might be relevant only in experiments involving the affected systems, other side effects of opioids can affect the general condition of an animal, and might therefore be of interest for many research fields. Opioid-induced respiratory depression and other opioid-related respiratory responses are well-known side effects of opioid treatment and are caused by the activation of opioid receptors expressed in the respiratory centers of the brain stem [53]. These effects might lead to complications during anesthesia and the post-anesthetic recovery period and have to be considered when designing analgesia and anesthesia protocols.

Conflicting results exist on whether opioids impair wound healing or not [8]. Chronic morphine administration lengthens time to wound closure in rats and mice by suppressing angiogenesis, whereas improved wound healing has been demonstrated in the rat after topical application of fentanyl, hydromorphone, and morphine [54]. Short-term treatment with buprenorphine or tramadol seems to have no negative effects on bone healing in rodents, while chronic treatment might be detrimental [8, 55].

Reduction of food intake and body weight gain are well-known side effects of opioids such as buprenorphine in mice and rats [56, 57]. These effects might be related to constipation and nausea. Opioid-induced constipation is a common effect of chronic opioid use. The mechanisms involve effects on the enteric nervous system that result in decreased intestinal fluid secretion and increased fluid absorption, as well as decreased motility of the small intestine and colon, leading to increased colonic transit time [58]. Opioids cause nausea and vomiting in humans. The pica behavior, also called allotriophagy or geophagy, is the rodent equivalent to the symptom of vomiting in other species. It involves eating non-nutritious substances, in most cases bedding or nesting material [59, 60]. A single injection of buprenorphine, for example, is sufficient to induce this uncontrolled eating behavior, which can be life-threating. Although pica is regularly reported after buprenorphine administration, especially in rats when higher doses are administered, detailed information on its clinical course is lacking. When pica behavior occurs, a reduction in opioid dose, or replacement with a non-opioid drug, might be necessary.

Opioids may affect animal behavior distinctly. Behavioral side effects of buprenorphine in mice include circling, tiptoe gate, straub tail, and an increase of activity that leads to a flattening of the circadian rhythmicity of the animals [56]. In contrast, in rats, buprenorphine has a sedating effect [61]. Opioids have many effects on sleep characteristics in humans, and effects on EEG recordings are also known for rodents [17]. It is important to take these potential confounding effects of opioids on many routinely used behavioral parameters into consideration when assessing analgetic efficacy and animal welfare.

3.2 Nonsteroidal Anti-Inflammatory Drugs

Nonsteroidal anti-inflammatory drugs (NSAIDs) can exert anti-inflammatory, analgetic, and antipyretic effects [62]. In the context of pain management, NSAIDs are administered to limit inflammation-associated pain in animals [63]. Respective effects can, for instance, be beneficial for perioperative pain management or in a model with induction of orthopedic pain. The main pharmacological effects of most NSAIDs are mediated by a reversible inhibition of cyclooxygenase 1 and 2 resulting in a limited production of different prostanoids including prostaglandin E2, which plays an important role in activation of nociceptors [62]. Thereby, the effects differ between drugs related to a different ratio in affinity to and inhibition of cyclooxygenase-1 and cyclooxygenase-2 [62]. In this context, it is important to note that species differences can exist in the selectivity of a drug to the respective COX isoforms, which can result in relevant differences in the quality of effects [62].

Whereas COX-1 is the primarily constitutive form relevant for several physiological effects of prostanoids, COX-2 is constitutively expressed in some organs including the kidney and brain and is induced by pro-inflammatory cytokines and mediators [64]. The subclass of coxibs has been developed as selective COX-2 inhibitors to more selectively target the inducible isoform [64].

When using NSAIDs in laboratory animals, one has to consider that desired effects as well as adverse effects may interfere with experimental readout parameters and with disease manifestation and course in models of different disorders. Respective effects need to be taken into account for drug selection, study design including the timeline of the experiments, and the interpretation of data. As a matter of course, the anti-inflammatory, analgetic, and antipyretic effects can be relevant depending on the readout parameters of the study [65]. Thereby it is of relevance that different NSAIDs can exert drug-specific effects. It has, for instance, been described that the impact of NSAIDs on neutrophil migration can be mediated by an interference with different signaling pathways [66]. In an experimental study, flunixin proved to exert beneficial effects in dogs with *Escherichia coli*-induced sepsis [67].

In general, disease manifestation or progression in all animal models of disorders with chronic, persistent, and excessive inflammatory processes can be affected and in some cases be ameliorated by the use of NSAIDs. This, for example, applies to models of neurodegenerative diseases, atherosclerosis, arthritis, and chronic inflammatory bowel disease, i.e., diseases for which COX-2 is discussed as a therapeutic target [68].

Related to the fact that the prostanoids exert various physiological effects, the reduction of prostanoid generation can have multiple detrimental consequences [64]. Again, it needs to be emphasized that the risk for these adverse effects and the intensity of the effects largely depend on the specific drug, the species, the dosing, and the duration of treatment [64]. Therefore, it is of utmost relevance to consider recommendations and guidelines including maximum doses, application intervals, and treatment duration.

A widely known adverse effect is the irritation of the gastrointestinal mucosa, which can progress to ulceration and hemorrhage, and can even result in death of the animals [62]. The irritation results from a reduction of the gastroprotective and vasodilatory prostaglandin E2, increased leukotriene production, and cumulation of drugs in mucosal cells [62]. If a long-term administration of NSAIDs is necessary, the co-administration of proton pump inhibitors can reduce the risk for severe gastrointestinal adverse effects. A higher risk for gastrointestinal irritation and ulceration needs to be considered in animal models of gastrointestinal disorders or in animals with exposure to stressors.

Related to the important role of prostaglandins for renal blood flow and kidney function, the pharmacological effects of NSAIDs can cause a retention of sodium, potassium, and water [69]. Development of renal papillary necrosis and interstitial nephritis is a rare consequence of NSAID exposure. However, in case of risk factors such as chronic renal insufficiency, cardiac insufficiency, liver dysfunction, and dehydration, NSAIDs can cause acute renal failure [62]. This fact should be considered for animal models with respective clinical conditions or disorders. Hypertonia can result from this effect on renal excretory function and a reduction in the production of vasodilatory prostaglandins [69].

Selected NSAIDs have a low to medium risk for hepatotoxicity [62]. However, a possible impact on liver-specific enzymes including aspartate and alanine aminotransferase needs to be generally considered.

Prostaglandins play an important role for parturition. Thus, NSAID administration can result in weakening of uterine contractions and can delay parturition [65]. Exposure to acetylsalicylic acid during gestation may imply a risk for hypocalcemia and fetal toxicity [70].

Related to differential effects on thromboxan 2 and prostacyclin 2 synthesis, an inhibition of COX-1 or COX-2 can result in a reduction or an increase in platelet aggregation, respectively, with contrasting consequences for the risk of thrombosis [64, 69]. A relevant negative impact on blood coagulation can in particular occur following exposure to the irreversible COX-1 inhibitor acetylsalicylic acid. Interestingly, this effect proved to depend on the species with sheep exhibiting an increased platelet aggregation in response to acetylsalicylic acid [71].

Finally, in vitro studies revealed a negative impact of some NSAIDs on the metabolism, remodeling, and healing processes of cartilage and bone [62, 72]. A putative delay in healing as a consequence of NSAID exposure should, for instance, be considered for drug selection in respective animal models with cartilage or bone defects [30]. Nevertheless, while long-term administration may delay bone and wound healing, it has been stated that NSAIDs may be used short-term in orthopedic and wound-healing models [8]. However, the study design should consider putative effects, and alternate analgetic drugs may be considered depending on the research hypothesis.

As a consequence of cyclooxygenase inhibition, higher levels of arachidonic acid are processed by the alternate pathway involving lipoxygenase [73]. This results in enhanced generation of leukotrienes, which can trigger bronchoconstriction and asthmatic reactions [73].

Depending on the research hypothesis and the study design, it can be of relevance for use in cancer models that COX-2 is often highly expressed in cancer cells with a contribution to cancer stem cell survival and that its inhibition can limit tumor angiogenesis and can improve therapeutic responses to cytostatic drugs or radiotherapy [74, 75].

In general, NSAIDs are unlikely to exert pronounced direct effects on behavior [76]. However, indirect effects cannot be excluded. This is supported by the fact that repeated flunixin administration without surgical intervention has been reported to lower activity levels in mice [5].

While some studies did not observe drug effects of flunixin on body weight in non-surgical control groups, GV-SOLAS recommendations (GV Solas Expert Information: Pain management for laboratory animals. 2015) describe a body weight loss in response to flunixin exposure in mice, and Tubbs et al. (2011) report a transient increase at the first day after initiation of treatment [77].

3.3 Metamizole/Dipyrone

The use of metamizole (dipyrone) has been recommended for management of mild to moderate pain [78]. Based on a spasmolytic effect, it may also be considered for more severe pain states in cases of visceral pain associated with smooth muscle spasms. The spasmolytic effect is based on an inhibition of kinin-induced spasms [78]. In the context of perioperative pain management, metamizole use can be applied in animals with abdominal surgery.

In general, metamizole is well tolerated with a low adverse effect potential [78]. However, fast intravenous administration can cause a pronounced vasodilatation with hypotension [78]. In a species-specific manner, metamizole can cause hypersalivation in cats [78]. In rare cases, chronic administration of metamizole in human patients has resulted in severe drug reactions with myelotoxic effects and blood dyscrasias (agranulocytosis, leukopenia), porphyria, or toxic epidermal necrolysis [79]. Animals seem to have a by far lower sensitivity to respective adverse effects. In rats an 8-week chronic exposure to metamizole failed to induce agranulocytosis [80].

The use of metamizole needs to consider that active metabolites are formed, which contribute to the consequence of drug administration [81]. For example, 4-methylaminoantipyrine (MAAP) has been reported to exert antiaggregatory effects when tested with human platelets [81].

In cats and neonates, toxicity has been reported due to metamizole formulations containing benzyl alcohol or phenol [78]. This example underlines the importance to carefully check all components of a drug formulation with regard to species-specific tolerability issues.

Cognitive deficits have been described following sub-chronic administration of pregabalin in Wistar rats [91].

In diabetic rat models it has been reported that gabapentin can ameliorate apoptosis and oxidative stress in the retina due to an inhibition of branched chain amino transferase and a limitation of glutamate excitotoxicity [92].

3.4 Gabapentinoids

The gabapentinoids gabapentin and pregabalin bind to $\alpha_2\delta$ subunits of presynaptic calcium channels and modulate release of the excitatory neurotransmitter glutamate [82]. While the compounds have originally been developed as antiepileptic drugs based on an anticonvulsant drug effect, both drugs proved to be efficacious in the treatment of neuropathic pain [83–85]. Effects have also been reported from a series of animal models with post-surgical pain and inflammation-associated pain [82]. More frequent adverse effects of gabapentin and pregabalin in humans include dizziness, ataxia, confusion, disorientation, changes in the emotional state, blurred vision, gastrointestinal effects with nausea, vomiting, diarrhea, or constipation, an increase in appetite associated with weight gain, edemas, leukopenia, rash, myalgia, and arthralgia [86]. Assessment in dogs pointed to only mild adverse effects with sedation and ataxia [87].

The acute anticonvulsant effect of gabapentinoids has been reported in seizure and epilepsy models in rats and mice [88]. However, to our knowledge no long-lasting disease-modifying effects have been described in respective models. Thus, a transient administration is unlikely to exert long-term effects in models of neurological disorders.

While one experimental study argued against a relevant impact of gabapentin or pregabalin on bone mineral density or strength in rats [89], a negative influence on bone formation parameters and an increase in bone resorption parameters were reported following gabapentin treatment in rats in another study [90].

3.5 Ketamine

Ketamine acts as a non-competitive NMDA receptor antagonist [93]. In a dose-dependent manner, the drug induces a dissociative anesthesia with analgesia, sleep, and catalepsy [93]. While ketamine has relevant effects on somatic pain, its effects on visceral pain are limited [93]. For surgical interventions ketamine is frequently combined with alpha$_2$-sympathomimetics [93]. For analgesia following surgery or in other clinical situations, it can be administered as a monotherapy to limit the perception of somatic pain [94, 95].

Catalepsy is characterized by an increased muscle tone, which can limit the animal's ability to show defensive movement. If administered without combination, ketamine can increase blood pressure and can exert effects on heart function [93]. As a consequence of the elevated blood pressure, animals may show an increased tendency to bleed. Activation of neuronal activity in selected brain regions can mediate hallucinogenic effects [96], which have been described as an unpleasant experience by human patients. In this context, it is of interest that prevention seems to be possible by pretreatment with a benzodiazepine. In some species (e.g., dogs) the CNS activation can be very pronounced resulting in the recommendation to use ketamine only in combination with a sedative drug such as an alpha$_2$-sympathomimetic or a benzodiazepine [93].

Considering possible adverse effects, ketamine should be used with caution or should be avoided in animals with tachycardic arrhythmias, coronary heart disorder, and lowered seizure susceptibility (e.g., following a brain insult or following epilepsy manifestation).

Immunomodulatory effects of ketamine with a limitation of increases in plasma TNF-alpha activity have been reported in dogs with experimentally induced endotoxemia [97].

Recently, an immediate antidepressant effect of ketamine has been demonstrated [98]. Thus, a possible impact on an animal's behavioral patterns should be considered for models of psychiatric disorders or neurological disorders with psychiatric comorbidities reflected by alterations in behavior in animals. In mouse models, ketamine proved to prevent stress-induced depression-like behavior [99].

3.6 Multimodal Analgesia

Despite the standard use of multimodal analgesia protocols in human patients, veterinary patients, and larger laboratory species, their use remains uncommon in mice and rats [3, 100, 101]. Multimodal analgesia is a concept that involves different classes of analgetics and/or different sites of drug administration. Administering a combination of two or more drugs with well-established, possibly complementary, pharmacokinetics and mechanism of action has been shown to result in a synergistic or additive effect [102].

Besides drugs with analgetic action, the use of adjuvant analgetics (drugs that are not designed primarily for pain relief) that might potentiate the effects of analgetics including antidepressants, anticonvulsants, local anesthetics, and steroids is possible [103, 104]. Local anesthetics are commonly used adjuvant analgetics in human patients or larger animal species. Combining long-acting local anesthesia in the wound area and non-opioid analgetics is, for example, a basic concept in human short-stay patients, and might reduce the need for systemic pain relief (see also below). For rodents, several effective multimodal analgesia protocols have been described, with examples including tramadol-carprofen [105] or fentanyl-trazodone-paracetamol [106].

The potential advantages of multimodal protocols over monotherapy are the maximization of analgetic effects and the minimization of side effects, as reduced amounts of each drug are needed [107]. Nevertheless, combinations of drugs might also have additive side effects, for example, the combination of acetylsalicylic acid and other NSAIDs escalates the effect on the gastrointestinal mucosa [36]. Thus, the pharmacokinetics, the side effect profile, and the potential interactions with test compounds have to be analyzed carefully for all drugs involved when used in animal experimentation.

3.7 Concept of Pre-emptive or Pre-operative Analgesia

Pre-emptive analgesia is the administration of an analgetic drug before the nociceptive insult to reduce sensitization of the pain pathways. This procedure is widely recommended when pain is expected during and after surgical or other invasive procedures because many anesthesia agents, such as isoflurane, do not induce analgesia. Pre-emptive analgesia has the potential to be more effective than a similar analgetic treatment initiated after surgery and to reduce the required analgesia dose. It can be considered a component of balanced anesthesia and should prevent the wind-up phenomenon and the development of secondary hyperalgesia. For this reason, it has a positive effect on pain perception after regaining consciousness; in addition, postoperative recovery can be improved [108]. It should be used in all chronic experiments (i.e., with re-awakening, recovery) whenever possible.

Nevertheless, common analgetics have side effects that might hamper anesthetic or surgical procedures, such as respiratory depression or increased risk of bleeding. If a partial μ-receptor agonist such as buprenorphine is used in premedication, the effect of a μ-receptor full agonist such as fentanyl is weakened due to the higher receptor affinity of buprenorphine.

4 Effects of Administration Routes

Desired and undesired effects of analgetics and anesthetics can largely depend on the administration mode. Additionally, the choice of administration route and interval can affect the animal's well-being. Oral administration of compounds can be generally carried out by oral gavage or by self-administration via drinking water or food. As an alternative, compounds can be injected intraperitoneally, subcutaneously, intramuscularly, or intravenously. In addition transdermal administration via patches has been described for different species including dogs, cats, and rabbits [109].

The selection of the administration mode needs to weigh the respective advantages and disadvantages. The decision should consider the frequency of handling and restraint necessary for repeated administration on one hand and the uncertainties in sufficient dosing associated with self-administration on the other hand [109]. Repeated injections or oral gavage of drugs require restraint of the animal, which can cause additional stress in small laboratory species [110] and might increase existing pain. This may be a substantial confounder of experimental data and may increase inter- and intra-animal variation [111].

To overcome these problems, and to assure continuous and stress-free administration of analgesia, depot formulations of analgesia for mice and rats have been developed for different drugs [109]. These formulations, due to their long release duration, significantly reduce the necessary frequency of drug administration. Respective formulations can on one hand limit the number of necessary injections and associated distress and can on the other hand result in a slow increase in plasma concentrations avoiding high peak concentrations. Thereby adverse effects can be limited, which occur in a concentration-dependent manner. According to recent reports sustained release formulations can improve the tolerability of buprenorphine in rats [112].

Voluntary oral administration of analgesia is another promising approach that avoids the negative effects of handling. Several routes of oral administration have been described, such as mixing analgetics with flavored gelatin [113], Nutella [114], regular diet [115], or (sweetened) drinking water [116]. These studies in mice and rats have shown that several analgetics are efficient when administered orally and voluntarily. Nevertheless, oral self-administration has been criticized as being less effective than subcutaneous treatment in rats [117]. Reduced bioavailability caused by metabolization of the drug before it reaches systemic circulation is a known obstacle of this administration route [118]. Moreover, latency to ingestion as well as the total amount ingested by the animals, especially during the resting phase, as well as gastrointestinal motility is difficult to anticipate and is clearly variable for each individual. Thus, voluntary ingestion protocols might be applicable only when pain is mild, or in combination with drug injections, at least during the resting phase of rodents [116].

It is important to note that drug resorption from transdermal patches can provide a continuous delivery for days, but can also significantly vary in an inter-individual manner with a pronounced influence of the preparation of the administration site, the skin thickness, and the regional temperature [109]. For instance, exposure to external heating devices as well as a rise in body temperature can accelerate resorption with the risk of intoxication.

As with oral administration, following intraperitoneal administration a first-pass effect needs to be considered for compounds that are metabolized and inactivated in the liver. Drugs that can cause gastrointestinal irritation may exert more pronounced adverse effects due to direct exposure of the mucosa to higher concentrations of the compound. Administration via any injection route also needs to consider the local tolerability as the compound and its formulation may cause skin or tissue irritation, which can even result in local necrosis. In this context, all components of a formulation need to be taken into account. Local anesthetic formulations can, for instance, contain vasoconstrictory compounds such as epinephrine or vasopressin analogues [119]. These vasoconstrictors result in an earlier onset and longer duration of action and limit the risk of resorptive intoxication. On the other hand, they need to be avoided in the area of terminal capillaries at the acra.

Different administration modes and formulations of drugs also result in a different time interval until therapeutic concentrations are reached at the target site. This needs to be considered when deciding about pretreatment times during study design.

5 Effects of Anesthetics, Hypnotic, and Sedative Drugs

5.1 Inhalation Anesthetics

Inhalation anesthetics can cause respiratory depression and can compromise the maintenance of airway patency [120]. Thus, controlled ventilation is of crucial relevance for prolonged exposure to inhalation anesthesia. Regurgitation can result from a reduction in the tone of the lower esophageal sphincter [121]. The respective risk can be limited by endotracheal intubation [121].

The most commonly used inhalation anesthetic isoflurane causes a decreased systemic vascular resistance with hypotension [121]. In a compensatory manner, heart rate can slightly increase [121]. While isoflurane acts as a bronchodilator, it can irritate and stimulate tracheal and bronchial reflexes and can trigger laryngospasm [121]. The vasodilatory effect of isoflurane can result in a slightly increased cerebral blood flow with a minor risk for increased intracranial pressure [121]. Despite this cerebrovascular effect isoflurane is considered a safe drug for surgery in patients with brain insults [121]. Thus, it can also be considered for craniotomy procedures in experimental animals.

Isoflurane exerts minor skeletal and smooth muscle relaxing effects [121]. Due to its effect on uterine muscles, it can interfere with labor during parturition [121]. In the kidney, isoflurane can transiently reduce renal blood flow and glomerular filtration during exposure [121]. In addition, an impact on hepatic blood flow can result in a transient minor impact on liver function assays [121].

Isoflurane can modulate immune system function. In mice, isoflurane limited the response to mechanical ventilation with a limitation of interleukin-1β production in the lung and of circulatory tumor-necrosis factor-alpha concentrations [122].

Isoflurane can exert neuroprotective effects that are of relevance for neuroscientific studies focusing on different disorders [33]. A neuroprotective effect with a limitation of excitotoxicity should, for instance, be considered for stroke and traumatic brain injury models [32].

Repeated isoflurane exposure in rat models of epilepsy development revealed a preventive, antiepileptogenic effect [123]. Depending on the rat model, isoflurane exposure attenuated blood-brain barrier dysfunction, neuronal cell loss, and neuroinflammation [123]. Respective effects need to be taken into account in neuroscientific studies.

Sevoflurane is applied for induction and maintenance anesthesia. It exerts hypotensive effects and can decrease cardiac output [121]. In contrast to other inhalation anesthetics, sevoflurane does not cause tachycardia [121]. Thus, it can be preferable in animals with a respective risk. While sevoflurane is not irritating to airways, exposure results in a reduction of minute ventilation due to a decrease in the respiratory volume [121]. The effects on the cerebral blood flow and on skeletal muscle function are comparable to those of isoflurane [121].

While the majority of effects of inhalation anesthetics is occurring in a transient manner during exposure, a controversial discussion exists about putative nephrotoxic effects of sevoflurane exposure [121]. The impact on renal function in rats, which has been first reported in 1975 by Cook and colleagues [124], seems to be related to generation of compound A, and maybe also additional compounds, by interaction of sevoflurane with a CO_2 absorbent [125, 126]. Recently, it has been described that sevoflurane anesthesia affects the renal metabolic and hemodynamic status to a lesser extent than a combination of midazolam, fluanisone, and fentanyl [127]. However, an increase in blood glucose levels has been reported in this study in rats [127]. In mice, no evidence for renal or hepatic toxicity was observed following single or repeated sevoflurane exposure; however, animals exhibited alterations in blood leukocyte counts, splenic lymphoid composition, and the immune response [128, 129].

Both isoflurane and sevoflurane attenuated the activation of hypoxia-inducible factor and of erythropoietin upregulation in response to hypoxic conditions in mice [130]. In contrast, sevoflurane proved to enhance hypoxia inducible factor 2α expression following ischemia/reperfusion injury of the kidney in mice [131].

Regarding post-surgical pain assessment, it is important to note that anesthetics can exert effects on the mouse pain grimace score. Following a 12-min exposure to isoflurane, mice exhibited increased grimace scores, which reoccurred following repeated exposure to the anesthetic [132]. A comparable effect has been reported following prolonged exposure to isoflurane in rats [132].

5.2 Injection Anesthetics

5.2.1 Propofol

Propofol is a fast- and short-acting injection anesthetic, which is applied intravenously or per infusion [93]. Its effects are predominantly mediated by an interaction with $GABA_A$ receptors [133]. In low doses propofol can exert sedative and anxiolytic effects [121]. The drug can reduce the cerebral metabolic rate of oxygen, cerebral and intraocular pressure. Based on vasodilatation and a mild negative ionotropic effect, propofol can lower blood pressure [121, 133]. Moreover, propofol exerts a respiratory depressant effect [121, 133]. In humans there is a very low risk for a propofol infusion syndrome, which is discussed to be related to an impact on the mitochondrial electron transport chain and can be associated with rhabdomyolysis and multiorgan failure [134]. Comparable reactions seem to be rare in animals. However, a recent case report described a comparable syndrome in a dog exposed to propofol infusion [135].

For experimental neuroscience research a possible neuroprotective effect of propofol with a reduction in excitotoxicity needs to be considered [32]. It has been emphasized that respective effects are of particular relevance for models of stroke and traumatic brain injury [32].

5.2.2 Barbiturates

Whereas classic barbiturates have been largely replaced by modern anesthetics, thiopental is still available as a short-acting injection anesthetic. Thiopental can lower the cerebral metabolic rate of oxygen as well as cerebral and intraocular pressure [93]. Based on peripheral vasoconstriction thiopental can increase blood pressure and the bleeding tendency during a surgical intervention [93]. Related to vagal nerve stimulation barbiturate exposure can cause increased salivation and bronchosecretion, bronchoconstriction, and laryngospasm [136]. Moreover, barbiturates act as respiratory depressants with a decrease in minute ventilation and volume and respiratory rate [93].

5.2.3 Etomidate

Etomidate is an ultrashort-acting injection anesthetic without relevant depressant effects on the respiratory and cardiovascular system [93]. Etomidate can trigger myoclonia and seizures [93], and should therefore be avoided in animals with lowered seizure thresholds (e.g., following a brain insult or following epilepsy manifestation). In addition, etomidate exerts pronounced effects on adrenal gland function with a suppression of hormone synthesis [93]. For etomidate it has been reported that it can reduce tumor blood flow in a similar way as a ketamine/xylazine combination, a fentanyl/fluanisone combination, or urethane [137].

5.2.4 Alphaxalone

Alphaxalone is a short-acting steroid anesthetic [93]. Newer formulations contain the solubilizer cyclodextrin, which seems to be well tolerated [138]. In other formulations with the two steroid compounds alphaxalone and alphadolone, Cremophor EL has been included as a solubilizing agent [93]. The latter acts as a histamine releaser resulting in anaphylactoid reactions including edema and laryngospasm [93]. Its use is contraindicated in dogs, which exhibit a high sensitivity to histamine release. Apart from this, alphaxalone has only minor adverse effects. These include a minor impact on respiration and on cardiovascular function with a slight vasodilatation and negative inotropic effect [93].

In vivo studies indicated that alphaxalone can exert beneficial effects on tumor growth. A delay in the growth of glioma cell grafts has been described in nude mice [139]. Thus, it might be important to control for respective drug effects in tumor studies.

5.2.5 Sedatives and Tranquilizers

In different animal species, $alpha_2$ sympathomimetics (e.g., xylazine, medetomidine, dexmedetomidine) are frequently used for surgical procedures in combination with benzodiazepines or the dissociative anesthetic ketamine [140]. The desired pharmacological effects comprise a sedative/hypnotic effect and an analgetic and muscle relaxant effect [140]. Following a short phase with a transient sympathomimetic effect associated with a short increase in arterial blood pressure, $alpha_2$ sympathomimetics reduce the central sympathetic tone resulting in hypotension, bradycardia, hypothermia, and respiratory depression [140]. An impact on gastrointestinal function can be observed with a decrease in gastroesophageal sphincter pressure and gastric reflux, emesis reported in dogs and cats, and an inhibitory effect on effect with a prolongation of gastrointestinal transit times in different species [140]. The most prominent effect on the endocrine system is a transient hypoinsulinemia resulting in hyperglycemia [140]. As a consequence of an increased myometrial tone, $alpha_2$ sympathomimetics can cause premature labor [136]. Mydriasis and reduced intraocular pressure can occur during exposure to $alpha_2$ sympathomimetics [141]. Moreover, an acute reversible transient lens opacification has been reported as a consequence of xylazine exposure in rats and mice [142].

The compounds differ regarding their selectivity toward $alpha_2$ receptors, and therefore the extent of their adverse effects is different [136].

Dexmedetomidine and ketamine have been reported to influence tumor growth in rodents [13].

Benzodiazepines are administered as anesthetic adjuncts due to their sedative and anesthetic-sparing effect [140]. In addition to their sedative effect, benzodiazepines exert potent anxiolytic, muscle relaxing, anticonvulsant, and appetite stimulating effects [136, 140]. Paradoxical agitation is possible following low doses [136]. Fast intravenous administration can exert relevant effects on the regulation of cardiovascular and respiratory function [136]. Exposure to benzodiazepines causes amnestic effects and reduces cognitive function [136]. Repeated exposure can result in dependence and tolerance [136]. Severe withdrawal symptoms can occur following abrupt termination of exposure [136].

5.2.6 Cooling

Depending on the cause and type of pain and its localization, cooling can be used as an adjunct therapeutic management approach in addition to anesthesia and analgesia [143–145]. However, despite earlier practice in small animals and neonates, it can never replace an anesthetic/analgetic regime for surgical interventions. In this context, it needs to be considered that noxious stimuli remain detectable in cooled tissue and that cooling can also induce hyperalgesia [146].

5.2.7 Local Anesthetics

Local anesthetic drugs can be used to limit or block activation of peripheral nociceptors, signal transduction along peripheral fibers of the nociceptive system, and processing of nociceptive signals at the level of the spinal cord [119]. Respective effects depend on the type of local anesthesia ranging from surface anesthesia, infiltration anesthesia, peripheral nerve block, or conduction anesthesia to epidural anesthesia. Resorption of local anesthetics from the tissue or a too high epidural anesthesia can affect cardiovascular function with hypotonia and bradycardia resulting in the risk of cardiovascular failure and death [119]. Restlessness and agitation represent first signs of an overdose and resorptive intoxication [119]. These CNS effects can progress to tremor and convulsions followed by CNS depression, which can be associated with respiratory depression and failure [119].

Clinical data from humans indicate that local anesthetics can cause antithrombotic effects

[147]. It might be necessary to consider respective effects in models with disturbance of blood coagulation. Bleeding during surgery can be limited by the use of formulations with vasoconstrictory compounds (e.g., epinephrine, norepinephrine, or the vasopressin analogue felypressin) [119]. These additives limit resorption, thereby reducing the risk of systemic effects, accelerating the onset of effects, prolonging the duration of action, and limiting bleeding [119]. Accidental intravenous administration of local anesthetic preparations with a vasoconstrictor results in stimulating effects on the cardiovascular system with hypertonia and tachycardic arrhythmias [119].

Local anesthesia agents block the depolarization in nociceptive neurons. This prevents the release of pro-inflammatory molecules, like prostaglandin and histamine, and therefore may result in an anti-inflammatory effect. Moreover, respective formulations may increase the risk for delayed wound healing and necrosis [119]. However, this mostly applies to areas with limited collateral circulation including the acra, where the administration of formulations with vasoconstrictors should be avoided.

In small rodents, local anesthesia can be used only as an improvement to analgesia, but cannot replace general anesthesia for surgical interventions, as any manipulation can induce stress in the animal.

5.2.8 Repeated Anesthesia

During sequential imaging studies or studies with repeated interventions requiring general anesthesia, animals are often exposed to repeated inhalation anesthesia.

Several studies have described that repeated exposure to isoflurane or sevoflurane can affect neuronal plasticity, cognitive function, and the electrophysiological correlate of learning and memory in rats [148]. Thereby, animals proved to be more susceptible during early development [149, 150]. Long-term effects of repeated inhalation anesthesia on neuronal survival, brain development, and cognitive development have been repeatedly reported following exposure in rat pups or during adolescence [151, 152]. However, in another study, repeated propofol anesthesia triggered neurodegeneration, whereas sevoflurane exposure remained without effects [153]. Interestingly, a study focused on an impact on the hippocampal ultrastructure demonstrated that the extent of the consequences might just be related to the cumulative exposure as a repeated 2-h exposure and a single 6-h exposure had comparable effects [154].

Immediate or delayed DNA damage in leukocytes, liver, kidney, and brain cells has been described, when mice were exposed to sevoflurane anesthesia for 2-h on 3 days [154].

As already mentioned above repetitive exposure to sevoflurane can exert immunomodulatory effects [129].

While the effects of repetitive inhalation anesthesia may be most relevant for the design of research studies related to its frequent use in sequential imaging studies, one group has also addressed the consequences of repeated administration of a ketamine and xylazine combination in mice. The authors observed an increased mouse pain grimace score and effects on trait anxiety-related behavior [155].

6 Impact of the Physical Condition and Disease Model on Pharmacokinetics of Drugs

In animal models, which are associated with a compromised renal or hepatic function, it needs to be considered that the excretion of drugs can be attenuated with a longer duration of action. In respective cases, it might be necessary to adjust the dosing or the administration intervals or to use alternate drugs.

Moreover, any model with a compromised bronchial and lung function due to alterations in bronchosecretion, an emphysema, or edema should be considered as a relative or absolute contraindication for inhalation anesthesia.

7 Implications for Study Design

Pain management includes the choice of anesthesia and analgesia agents, their dose, administration method, duration and frequency of treatment, and a pain-monitoring scheme for each individual animal. It is therefore an important part of experimental design, and determining the appropriate protocol is mandatory when planning animal experiments.

A possible impact on readout parameters of a scientific study should not only be considered for the choice of the anesthetic and analgetic regime but also for the time line of the study. In case of concerns about an influence on parameters of interest in the study, the time plan can be very important. Therefore, instead of avoiding a specific anesthetic or analgetic compound, which may serve as a confounding factor, it may also be possible to adjust and extend the time span between a surgical intervention and the assessment of the study parameters. Thereby, one can avoid an impact of acute effects of anesthetics and analgetics on the data obtained. On the other hand, respective decisions about the time planning need to consider the cumulative burden for the animals, which is relevant when the animal model is associated with continuous distress or pain.

Depending on the research hypothesis and the readout parameters, drug-exposed control groups can be crucial for the interpretation of data. Again, decisions about the necessity for respective control groups require careful considerations focused on the reduction principle of the 3Rs concept.

8 Conclusions

Pain in animal experimentation is a major welfare issue, which must be minimized for ethical and legal reasons (Fig. 2). Additionally, unrelieved pain may have substantial and poorly controllable effects. It may affect complex behavioral traits such as circadian rhythmicity or goal-directed behaviors via motivational changes, may change sensory capacities of animals via allodynia and hyperalgesia, or affect many physiological and endocrine systems via HPA activation. Thus, untreated pain carries the potential to increase the variability of research data significantly, meaning that pain relief has also an important scientific and methodological dimension (Fig. 2).

Analgesia and anesthesia are two of the many experimental interventions applied to laboratory animals, and everyone involved with in vivo experiments should be aware of their potential effects. Nevertheless, if analgesia and anesthesia protocols are chosen with care (Fig. 2), effects are controllable and, to a certain extent, standardizable. If information on effects of new analgesia and anesthesia protocols in specific experiments are missing, the inclusion of an analgesia and/or anesthesia control group might be advisable (Fig. 2). The publications based on such applied approaches can provide valuable insights for the scientific community working with laboratory animals. It should be noted that an important prerequisite for reproducible animal experiments is the proper and complete reporting of every analgetic and anesthetic intervention.

Although standardized anesthesia and analgesia protocols are highly appreciated, both need continuous learning and require assessment and adjustment for individual animals, even for animals undergoing similar procedures. Standard, rule-of-thumb protocols are often not appropriate. In addition to promoting animal welfare, providing laboratory animals with optimal analgesia and anesthesia might also improve the clinical relevance of animal models, as customized anesthesia and analgesia protocols are more reflective of the medical treatment of human patients.

It is important to keep in mind that there might be distinct sex differences in regard to pain perception and the effects of analgesia or anesthesia in many species (see, e.g., [156]) that have not been discussed in this chapter.

Any pain management plan has to be accompanied by a suitable pain assessment and monitoring plan. Score sheets may help to formalize and standardize the assessment and monitoring of pain. Score sheets should deploy meaningful parameters, such as robust and specific signs of pain, and signs that measure the actual, specific effect on the system targeted by the experimental manipulation, as well as more general welfare or health measures. In addition to classical clinical signs, such as physiological symptoms and outer appearance, there are also several ethological indicators of pain that have been introduced for

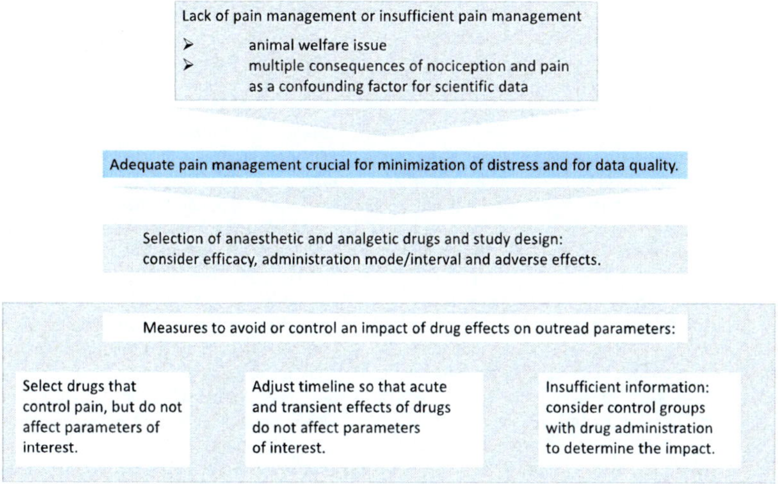

Fig. 2 Overview of the scientific and methodological dimensions of pain management in animal experiments

many laboratory species in the last decades. Indicators should be tested for their sensitivity (the ability to correctly identify animals with pain) and specificity (the ability to identify those without pain) [157]. Pain assessment should be frequent during expected pain peaks, for example, during the first 12-h to first days after surgery or during the late stage of painful progressing diseases. The mode of detection of residual pain and the maximum scores that will trigger any following action should be established in advance and be followed up by adequate remedial measures (such as providing additional rescue analgesia or termination of the experiment).

In summary, reproducibility and transparency are basic principles of science and prerequisites for the scientific and ethical justification of animal experimentation. Adequate anesthesia, pain monitoring, and pain treatment regimens have to be reported in publications and may contribute to better transparency and reproducibility. Thus, they may be able to increase scientific quality and reduce unnecessary suffering and animal numbers.

Literature

1. IASP. subcommittee on taxonomy. Pain terms. A list with definitions and notes on usage. 1979;6(3):249–52.
2. IASP. Classification of chronic pain. 1994.
3. Carbone L, Austin J. Pain and laboratory animals: publication practices for better data reproducibility and better animal welfare. PLoS One. 2016;11(5):e0155001.
4. Molony V, Kent JE. Assessment of acute pain in farm animals using behavioral and physiological measurements. J Anim Sci. 1997;75(1):266–72.
5. Arras M, Rettich A, Cinelli P, Kasermann HP, Burki K. Assessment of post-laparotomy pain in laboratory mice by telemetric recording of heart rate and heart rate variability. BMC Vet Res. 2007;3(1):16.
6. Conzemius MG, Hill CM, Sammarco JL, Perkowski SZ. Correlation between subjective and objective measures used to determine severity of postoperative pain in dogs. J Am Vet Med Assoc. 1997;210(11):1619–22.
7. Gehrmann J, Hammer PE, Maguire CT, Wakimoto H, Triedman JK, Berul CI. Phenotypic screening for heart rate variability in the mouse. Am J Physiol Heart C. 2000;279(2):H733–H40.
8. Huss MK, Felt SA, Pacharinsak C. Influence of pain and analgesia on orthopedic and wound-healing models in rats and mice. Comp Med. 2019;69(6):535–45.
9. Henke J, Erhardt W. Schmerzmanagement beim Klein- und Heimtier: ENKE. Stuttgart; 2001.
10. Carstens E, Moberg GP. Recognizing pain and distress in laboratory animals. ILAR J. 2000;41(2):62–71.
11. DeMarco GJ, Nunamaker EA. A review of the effects of pain and analgesia on immune system function and inflammation: relevance for preclinical studies. Comp Med. 2019;69(6):520–34.
12. Page GG. The immune-suppressive effects of pain. Adv Exp Med Biol. 2003;521:117–25.

13. Taylor DK. Influence of pain and analgesia on cancer research studies. Comp Med. 2019;69(6):501–9.
14. Jirkof P, Cesarovic N, Rettich A, Nicholls F, Seifert B, Arras M. Burrowing behavior as an indicator of post-laparotomy pain in mice. Front Behav Neurosci. 2010;4:165.
15. Jirkof P, Cesarovic N, Rettich A, Fleischmann T, Arras M. Individual housing of female mice: influence on postsurgical behaviour and recovery. Lab Anim. 2012;46(4):325–34.
16. Jirkof P, Fleischmann T, Cesarovic N, Rettich A, Vogel J, Arras M. Assessment of postsurgical distress and pain in laboratory mice by nest complexity scoring. Lab Anim. 2013;47(3):153–61.
17. Toth LA. Interacting influences of sleep, pain, and analgesic medications on sleep studies in rodents. Comp Med. 2019;69(6):571–8.
18. Jirkof P, Rudeck J, Lewejohann L. Assessing affective state in laboratory rodents to promote animal welfare-what is the progress in applied refinement research? Animals (Basel). 2019;9(12)
19. Bell A. The neurobiology of acute pain. Vet J. 2018;237:55–62.
20. McKune CM, Murrell JC, Nolan AM, White KL, Wright BD, et al. Chapter 29: Nociception and pain. In: Veterinary anesthesia and analgesia, Wiley-Blackwell; 2015. p. 584–627.
21. Ji RR, Nackley A, Huh Y, Terrando N, Maixner W. Neuroinflammation and central sensitization in chronic and widespread pain. Anesthesiology. 2018;129(2):343–66.
22. Pogatzki-Zahn E, Segelcke D, Zahn P. Mechanisms of acute and chronic pain after surgery: update from findings in experimental animal models. Curr Opin Anaesthesiol. 2018;31(5):575–85.
23. Pogatzki-Zahn EM, Zahn PK. From preemptive to preventive analgesia. Curr Opin Anaesthesiol. 2006;19(5):551–5.
24. Kehlet H, Jensen TS, Woolf CJ. Persistent postsurgical pain: risk factors and prevention. Lancet. 2006;367(9522):1618–25.
25. Clutton RE. A review of factors affecting analgesic selection in large animals undergoing translational research. Vet J. 2018;236:12–22.
26. Flecknell P. Analgesics in small mammals. Vet Clin North Am Exot Anim Pract. 2018;21(1):83–103.
27. Orr PM, Shank BC, Black AC. The role of pain classification systems in pain management. Crit Care Nurs Clin North Am. 2017;29(4):407–18.
28. Wright ME, Rizzolo D. An update on the pharmacologic management and treatment of neuropathic pain. J Am Acad PAs. 2017;30(3):13–7.
29. Gebhart GF, Bielefeldt K. Physiology of visceral pain. Compr Physiol. 2016;6(4):1609–33.
30. KuKanich B, Wiese AJ. Chapter 11: Opioids. In: Grimm KA, Lamont LA, Tranquilli WJ, et al., editors. Veterinary anesthesia and analgesia; 2015. p. 207–27.
31. Nowoczyn M, Marie N, Coulbault L, Hervault M, Davis A, Hanouz JL, et al. Remifentanil produces cross-desensitization and tolerance with morphine on the mu-opioid receptor. Neuropharmacology. 2013;73:368–79.
32. Larson CM, Wilcox GL, Fairbanks CA. Defining and managing pain in stroke and traumatic brain injury research. Comp Med. 2019;69(6):510–9.
33. Hoffmann U, Sheng H, Ayata C, Warner DS. Anesthesia in experimental stroke research. Transl Stroke Res. 2016;7(5):358–67.
34. Williams JT, Ingram SL, Henderson G, Chavkin C, von Zastrow M, Schulz S, et al. Regulation of mu-opioid receptors: desensitization, phosphorylation, internalization, and tolerance. Pharmacol Rev. 2013;65(1):223–54.
35. Sehgal N, Smith HS, Manchikanti L. Peripherally acting opioids and clinical implications for pain control. Pain Physician. 2011;14(3):249–58.
36. Aronson J. Meyler's side effects of analgesics and anti-inflammatory drugs. 1st ed: Elsevier; 2010.
37. Rivat C, Ballantyne J. The dark side of opioids in pain management: basic science explains clinical observation. PAIN Rep. 2016;1:e570.
38. King T, Ossipov MH, Vanderah TW, Porreca F, Lai J. Is paradoxical pain induced by sustained opioid exposure an underlying mechanism of opioid antinociceptive tolerance? Neurosignals. 2005;14(4):194–205.
39. Wala EP, Holtman JR Jr. Buprenorphine-induced hyperalgesia in the rat. Eur J Pharmacol. 2011;651(1–3):89–95.
40. Lyons PJ, Rivosecchi RM, Nery JP, Kane-Gill SL. Fentanyl-induced hyperalgesia in acute pain management. J Pain Palliat Care Pharmacother. 2015;29(2):153–60.
41. Crain SM, Shen KF. Acute thermal hyperalgesia elicited by low-dose morphine in normal mice is blocked by ultra-low-dose naltrexone, unmasking potent opioid analgesia. Brain Res. 2001;888(1):75–82.
42. Carpenter KC, Hakenjos JM, Fry CD, Nemzek JA. The influence of pain and analgesia in rodent models of sepsis. Comp Med. 2019;69(6):546–54.
43. Sacerdote P. Opioid-induced immunosuppression. Curr Opin Support Palliat Care. 2008;2(1):14–8.
44. Al-Hashimi M, Scott SW, Thompson JP, Lambert DG. Opioids and immune modulation: more questions than answers. Br J Anaesth. 2013;111(1):80–8.
45. Xia M, Tong JH, Zhou ZQ, Duan ML, Xu JG, Zeng HJ, et al. Tramadol inhibits proliferation, migration and invasion via alpha2-adrenoceptor signaling in breast cancer cells. Eur Rev Med Pharmacol Sci. 2016;20(1):157–65.
46. Zhang XL, Chen ML, Zhou SL. Fentanyl inhibits proliferation and invasion of colorectal cancer via beta-catenin. Int J Clin Exp Pathol. 2015;8(1):227–35.

47. Sasamura T, Nakamura S, Iida Y, Fujii H, Murata J, Saiki I, et al. Morphine analgesia suppresses tumor growth and metastasis in a mouse model of cancer pain produced by orthotopic tumor inoculation. Eur J Pharmacol. 2002;441(3):185–91.
48. Bimonte S, Barbieri A, Rea D, Palma G, Luciano A, Cuomo A, et al. Morphine promotes tumor angiogenesis and increases breast cancer progression. Biomed Res Int. 2015;2015:161508.
49. Tanaka K, Kersten JR, Riess ML. Opioid-induced cardioprotection. Curr Pharm Des. 2014;20(36):5696–705.
50. Xu YC, Li RP, Xue FS, Cui XL, Wang SY, Liu GP, et al. Kappa-opioid receptors are involved in enhanced cardioprotection by combined fentanyl and limb remote ischemic postconditioning. J Anesth. 2015;29(4):535–43.
51. Brennan MJ. The effect of opioid therapy on endocrine function. Am J Med. 2013;126(3 Suppl 1):S12–8.
52. Goulding DR, Myers PH, Goulding EH, Blankenship TL, Grant MF, Forsythe DB. The effects of perioperative analgesia on litter size in Crl:CD1(ICR) mice undergoing embryo transfer. J Am Assoc Lab Anim. 2010;49(4):423–6.
53. van der Schier R, Roozekrans M, van Velzen M, Dahan A, Niesters M. Opioid-induced respiratory depression: reversal by non-opioid drugs. F1000Prime Rep. 2014;6:79.
54. McIntyre MK, Clifford JL, Maani CV, Burmeister DM. Progress of clinical practice on the management of burn-associated pain: lessons from animal models. Burns. 2016;42(6):1161–72.
55. Jirkof P, Durst M, Klopfleisch R, Palme R, Thone-Reineke C, Buttgereit F, et al. Administration of tramadol or buprenorphine via the drinking water for post-operative analgesia in a mouse-osteotomy model. Sci Rep. 2019;9(1):10749.
56. Jirkof P, Tourvieille A, Cinelli P, Arras M. Buprenorphine for pain relief in mice: repeated injections vs sustained-release depot formulation. Lab Anim. 2015;49(3):177–87.
57. Bomzon A. Are repeated doses of buprenorphine detrimental to postoperative recovery after laparotomy in rats? Comp Med. 2006;56(2):114–8.
58. Webster LR, Camilleri M, Finn A. Opioid-induced constipation: rationale for the role of norbuprenorphine in buprenorphine-treated individuals. Subst Abus Rehabil. 2016;7:81–6.
59. Clark JA, Myers PH, Goelz MF, Thigpen JE, Forsythe DB. Pica behavior associated with buprenorphine administration in the rat. Lab Anim Sci. 1997;47(3):300–3.
60. Takeda N, Hasegawa S, Morita M, Matsunaga T. Pica in rats is analogous to Emesis – an animal-model in Emesis research. Pharmacol Biochem Be. 1993;45(4):817–21.
61. Johnson RA. Voluntary running-wheel activity, arterial blood gases, and thermal antinociception in rats after 3 buprenorphine formulations. J Am Assoc Lab Anim Sci. 2016;55(3):306–11.
62. Papich MG, Messenger K. Chapter 12: Non-steroidal anti-inflammatory drugs. In: Grimm KA, Lamont LA, Tranquilli WJ, et al., editors. Veterinary anesthesia and analgesia; 2015. p. 227–44.
63. Monteiro B, Steagall PV. Antiinflammatory drugs. Vet Clin North Am Small Anim Pract. 2019;49(6):993–1011.
64. Patrignani P, Patrono C. Cyclooxygenase inhibitors: from pharmacology to clinical read-outs. Biochim Biophys Acta. 2015;1851(4):422–32.
65. Kohn DF, Martin TE, Foley PL, Morris TH, Swindle MM, Vogler GA, et al. Guidelines for the assessment and management of pain in rodents and rabbits. J Am Assoc Lab Anim. 2007;46(2):97–108.
66. Bertolotto M, Contini P, Ottonello L, Pende A, Dallegri F, Montecucco F. Neutrophil migration towards C5a and CXCL8 is prevented by non-steroidal anti-inflammatory drugs via inhibition of different pathways. Br J Pharmacol. 2014;171(14):3376–93.
67. Hardie E, Rawlings C, Shotts JE, Waltman D, Rakich P. Escherichia coli-induced lung and liver dysfunction in dogs: effects of flunixin meglumine treatment. Am J Vet Res. 1987;48(1):56–62.
68. Ferrer MD, Busquets-Cortes C, Capo X, Tejada S, Tur JA, Pons A, et al. Cyclooxygenase-2 inhibitors as a therapeutic target in inflammatory diseases. Curr Med Chem. 2019;26(18):3225–41.
69. Curiel RV, Katz JD. Mitigating the cardiovascular and renal effects of NSAIDs. Pain Med. 2013;14(Suppl 1):S23–8.
70. Saito H, Yokoyama A, Takeno S, Sakai T, Ueno K, Masumura H, et al. Fetal toxicity and hypocalcemia induced by acetylsalicylic acid analogues. Res Commun Chem Pathol Pharmacol. 1982;38(2):209–20.
71. Spanos HG. Aspirin fails to inhibit platelet aggregation in sheep. Thromb Res. 1993;72(3):175–82.
72. O'Connor JP, Lysz T. Celecoxib, NSAIDs and the skeleton. Drugs Today. 2008;44(9):693.
73. Wöhrl S. NSAID hypersensitivity–recommendations for diagnostic work up and patient management. Allergo J Int. 2018;27(4):114–21.
74. Pang LY, Hurst EA, Argyle DJ. Cyclooxygenase-2: a role in cancer stem cell survival and repopulation of cancer cells during therapy. Stem Cells Int. 2016;2016:1.
75. Todoric J, Antonucci L, Karin M. Targeting inflammation in cancer prevention and therapy. Cancer Prev Res. 2016;9(12):895–905.
76. Roughan JV, Flecknell PA. Behavioural effects of laparotomy and analgesic effects of ketoprofen and carprofen in rats. Pain. 2001;90(1–2):65–74.
77. Tubbs JT, Kissling GE, Travlos GS, Goulding DR, Clark JA, King-Herbert AP, et al. Effects of buprenorphine, meloxicam, and flunixin meglumine as postoperative analgesia in mice. J Am Assoc Lab Anim. 2011;50(2):185–91.

78. Tacke S, Henke J, Erhardt W. Metamizol (dipyrone) for pain therapy. Tierarztl Prax Ausg K Klientiere Heimtiere. 2008;36(01):19–25.
79. Blaser LS, Tramonti A, Egger P, Haschke M, Krähenbühl S, Bravo AER. Hematological safety of metamizole: retrospective analysis of WHO and Swiss spontaneous safety reports. Eur J Clin Pharmacol. 2015;71(2):209–17.
80. Novak AF, Ferguson N. Attempts at induced agranulocytosis in rats using dipyrone. J Pharm Sci. 1966;55(11):1306–8.
81. Weithmann K, Alpermann H. Biochemical and pharmacological effects of dipyrone and its metabolites in model systems related to arachidonic acid cascade. Arzneimittelforschung. 1985;35(6):947–52.
82. Chincholkar M. Analgesic mechanisms of gabapentinoids and effects in experimental pain models: a narrative review. Br J Anaesth. 2018;120(6):1315–34.
83. Senderovich H, Jeyapragasan G. Is there a role for combined use of gabapentin and pregabalin in pain control? Too good to be true? Curr Med Res Opin. 2018;34(4):677–82.
84. Guay DR. Pregabalin in neuropathic pain: a more "pharmaceutically elegant" gabapentin? Am J Geriatr Pharmacother. 2005;3(4):274–87.
85. Waszkielewicz A, Gunia A, Sloczynska K, Marona H. Evaluation of anticonvulsants for possible use in neuropathic pain. Curr Med Chem. 2011;18(28):4344–58.
86. Baftiu A, Lima MH, Svendsen K, Larsson PG, Johannessen SI, Landmark CJ. Safety aspects of antiepileptic drugs—a population-based study of adverse effects relative to changes in utilisation. Eur J Clin Pharmacol. 2019;75(8):1153–60.
87. Platt S, Adams V, Garosi L, Abramson C, Penderis J, De Stefani A, et al. Treatment with gabapentin of 11 dogs with refractory idiopathic epilepsy. Vet Rec. 2006;159(26):881–4.
88. Vartanian MG, Radulovic LL, Kinsora JJ, Serpa KA, Vergnes M, Bertram E, et al. Activity profile of pregabalin in rodent models of epilepsy and ataxia. Epilepsy Res. 2006;68(3):189–205.
89. Simko J, Karesova I, Kremlacek J, Eva Z, Horacek J, Fekete S, et al. The effect of gabapentin and pregabalin on bone turnover and bone strength: a prospective study in Wistar rats. Pharmacol Rep. 2019;71(6):1213–8.
90. Kanda J, Izumo N, Kobayashi Y, Onodera K, Shimakura T, Yamamoto N, et al. Effects of the antiepileptic drugs phenytoin, gabapentin, and levetiracetam on bone strength, bone mass, and bone turnover in rats. Biol Pharm Bull. 2017;40(11):1934–40.
91. Salimzade A, Hosseini-Sharifabad A, Rabbani M. Comparative effects of chronic administrations of gabapentin, pregabalin and baclofen on rat memory using object recognition test. Res Pharm Sci. 2017;12(3):204.
92. Ola MS, Alhomida AS, LaNoue KF. Gabapentin attenuates oxidative stress and apoptosis in the diabetic rat retina. Neurotox Res. 2019;36(1):81–90.
93. Berry SH. Chapter 15: Injectable anesthetics. In: Grimm KA, Lamont LA, Tranquilli WJ, Greene SA, et al., editors. Veterinary anesthesia and analgesia; 2015. p. 277–97.
94. Persson J. Wherefore ketamine? Curr Opin Anesthesiol. 2010;23(4):455–60.
95. Svenson JE, Abernathy MK. Ketamine for prehospital use: new look at an old drug. Am J Emerg Med. 2007;25(8):977–80.
96. Sellers EM, Romach MK, Leiderman DB. Studies with psychedelic drugs in human volunteers. Neuropharmacology. 2018;142:116–34.
97. DeClue AE, Cohn LA, Lechner ES, Bryan ME, Dodam JR. Effects of subanesthetic doses of ketamine on hemodynamic and immunologic variables in dogs with experimentally induced endotoxemia. Am J Vet Res. 2008;69(2):228–32.
98. Zanos P, Gould TD. Mechanisms of ketamine action as an antidepressant. Mol Psychiatry. 2018;23(4):801–11.
99. Brachman RA, McGowan JC, Perusini JN, Lim SC, Pham TH, Faye C, et al. Ketamine as a prophylactic against stress-induced depressive-like behavior. Biol Psychiatry. 2016;79(9):776–86.
100. Herrmann K, Flecknell P. Retrospective review of anesthetic and analgesic regimens used in animal research proposals. ALTEX. 2019;36(1):65–80.
101. Flecknell P. Rodent analgesia: assessment and therapeutics. Vet J. 2018;232:70–7.
102. Schug SA. Combination analgesia in 2005 – a rational approach: focus on paracetamol-tramadol. Clin Rheumatol. 2006;25(Suppl 1):S16–21.
103. Fishbain D. Evidence-based data on pain relief with antidepressants. Ann Med. 2000;32(5):305–16.
104. Mitra R, Jones S. Adjuvant analgesics in cancer pain: a review. Am J Hosp Palliat Me. 2012;29(1):70–9.
105. Cannon CZ, Kissling GE, Goulding DR, King-Herbert AP, Blankenship-Paris T. Analgesic effects of tramadol, carprofen or multimodal analgesia in rats undergoing ventral laparotomy. Lab Anim. 2011;40(3):85–93.
106. Fernandez-Duenas V, Poveda R, Fernandez A, Sanchez S, Planas E, Ciruela F. Fentanyl-trazodone-paracetamol triple drug combination: multimodal analgesia in a mouse model of visceral pain. Pharmacol Biochem Behav. 2011;98(3):331–6.
107. Wickerts L, Warren Stomberg M, Brattwall M, Jakobsson J. Coxibs: is there a benefit when compared to traditional non-selective NSAIDs in postoperative pain management? Minerva Anestesiol. 2011;77(11):1084–98.
108. Clark L. Pre-emptive or preventive analgesia – lessons from the human literature? Vet Anaesth Analg. 2014;41(2):109–12.

109. Foley PL. Current options for providing sustained analgesia to laboratory animals. Lab Anim. 2014;43(10):364–71.
110. Cinelli P, Rettich A, Seifert B, Burki K, Arras M. Comparative analysis and physiological impact of different tissue biopsy methodologies used for the genotyping of laboratory mice. Lab Anim. 2007;41(2):174–84.
111. Moberg GP. When does stress become distress? Lab Anim. 1999;28(4):22–6.
112. Foley PL, Liang H, Crichlow AR. Evaluation of a sustained-release formulation of buprenorphine for analgesia in rats. J Am Assoc Lab Anim. 2011;50(2):198–204.
113. Liles JH, Flecknell PA, Roughan J, Cruz-Madorran I. Influence of oral buprenorphine, oral naltrexone or morphine on the effects of laparotomy in the rat. Lab Anim. 1998;32(2):149–61.
114. Goldkuhl R, Jacobsen KR, Kalliokoski O, Hau J, Abelson KS. Plasma concentrations of corticosterone and buprenorphine in rats subjected to jugular vein catheterization. Lab Anim. 2010;44(4):337–43.
115. Molina-Cimadevila MJ, Segura S, Merino C, Ruiz-Reig N, Andres B, de Madaria E. Oral self-administration of buprenorphine in the diet for analgesia in mice. Lab Anim. 2014;48(3):216–24.
116. Sauer M, Fleischmann T, Lipiski M, Arrasa M, Jirkof P. Buprenorphine via drinking water and combined oral-injection protocols for pain relief in mice. Appl Anim Behav Sci. 2016.
117. Thompson AC, DiPirro JM, Sylvester AR, Martin LB, Kristal MB. Lack of analgesic efficacy in female rats of the commonly recommended oral dose of buprenorphine. J Am Assoc Lab Anim Sci. 2006;45(6):13–6.
118. Brewster D, Humphrey MJ, Mcleavy MA. The systemic bioavailability of buprenorphine by various routes of administration. J Pharm Pharmacol. 1981;33(8):500–6.
119. Garcia ER. Chapter 17: Local anesthetics. In: Grimm KA, Lamont LA, Tranquilli WJ, Greene SA, et al., editors. Veterinary anesthesia and analgesia; 2015. p. 332–57.
120. Steffey EP, Mama KR, Brosnan RJ. Chapter 16: Inhalation anesthetics. In: Grimm KA, Lamont LA, et al., editors. Veterinary anesthesia and analgesia; 2015. p. 297–332.
121. Evers A, Crowder A, Balser J. Chapter 13: General anesthetics. In: Brunton L, Lazo J, et al., editors. Goodman and Gilman's The pharmacological basis of therapeutics; 2006. p. 341–69.
122. Vaneker M, Santosa J, Heunks L, Halbertsma F, Snijdelaar D, Van Egmond J, et al. Isoflurane attenuates pulmonary interleukin-1β and systemic tumor necrosis factor-α following mechanical ventilation in healthy mice. Acta Anaesthesiol Scand. 2009;53(6):742–8.
123. Bar-Klein G, Klee R, Brandt C, Bankstahl M, Bascuñana P, Töllner K, et al. Isoflurane prevents acquired epilepsy in rat models of temporal lobe epilepsy. Ann Neurol. 2016;80(6):896–908.
124. Cook TL, Beppu WJ, Hitt BA, Kosek JC, Mazze RI. Renal effects and metabolism of sevoflurane in fisher 3444 rats: an in-vivo and in-vitro comparison with methoxyflurane. Anesthesiology. 1975;43(1):70–7.
125. Stabernack CR, Eger EI, Warnken UH, Förster H, Hanks DK, Ferrell LD. Sevoflurane degradation by carbon dioxide absorbents may produce more than one nephrotoxic compound in rats. Can J Anaesth. 2003;50(3):249–52.
126. Kharasch ED, Schroeder JL, Sheffels P, Liggitt HD. Influence of sevoflurane on the metabolism and renal effects of compound a in rats. Anesthesiol J Am Soc Anesthesiol. 2005;103(6):1183–8.
127. Qi H, Mariager CO, Lindhardt J, Nielsen PM, Stodkilde-Jorgensen H, Laustsen C. Effects of anesthesia on renal function and metabolism in rats assessed by hyperpolarized MRI. Magn Reson Med. 2018;80(5):2073–80.
128. Puig N, Ferrero P, Bay M, Hidalgo G, Valenti J, Amerio N, et al. Effects of sevoflurane general anesthesia: immunological studies in mice. Int Immunopharmacol. 2002;2(1):95–104.
129. Elena G, Amerio N, Ferrero P, Bay M, Valenti J, Colucci D, et al. Effects of repetitive sevoflurane anaesthesia on immune response, select biochemical parameters and organ histology in mice. Lab Anim. 2003;37(3):193–203.
130. Tanaka T, Kai S, Koyama T, Daijo H, Adachi T, Fukuda K, et al. General anesthetics inhibit erythropoietin induction under hypoxic conditions in the mouse brain. PloS One. 2011;6:12.
131. Zheng B, Zhan Q, Chen J, Xu H, He Z. Sevoflurane pretreatment enhance HIF-2α expression in mice after renal ischemia/reperfusion injury. Int J Clin Exp Pathol. 2015;8(10):13114.
132. Miller AL, Golledge HD, Leach MC. The influence of isoflurane anaesthesia on the Rat Grimace Scale. PloS One. 2016;11:11.
133. Trapani G, Altomare C, Sanna E, Biggio G, Liso G. Propofol in anesthesia. Mechanism of action, structure-activity relationships, and drug delivery. Curr Med Chem. 2000;7(2):249–71.
134. Sumi C, Okamoto A, Tanaka H, Nishi K, Kusunoki M, Shoji T, et al. Propofol induces a metabolic switch to glycolysis and cell death in a mitochondrial electron transport chain-dependent manner. PLoS One. 2018;13:2.
135. Mallard JM, Rieser TM, Peterson NW. Propofol infusion-like syndrome in a dog. Can Vet J. 2018;59(11):1216.
136. Ammer H, Potschka H, Hrsg: Löscher W, Richter A. Lehrbuch der Pharmakologie und Toxikologie für die Veterinärmedizin; Chapter 4: Pharmakologie des zentralen Nervensystems (ZNS). 2016:125–180

137. Menke H, Vaupel P. Effect of injectable or inhalational anesthetics and of neuroleptic, neuroleptanalgesic, and sedative agents on tumor blood flow. Radiat Res. 1988;114(1):64–76.
138. Goodchild CS, Serrao JM, Kolosov A, Boyd BJ. Alphaxalone reformulated: a water-soluble intravenous anesthetic preparation in sulfobutyl-ether-β-cyclodextrin. Anesth Analg. 2015;120(5):1025–31.
139. Sun H, Zheng X, Zhou Y, Zhu W, Ou Y, Shu M, et al. Alphaxalone inhibits growth, migration and invasion of rat C6 malignant glioma cells. Steroids. 2013;78(10):1041–5.
140. Rankin DC. Chapter 10: Sedatives and tranquilizers. In: Grimm KA, Lamont LA, Tranquilli WJ, Greene SA, et al., editors. Veterinary anesthesia and analgesia; 2015. p. 196–207.
141. Hsu WH, Lee P, Betts DM. Xylazine-induced mydriasis in rats and its antagonism by α-adrenergic blocking agents. J Vet Pharmacol Ther. 1981;4(2):97–101.
142. Calderone L, Grimes P, Shalev M. Acute reversible cataract induced by xylazine and by ketamine-xylazine anesthesia in rats and mice. Exp Eye Res. 1986;42(4):331–7.
143. McKemy DD. The molecular and cellular basis of cold sensation. ACS Chem Neurosci. 2013;4(2):238–47.
144. Chughtai M, Elmallah RD, Mistry JB, Bhave A, Cherian JJ, McGinn TL, et al. Nonpharmacologic pain management and muscle strengthening following total knee arthroplasty. J Knee Surg. 2016;29(03):194–200.
145. Raggio BS, Barton BM, Grant MC, McCoul ED. Intraoperative cryoanalgesia for reducing post-tonsillectomy pain: a systemic review. Ann Otol Rhinol Laryngol. 2018;127(6):395–401.
146. Foulkes T, Wood J. Mechanisms of cold pain. Channels. 2007;1(3):154–60.
147. Lo B, Hönemann CW, Kohrs R, Hollmann MW, Polanowska-Grabowska RK, Gear AR, et al. Local anesthetic actions on thromboxane-induced platelet aggregation. Anesth Analg. 2001;93(5):1240–5.
148. Long I, Robert P, Aroniadou-Anderjaska V, Prager EM, Pidoplichko VI, Figueiredo TH, et al. Repeated isoflurane exposures impair long-term potentiation and increase basal gabaergic activity in the basolateral amygdala. Neural Plast. 2016;2016
149. Zhu C, Gao J, Karlsson N, Li Q, Zhang Y, Huang Z, et al. Isoflurane anesthesia induced persistent, progressive memory impairment, caused a loss of neural stem cells, and reduced neurogenesis in young, but not adult, rodents. J Cereb Blood Flow Metab. 2010;30(5):1017–30.
150. Huang H, Liu C-M, Sun J, Jin W-J, Wu Y-Q, Chen J. Repeated 2% sevoflurane administration in 7-and 60-day-old rats. Anaesthesist. 2017;66(11):850–7.
151. Makaryus R, Lee H, Feng T, Park J-H, Nedergaard M, Jacob Z, et al. Brain maturation in neonatal rodents is impeded by sevoflurane anesthesia. Anesthesiology. 2015;123(3):557.
152. Shen X, Liu Y, Xu S, Zhao Q, Guo X, Shen R, et al. Early life exposure to sevoflurane impairs adulthood spatial memory in the rat. Neurotoxicology. 2013;39:45–56.
153. Bercker S, Bert B, Bittigau P, Felderhoff-Müser U, Bührer C, Ikonomidou C, et al. Neurodegeneration in newborn rats following propofol and sevoflurane anesthesia. Neurotox Res. 2009;16(2):140–7.
154. Amrock LG, Starner ML, Murphy KL, Baxter MG. Long-term effects of single or multiple neonatal sevoflurane exposures on rat hippocampal ultrastructure. Anesthesiology. 2015;122(1):87–95.
155. Hohlbaum K, Bert B, Dietze S, Palme R, Fink H, Thöne-Reineke C. Impact of repeated anesthesia with ketamine and xylazine on the well-being of C57BL/6JRj mice. PloS One. 2018;13:9.
156. Smith JC. A review of strain and sex differences in response to pain and analgesia in mice. Comp Med. 2019;69(6):490–500.
157. Golledge H, Jirkof P. Score sheets and analgesia. Lab Anim. 2016;50(6):411–3.

Part II

Statistics: Basics and Explanation of Different Designs and Tests

Why Do We Need a Statistical Experiment Design?

Michael Parkinson and Carlos Oscar Sánchez Sorzano

In order to develop new treatments for diseases, high-fidelity models are required (Russell WMS, Burch RL. (1959)) to advance our understanding to the stage where human trials can begin. We have to strike a harm/benefit balance, and these are now enshrined in the 3R's principles of the European directive 2010/63/EU which is enacted in the laws of European countries. Good experimental design which will allow us to achieve this is therefore not only morally good but legally required.

These chapters address the second R, reduction.

1 Statistical Experiment Design

We need to address a number of areas to produce well-designed experiments:

1. Design: Having justified our research question, we need to consider:
   - Fidelity of the model.
   - What to measure.
   - Treatments and controls.
   - The statistical test.
   - The size of difference we want to detect. There are two issues here: Firstly, will we be able to detect an expected difference, and, secondly, is that difference biologically relevant?
2. How many replicates?: There is no point in doing research that will not work. Every time that we carry out an experiment, we want to have a reasonable expectation of seeing a statistically significant result; the expectation of seeing a statistically significant result is the power of the experiment. Reasonable is typically defined as 0.8–0.9. The power of your experiment is related to your treatment differences, the variability, and the sample size. All other things being equal, the bigger the treatment difference, and the smaller the variability, and the larger the sample size, the bigger the power.
3. Experimental layout design: You should avoid confounding, which is where something other than your treatment affects what you are measuring. If it is applied asymmetrically, this could lead to false results which could stop the development of a promising drug or lead you down a blind alley. Applied to all treat-

M. Parkinson
School of Biotechnology, Dublin City University, Dublin, Ireland
e-mail: michael.parkinson@dcu.ie

C. O. S. Sorzano (✉)
Natl. Center of Biotechnology (CSIC), Madrid, Spain
e-mail: coss@cnb.csic.es

© Springer Nature Switzerland AG 2021

J. M. Sánchez Morgado, A. Brønstad (eds.), *Experimental Design and Reproducibility in Preclinical Animal Studies*, Laboratory Animal Science and Medicine 1,
https://doi.org/10.1007/978-3-030-66147-2_6

ments, it will increase the variability requiring a larger sample size. As an example, there is often batch-to-batch variability. To minimize confounding we need first to identify possible confounding factors and then design the experiment to either increase the homogeneity for that confounding factor (e.g., by doing the whole experiment with one batch of animals) or if this is not possible to block out the confounding factor, for example, if you need ten replicates but cannot manage the whole experiment in one batch, to do five replicates of each treatment combination in batch 1 and 5 replicates in a second batch. The batch-to-batch difference may then be factored out as part of the experimental design.

Blocking like this is very efficient as several sources of variability can be incorporated into the one block. For example, if I need to carry out an experiment in two batches, I could do the first batch of the experiment this week with the first batch of animals and the first batch of drug, and a colleague could carry out the experiment on a second batch of animals with a second batch of drug. The person to person, animal batch to batch, and drug batch to batch variability can then all be factored out in the same block. Given that it can be difficult to identify confounding variables, it is important to plan your experiment to avoid designing in confounding factors. For example, two researchers work together in cancer research to make up batches of cells and to inject them subcutaneously into the animal. One makes the batches of cells, and the other injects them. However, to gain experience they swap halfway with the result that all the control cells were prepared by researcher A and all the treatment cells prepared by researcher B. We should *control what we can, block what can't be controlled, and randomize whatever sources of variability are left*.

Only by being very systematic in what we can do, we control the variability in the experiment sufficiently to minimize confounding. There is no downside to good experimental design. It is clear from the literature that many studies are not well designed or reported in such a way that they could be replicated. In 2009 an NC3Rs-commissioned review analyzed 271 randomly chosen peer-reviewed publications. The results were an eye-opener: only one in eight reported randomization and only one in seven reported blinding, over one in three failed to include three important pieces of information, the research hypothesis, and the number of animals used and their characteristics. This led them to develop the ARRIVE guidelines which is an excellent tool to help in experimental design and the reporting of animal experiments ([18]; see Table 1). The experimental design is therefore critical, and design and analysis need to be built in to the experiment [10, 11]. To enforce application of the ARRIVE guidelines and to facilitate reporting of experimental design, the NC3Rs also developed the Experimental Design Assistant.

2 Pilot, Exploratory, and Confirmatory Experiments

Depending on what we hope to achieve, we may carry out **pilot**, **exploratory**, and **confirmatory** experiments.

Pilot experiments are small studies (with 1–30 subjects) which aim to determine the parameters of an experiment. With a novel problem, we are often faced with having very little information on a model such as the size of effects or the most effective drug concentrations to use. Pilot experiments can allow us to practice techniques and knock all the rough edges off the methodology. Prosaically, the place to screw up is not in a full-scale experiment but in a small pilot. While pilot experiments can give us a "ball park" figure for sample size based on estimates of treatment effect and variability, they are not really suitable to give a robust calculation of the sample size [25]. There are two good places to get this information: related experiments in the scientific literature and prior data from the researcher's own laboratory.

Exploratory experiments can be used to generate and refine research hypotheses, for example, many microarray gene expression experiments looking at the expression level of thousands of genes. One of the major problems with this ap-

Table 1 Items in the ARRIVE guidelines related to the statistical design, analysis, and report

Item 6. Study design	For each experiment, give brief details of the study design, including: (a) The number of experimental and control groups (b) Any steps taken to minimize the effects of subjective bias when allocating animals to treatment (e.g., randomization procedure) and when assessing results (e.g., if done, describe who was blinded and when) (See Sect. 4.) (c) The experimental unit (e.g., a single animal, group, or cage of animals) (See Sect. 3.) A time-line diagram or flow chart can be useful to illustrate how complex study designs were carried out
Item 10. Sample size	(a) Specify the total number of animals used in each experiment and the number of animals in each experimental group (b) Explain how the number of animals was decided. Provide details of any sample size calculation used (See Sect. 7 and chapter "Statistical Tests and Sample Size Calculations".) (c) Indicate the number of independent replications of each experiment, if relevant (See Sect. 6.2.)
Item 11. Allocating animals to experimental groups	(a) Give full details of how animals were allocated to experimental groups, including randomization or matching if done (See Sects. 4 and 5.7 and chapter "Design of Experiments".) (b) Describe the order in which the animals in the different experimental groups were treated and assessed
Item 13. Statistical methods	(a) Provide details of the statistical methods used for each analysis (b) Specify the unit of analysis for each dataset (e.g., single animal, group of animals, single neuron) (See Sect. 3.) (c) Describe any methods used to assess whether the data met the assumptions of the statistical approach
Item 14. Baseline data	For each experimental group, report relevant characteristics and health status of animals (e.g., weight, microbiological status, and drug- or test-naïve) before treatment or testing (this information can often be tabulated) (See Sect. 5.7.)
Item 15. Numbers analyzed	(a) Report the number of animals in each group included in each analysis. Report absolute numbers (e.g. 10/20, not 50%) (b) If any animals or data were not included in the analysis, explain why (See Sect. 5.4 .)
Item 16. Outcomes and estimation	Report the results for each analysis carried out, with a measure of precision (e.g., standard error or confidence interval) (See Sect. 6.2.)

proach is the generation of false positives. We normally set our significance level at $p = 0.05$. By definition this is going to generate false positives in 1 in 20 of our tests. By not setting out our research hypothesis up front but developing it after seeing the data, we are choosing from literally thousands of potential research hypotheses; some of our data is going to fit. Our eyes are very good at seeing patterns whether they are real or not, and with enough false positives, we can generate illusory hypotheses. It is therefore important that the generated or refined research hypothesis be confirmed in a confirmatory experiment.

Confirmatory experiments Once we have generated or refined a research hypothesis, we can test this in a very strict and formalized manner. This normally compares two or more groups where we aim to disprove a null hypothesis (usually the absence of any effect). If we fail to disprove it, it does not mean that the alternative hypothesis is not true (e.g., that our drug does affect tumor growth) but that there is insufficient evidence for it. It could be that either there is a background of too much variability or the true effect of drug is small and difficult to pick up, or we may simply not have used enough samples.

There are thus three ways that we can improve the power of the experiment (the chance of seeing a statistically significant result if there is a real difference):

- *Increasing the number of animals.*
- *Decreasing the variance of measurements.* Variance can be reduced by either making the experimental material more homogeneous or by factoring out confounding factors and "nuisance variables."
- *Increasing treatment effect.* Treatment effect may be optimized by pilot experiments with varying doses.

Statistically we are comparing the differences seen between experimental units. If these are not independent, there is the potential for confounding of the experiment. For example, if two different drugs are given to two batches of five mice, putting all five controls in one cage and all the treatment in a separate cage causes confounding. We are unsure whether the result we are seeing is due to a real drug effect or to cage effects; the controls could have been fighting, there could be a subclinical infection, water bottles might have leaked, and animals become dehydrated.

Bias is potentially fatal to your experiment. There are two ways to control bias, randomization of the experimental subjects and blinding of the experimenter to treatment.

Ideally we would like to maximize the scope of experiments to maximize external validity. This could be done by using a very heterogeneous sample, but this will increase variability making it more difficult to repeat and with consequent low internal validity. Far better is to identify the varying factors and build them in to a factorial design.

It is therefore a big mistake to do the experiment first and then plan the statistical analysis later; we can only build in scope if we can identify the factors first. In some instances it may not be possible to do any statistical analysis. To work out how many replicates are required, we can carry out a power analysis, and this is based on a statistical design. Therefore before starting the analysis, we should plan for its statistical analysis (absolutely required for good laboratory practices, Kilkenny et al. [18], Macleod et al. [19]). Each experiment should be planned based on the results from the previous one to use the newly acquired knowledge to refine the next experiment.

3 Independence Between Individuals: Experimental Units

The experimental unit is the smallest experimental unit such that any two experimental that can receive a different treatment. The concept of experimental unit is better illustrated by examples:

- We have a drug which we feel may affect body weight of rats and want to test this. We have a control which has a vehicle rather than the drug and three concentrations of the drug we want to test. We have decided on five animals per treatment. How we give the drug to the rats and how we group them will affect the sample size needed.
- If we have one cage of five rats per treatment, irrespective of how we give the drug, we have one replicate of each since whatever happens in the cage affects all animals in the same way. To get our five replicates, we would need five cages per treatment so five animals per cage × five cages per treatment × four treatments = 100 animals. We will get some savings in animals since the average weight of five animals per cage will give us a better estimate of the true value than a single value so we should revisit our power calculation with the revised (and smaller) estimate of variability, but we are still talking about a lot of animals. The same rationale as the cage applies to litters. Typically the treatment is applied to the mother so whatever happens to the mother affects all neonates, which all receive the same treatment. If we do carry out the treatments using litters of animals, then to block by litter and apply the

different treatments to one member of the litter is a useful way to optimize the experimental design and factor our variability.

- If we inject the drug and put one animal of each treatment in the one cage, we have one replicate of each treatment per cage. Five replicate cages × four treatments = 20 animals. If we suspect cage effects, then we have the option of blocking by cage to factor out the cage effects.
- If the analysis is nondestructive (e.g., measurement of body weight), then we have the option of carrying out all four treatments on one animal. We have to make sure that there is no carry-over from one treatment to another, and we need to take into account the order effects, but if this can be done, then the animal at each time point becomes the experimental unit. We have one cage of five animals measured at four different times = five animals. We also have the advantage that the animal-to-animal variability, which typically may be half of the total variability in the experiment, can be blocked out since every animal is getting every treatment. If we suspect animal-to-animal variability, we can block by animal.
- The same rationale applies to treatments carried out at the same time but on different parts of the animal. For example, if we were interested in the effect of an anti-inflammatory on skin inflammation, we could induce inflammation in patches of the skin and apply a different treatment to each patch. Each animal has two ears, two eyes, two lungs, and two pairs of legs. It would be possible to treat one and use the other as a control. For example, pneumothorax (collapsed lung) is a common result of lung biopsies. If we had a new treatment, we could apply the new treatment to one lung and the comparison treatment to the other.
- We have to be careful about pseudoreplication. Simply measuring the same thing multiple times on the same animal does not give us any additional replication as we are measuring the same thing on the same animal. Where there is appreciable measurement variability, this can be useful to reduce measurement error as we can use the average of the measurements which should be a better estimate of the true value than a single measurement.
- Where measurements are related, for example, in a time series carried out on the same animal, then we need to factor in the time in a repeated measures design rather than just lumping all the measurements in to the analysis as separate replicates.

4 Avoiding Bias: Blocking, Randomization, and Blinding

Bias is potentially a fatal flaw in an experiment (see Sect. 1). However, there are many causes of bias, all of them important in general biomedical research because they can increase variability and lead to confounding:

- Omitted-variable bias is caused by not including a variable when it has a significant influence on the measurements.
- Selection bias is caused by some individuals being more likely to be selected than others.
- Performance bias is subconsciously caused by the vested interest of researchers.
- Observer bias is caused when there is subjectivity in scoring, for example, in histology. Blinding of observer to treatment is the best solution.
- Exclusion bias is caused by a systematic exclusion of measurements. For example, outliers may be thoroughly examined and excluded in a biased way depending on their origin, while points in the body of the data are not examined.
- Attrition bias is caused by losses due to treatment. All experiments should include humane endpoints, and differences in treatment effect may lead to animals being lost "not at random." This is especially problematical but may be solved by using analysis based on time to endpoint like survival analysis or derived measures such as tumor-specific growth rate rather than tumor size at a specific time.

There are other types of less technical biases like publication bias (it is far easier to report positive results than negative results, which are seldom reported [20, 22]). Given that it is unethical to repeat studies which have already been carried out, it would be very useful to have access to this "grey" literature. Experimental bias is one of the main sources of incorrect conclusions and lack of repeatability and has been extensively studied in random clinical trials [13], case-control studies [23], and experiments with animals [26]. Hooijmans et al. [14] and Zeng et al. [28] provide useful guidelines to try to avoid, or at least identify, bias in biomedical research with laboratory animals.

The main tools to fight bias are blocking, randomization, blinding, and good reporting:

1. **Blocking**: Each of the blocks is essentially a mini-experiment, in which all treatments (i.e., control and treatment) are applied. The effect of blocks can then be factored out in the statistical analysis. If the potential biasing factor is a variable, for example, animal age, it can be incorporated into the analysis as a covariate.

   Given that most animals are social, sometimes animals are housed with a companion animal that is not part of the study. In experiments with chemical reactants, batch can be an important source of confounding, for example, tenfold differences in binding affinity were seen for an immunological test based on the batch of reagent. Experiments performed with microarrays are particularly sensitive to these effects [17].

   Given that instrumentation can drift over time, it is important ideally to use the same instrument at the same time for sample measurements of all treatments and to make sure that this is properly calibrated.

2. **Randomization** is the process of randomly allocating the experimental units to the treatment(s) or control. The best insurance against bias is to identify the source of the bias and block it out as this not only accounts for the biasing factor but reduces its effects on overall variability. There are however many sources of variability in every experiment, and it is not possible to account for all of these. The best insurance then against bias is to spread out the biasing factor as evenly as possible by randomly allocating individuals to treatment and the order of all procedures.

   Stratified randomization is randomization within each block. For example, if we are using litters of animals, we can randomly assign individuals within each litter. This is especially important where we anticipate outliers in the starting population to prevent them being assigned to one treatment, for example, a subpopulation of older animals. Splitting the population into cohorts based on baseline characteristics is a useful strategy for stratification before randomization.

3. **Blinding** hides the treatment information to the patient (single blinding), the patient and the experimenter (double blinding), or the patient, the experimenter, and the data analyst (triple blinding). With laboratory animals, single blinding is normally unnecessary. However, if possible, blinding the experimenter from the treatment he or she is applying or evaluating drastically improves the fairness of the experiment. Bebarta et al. [2] evaluated the outcome of 290 research studies with animals. Those studies lacking randomization, blinding, or both were significantly more likely to report positive outcomes. Blinding directly addresses performance and observer bias.

4. **Good reporting**. Unfortunately, except for a few cases like survival analysis, there is no ideal technical solution for exclusion or attrition bias. At least, good reporting of the experiment and its data filtering and processing may help the reader evaluate the quality of the reported results. In this regard, Hooijmans et al. [14], Kilkenny et al. [18], Zeng et al. [28] provide a guideline to experiment reporting that should minimize this kind of bias.

5 Reducing Variance: Variable and Population Selection, Experimental Conditions, Averaging, and Blocking

Virtually all biological measures show variability with variation due to different individuals plus measurement noise. Given that overall error is biological error plus measurement error, reducing measurement error will reduce the overall error.

Given that sample size will depend upon how many standard deviations your treatment is from control generally higher variability will require a larger sample size for detecting the same treatment effect or for a fixed sample size, higher variability will reduce the power to detect a given treatment effect. These ideas are further discussed in Sect. 6.

5.1 Variable Selection

As we will see in chapter "Statistical Tests and Sample Size Calculations", the calculation of the sample size depends on the information brought in by each one of the experimental units and the noise of our measurements. Generally speaking, the information order of variables would be categorical, ordinal, discrete, and continuous. For example, if we are studying the presence of macrophages in a given microscopy field, the following measurements would bring an increasing amount of information: (1) absence or presence of macrophages (categorical), (2) qualitative number of macrophages (ordinal: none; one or two; three, four, or five; more than five), (3) quantitative number of macrophages (0, 1, 2, 3, ...(discrete)); and (4) area occupied by the macrophages in the field (continuous). If possible, we should work with as informative variables as possible.

Some discrete variables may be treated as (almost) "continuous" for the purposes of statistical analysis. For instance, we may measure the severity of arthritis of a single paw in a scale from 0 to 4. Each animal receives a score that is the sum of the scores of the four paws.

It is common practice to 'normalize to control' basically dividing one measurement by another to produce a ratio. This may solve one problem of differences in baseline but typically introduces others. One problem with this approach is that the original data, and all its variation becomes hidden. An animal may spend a quarter of its active time searching for food, but this could be 2 min out of 8 min or 200 min out of 800 min.

Ideally we should minimize variability. For example, if we are interested in an appetite suppressant, it would be less variable to measure weight gain rather than food intake.

5.2 Population Selection

Experiments can be performed on mixed stocks, outbred stocks, and inbred strains [5]. For our experiments we have two conflicting aims, one of maximizing the scope of the results so that we can maximize repeatability and one of minimizing the variability so that we use the minimum number of animals. The greater the variability, the greater the number of animals needed, so mixed stocks of animals which is the equivalent of the genetic variability encountered in large human populations (like a whole country) are very rarely used for animal experiments as the number of animals needed is too large. This leaves us with outbred stocks and inbred stocks. Outbred stocks would be equivalent of small human communities with little interaction with other communities (like Lapland), and with the exception of research on quantitative trait loci, the experimental use of outbred stocks is discouraged [5] as variability is much larger than in inbred strains. Inbred or hybrid F1 strains are genetically identical like human identical twins, and variability is much lower than in outbred strains. This is a double-edged sword in that although we can have reduced variability we also have lower scope.

We can get all the benefits of reduced variability but maintain the scope if we use several independent inbred strains. As an example Jay Jr [16] analyzed the effect of the drug hexobarbital on sleeping time of mice. To get the same, statistical power would need between 2 and 3 times more outbred animals than if we use a mix of five inbred strains. How we carry out the experiment may also affect variability, and there is evidence Chvedoff et al. [6] that variability increases with the number of mice per cage.

5.3 Experimental Conditions

Increasing scope should make our results more robust; however just because we can replicate the results in our own laboratory does not necessarily mean that our results will be exactly reproducible in another laboratory. Crabbe et al. [7] repeated the same experiment with eight mouse strains in three different locations: Portland, Edmonton, and Albany. Despite controlling for many experimental variables, they found significant differences in body weight and behavioral tests in the three experimental sites.

5.4 Population Scope, Outliers, and Lack of Independence

We should always be mindful of the balance between variability and scope. Typically, we would make our experimental conditions as homogeneous as possible to reduce variability and should report the experimental conditions accurately and comprehensively to facilitate reproducibility.

We have to be careful to differentiate between experimental error, which is the animal-to-animal variability, and measurement error, which is the variability of repeated measurements on the same animal. Experiments with large numbers of observations from a small number of animals (e.g., measuring 1,000 observations of gene copy number in five animals) should be handled with care. These experiment give a precise estimate from each single animal and so minimize measurement error, and it is tempting to lump all the observations into one statistical analysis. However if we get 1,000 observations on 5 animals, we have a really good estimate on 5 animals, so actually 5 replicates and not 5,000 replicates.

Ideally we want to remove invalid points. If the invalid point lies in the body of the distribution, it is impossible to identify. Fortunately, if it is in the body of the distribution, it is not going to bias the results of a great deal. The invalid points that cause the most problems and that we can readily identify occur as outliers. These pull the average strongly toward them and are also unduly influential on the variability of the data. We need to decide what to do with outliers. They can be removed, left in, or treated separately. What we should do depends upon the nature of those outliers:

- Firstly check for measurement error. If obvious (e.g., a mouse that weighs 25 kg), go back to the original data and check. Sometimes the original data is still available, or the error is obvious (e.g., a missing decimal point) and can be fixed; otherwise delete them.
- Is there an obvious error in the application of the treatment (e.g., missing a vein during the injection)? It is probably safest to do the analysis twice, once with the outliers left in and once with them removed. We do not want to artificially inflate the variability and move the average, but others may make the same mistake that we did but then choose to leave them in. We could choose to treat the outliers as a separate subpopulation.
- Is there more than one peak in your data, for example, 70% has a strong response to treatment and 30% has little or no response? If so, you've got subpopulations, each having a different response. We should analyze the subpopulations separately and draw conclusions for each. We can use Stratified sampling if we can predict subpopulations in our data. The interested reader is referred to Thompson [27, Chap. 11].
- Is your data normally distributed? Data which is log normal (e.g., plasma hormone concentrations) will tend to have a tail on the high side, and this can lead to outliers. If this is suspected, then to transform the data (log or square root usually works) will typically remove outliers.

The presence of subpopulations can lead to incorrect conclusions. Figure 1 shows the result

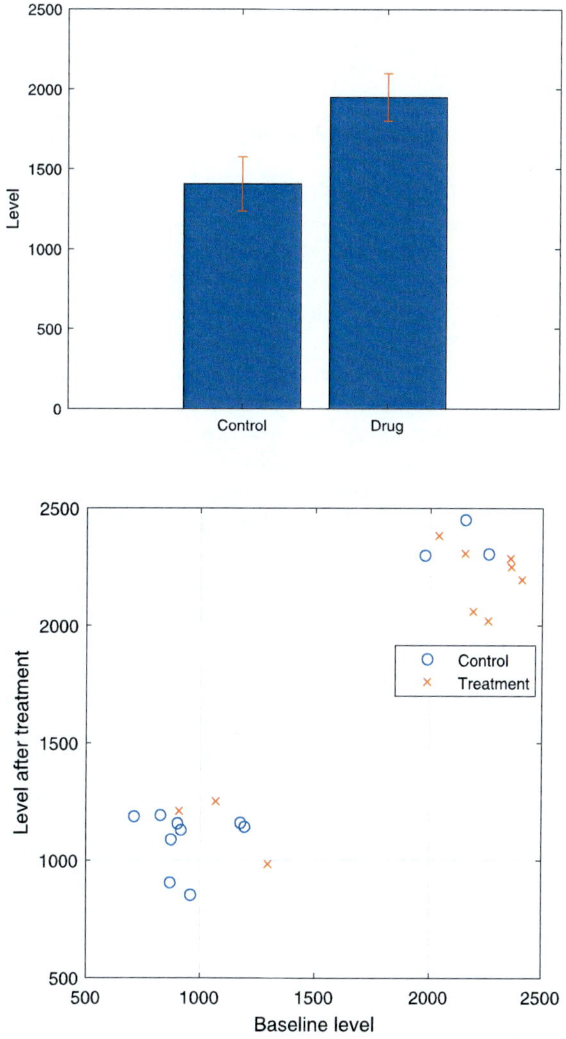

Fig. 1 Effect of the presence of subpopulations (see text)

of a study. From the plot at the top of Fig. 1 which shows means with standard error, we would conclude that the drug caused a significant increase over control. However, if we break the analysis down by the baseline level (see Fig. 1, bottom), we can see two different subpopulations with most of the treatment groups randomly assigned to the high baseline group and with no apparent effect of treatment in the two subpopulations.

An artificially low variance can be caused by violating the assumption of independence of the samples, either between groups or within a group. Independence between groups would be violated if the same individual participated in more than one group.

Independence within a group could be violated by collecting multiple samples from the same individual as we have seen earlier. These are technical replicates. They can be averaged to produce a single, more reproducible measurement, or we may integrate the measurements into a repeated measures ANOVA. This essentially blocks by individual. We need to be careful when making our material more homogeneous that we maintain as much scope as possible so that the results are more reproducible.

5.5 Averaging and Pooling

The value we observe for a measurement is the sum of the true value plus noise. The noise in an experiment is due to both biological variability and measurement error (which can be reduced by averaging a number of "technical replicates"). How many biological replicates and how many technical replicates we use depend upon the inherent variability and cost of each. For example, if we have a lot of variability in measurement, for example, cell counts, which is cheap to measure, we would be wise to carry out a number of cell counts and get an average. If there is a lot of animal-to-animal variability, then repeated measures techniques where the same measurement is measured multiple times on the same animal can give better estimates of average.

If we have more than one source of noise, we assume that the total effect is additive. However, not all measurement errors or sources of variability are additive. If the average follows a log distribution, then the noise will be similarly distributed. For this reason, in many fields, like microarray analysis [21], technical replicates are averaged using a geometric mean.

5.6 Blocking

Differences in our samples can be due to treatment or the combined variation induced by all other experimental variables. We can think in terms of a signal-to-noise ratio. The bigger the signal and the smaller the noise, the easier it is to show statistical significance. A good way to make our experiments more powerful and efficient is to identify sources of variability and block them out. This is at the core of the analysis of variance (ANOVA), analysis of covariance (ANCOVA), and generalized linear models (GLMs).

If we know the factor has an effect, for example, that there really are batch-to-batch differences, then it really makes sense to block this effect out in our experiments. If we suspect an effect, then we might still block. Blocking is an efficient form of "research insurance." Batch may or may not make a difference in our measurements, but if it does, by blocking, we will be able to remove its effect from the unexplained variance. Whatever factors we feel may affect an experimental outcome can be blocked. For example, if I cannot carry out an experiment on the effect of botulinum neurotoxins on pain in a rodent model all in one batch because there is too much work to do, I can split it into blocks. In Block 1 I have one surgeon inducing the pain by leg surgery on one batch of animals, and I measure the pain. A month later, in Block 2 I have a different surgeon inducing the pain in a second batch of animals, and I have to be away at a conference so a colleague will measure the pain. The surgeon-to-surgeon, batch-to-batch, week-to-week, and experimenter-to-experimenter variability is all taken out in one set of blocks. Blocking variables are therefore extremely "cheap" in terms of an extra number of animals for our experiment.

Sometimes there are quantitative factors like baseline measurements which we can be factored out. Rather than blocks or factors, these are called covariates, and factoring these out brings the same kind of benefits : removing unexplained variance. Our statistical analysis will then be even more sensitive to differences caused by our treatment. With the same number of animals, we will increase our statistical power. Or alternatively, for the same statistical power, we may reduce the number of animals in the experiment.

5.7 Paired Samples

Paired samples can be seen as a special case of blocking in which individuals serve as their own controls. There are a number of ways of doing this, for example, in experiments in which we can measure before and after applying the treatment or we can measure the response of the left and right eyes to different treatments or experiments with twins, siblings, or matched pairs (looking for another individual with similar characteristics). Crossover designs in which an individual is given a treatment for a period, followed by a "washout" period and then another treatment in another period are also analyzed as paired samples. However, care needs to be taken that the individual really reverts to its initial condition after the first treatment and that there are no "order" effects. For example, in measuring weight gain, the animal is likely to be larger in the second period and likely therefore to have a greater absolute weight gain.

Repeated measurements can be seen as an extension of paired samples. An animal is given a treatment and, then, measured multiple times, at different parts of its body or at different tasks. The different time points can be compared to the initial measurement at $t = 0$. Typically repeated measures are treated as a split-plot design in which the subject is the factor "hard to change."

By computing the difference between the two measurements, we remove the intersubject variability. Given that the two treatments are carried out on the same animal, we also halve the number of animals.

For two samples we typically would use a paired t-test rather than a two-sample t-test. There are non-parametric equivalents such as the Wilcoxon signed-rank test.

5.8 Blocking and Randomization

We may combine the benefits of blocking and randomization by first blocking and then randomizing within a block.

We could finish this section on blocking and randomization with a *statistical mantra* for experiment design: "*Control what you can, block what you cannot, and randomize the rest.*" We can control our treatments, we can block those variables that we think may have an impact on the variability of the observations, and the rest should be randomized (e.g., position of the cages in the animal house racks, the order of feeding and treating, the person applying the treatment, the person performing the measurements, the order of measuring, etc.).

▶ Important remarks

1. Control what you can, block what you cannot, and randomize the rest.

6 Automating Decision-Making: Hypothesis Testing

In God we trust, all others must bring data. (Anonymous)

In research we are typically trying to establish if our treatment has an effect, for example, a drug affects blood pressure. There are two complementary possibilities: the drug has an effect, which we call the alternative hypothesis, or the drug has no effect which is called the null hypothesis which has to accommodate all the other possibilities. How we specify these is very important to the efficiency of the statistical test. If we do not know what is going to happen, then we need to carry out what is called a two-tailed test. In a two-tailed test, the alternative hypothesis is that the drug has an effect (it could either reduce blood pressure or it could increase blood pressure), and the complementary null hypothesis is that the drug has no effect. If we anticipate a change with treatment in one direction only (e.g., our new drug is a new variant of a family of drugs which all reduce blood pressure, so we are expecting the new drug to either have no effect or to reduce blood pressure), we need to carry out what is called a one-tailed test. The drug may decrease or not the blood pressure (unexpectedly, it may even increase it); but we are only interested in identifying those drugs for which the drug decreases the blood pressure. In a one-tailed test, the alternative hypothesis in this case would be that the drug reduces blood pressure. The null hypothesis is that the drug either has no effect or increases blood pressure. The one-tailed test only looks at differences in one direction so needs a smaller number of animals for the same statistical significance. For any experiment there is variability, and this means that we can never be absolutely sure that the average for our treatment is really different from the control. It could be that the difference we are seeing is real but too small to pick up with the sample size that we are using. For this reason we can never accept the alternative hypothesis but rather try to disprove the null hypothesis. We need a way to decide if we can reject the null hypothesis. The best that we can do is to set arbitrary limits (typically a chance of 1 in 20 = 0.05) to a difference of this big happening by chance (the p-value). This is the whole basis of statistical significance testing.

One thing that is important and that a large proportion of researchers ignore is that every statistical test has assumptions that affect the p-value. For example, the t-test which is commonly used to compare a treatment to a standard or a control assumes that the distribution of sample averages is normally distributed (a histogram of the sample averages would look like a bell-shaped curve with a very specific fall-off). The p-value is based on putting limits on this curve to cut off certain values in the tail(s). If the data is not normally distributed, then you can see that this is all screwed up. Small deviations are going to produce small errors, and large deviations are going to produce large errors and may make the test of little value. It is therefore important when carrying out statistical tests that one tests the assumptions around that test.

These are examples of superiority tests (one-tailed tests) and significance tests (two-tailed tests). Superiority and significance tests are the most common ones used in animal research. However, there are other classes of tests which are used more in quality control. For instance, equivalence tests are typically used when we want to test if two treatments can be considered to be the same.

Example 1 We are testing a batch of botox to see if it conforms to standard. Note that rather than trying to disprove the null hypothesis as we did for significance testing and superiority testing, we are now trying to disprove the alternative hypothesis instead. This alternative hypothesis, rather than having a single value, will typically have upper and lower bounds of acceptability. For this reason tests of equivalence typically require much larger numbers of animals for the same statistical significance than the superiority and statistical tests which we typically would use for research.

$$H_0 : \pi_{batch} \neq \pi_{reference}$$
$$H_a : \pi_{batch} = \pi_{reference}$$

Example 2 If, for example, we are developing a new HepC vaccine, we want it to work at least as well as the reference vaccine. In this case the hypotheses are

$$H_0 : \pi_{new} > \pi_{reference}$$
$$H_a : \pi_{new} \leq \pi_{reference}$$

These non-inferiority tests (our new drug is at least as good as the reference), and the way to calculate the p-value and the number of animals is different from the significance tests in much the same way as the equivalence test.

Given that equivalence tests and non-inferiority tests require much larger numbers of animals than superiority tests and significance tests and that two-tailed tests need more animals than one-tailed tests, it is vitally important to specify the correct test as our understanding of the statistical significance will be hugely compromised if we use the wrong test. In animal research, we need the right test, and we also need the right number of animals. This is going to be based on the the effect size, which is the difference between treatment and control.

▶ Important Remarks

2. The smaller the difference we want to detect (the effect size), the larger the number of experimental units required for the experiment.
3. We can reject or not the null hypothesis.
4. Failing to reject the null hypothesis does not make it true.

6.1 An Intuitive Introduction to Hypothesis Testing

This section gives a nontechnical insight into the hypothesis testing procedure. The reader is referred to Ellenberg [9] for an excellent general public book on statistical, and mathematical in general, thinking. Ellenberg manages to smoothly introduce the reader into many complex statistical concepts.

The goal of hypothesis testing is to disprove the null hypothesis. Suppose we have a new drug that we feel should reduce blood pressure and we want to find out if there is a reasonable probability that it does so. The alternative hypothesis is therefore that drug reduces blood pressure, and the null hypothesis, which has to cover all other possibilities, is that either the drug does not have any effect, or it increases blood pressure. We treat 16 individuals with the drug and measure their blood pressure before and after treatment. This kind of design is an efficient design called a crossover design. Basically for each individual, we are working on the difference between the before and after treatments and are using the "before" measurement as a control for the drug treatment rather than having one pool of individuals treated with the drug and a separate pool of individuals given a placebo. By doing this we are removing the person-to-person variability in blood pressure before being given the drug. It also halves the number of individuals that we need. We are using it here because it makes the explanation of hypothesis testing slightly more simple. We have an average effect size (before blood pressure–after blood pressure). If the drug had no effect, then we would expect the before and after blood pressure to be the same (zero reduction in blood pressure), so we're comparing what we find as an average effect size (say 10 mm Hg reduction on average in blood pressure) against zero (drug has no effect). Not all individuals will show the same reduction in blood pressure so we also need to consider a measure of variability. We can measure this variability by the standard deviation (say 20 mg Hg). We have just taken a sample of 16 individuals so rather than working with the distribution of individual values, we are working on a distribution of sample averages; it stands to reason that an average of 16 individuals is going to give us a better average value than the individual values themselves, and the more samples, the better the average. The standard deviation of this distribution of sample averages, which we call the standard error = standard deviation/square root of sample size. In our example 20 mm Hg/square root of 16 $= 20/4 = 5$ mm Hg. Where do we put our cutoff point that dictates that we can reject the null hypothesis that the drug has no effect or increases blood pressure? Well we want to put the cutoff at that point that cuts off 5% of the distribution into the one tail on the low side. The theoretical distribution of the normal curve (z-distribution) that cuts 5% off in one tail is at 1.65 standard errors away from the mean, so $1.65 \times (-5\text{mm Hg}) = -8.25$ mm Hg. Our average was lower than this at -10 mm Hg so we have a statistically significant reduction in average blood pressure with our drug. Note that the expression "statistically significant" does not mean "practically important," but rather that its effect is clearly different from the effect expected under the null hypothesis. For example, with a very large sample size (say 100 individuals), we could have detected as significant a very small reduction in blood pressure that may not be practically useful.

The significance level that we use, $p = 0.05$, is going to give a false positive in 5% of our experiments even if our drug does not have any effect. We therefore have to be careful with the 0.05 threshold of the classical statistical testing where we are screening many samples; for example, 10,000 readings from a gene array will generate on average 500 false positives. The more tests we do and the smaller the sample size in those tests, the more likely we are to generate false positives, and in recent years, there has been a concern about the reproducibility of research studies. There are systemic reasons for this like small experimental groups, the pressure to publish significant results, the fact that negative results cannot normally be published, the fact that the same or similar problems are studied by many groups worldwide, and, just by chance, one of them gets a significant result, the fact that results tend to be published only once (if it is a positive result, a second, third, …group cannot normally publish the confirmation of the result; and if it is a negative result, it is more difficult to publish because it goes against the "established, peer-reviewed" previous result), the researcher's freedom to choose the data to analyze and the analysis technique [15, 24], etc.

We need to be mindful with a statistical significance level of $p = 0.05$ that 1 in 20 experiments will generate statistically significant findings purely by chance.

6.2 Statistical Power and Confidence

The chance of getting a false positive is defined by the significance level (typically $p = 0.05$) and the chance of getting a false negative by the power of the test (typically set to 0.8 to 0.9).

For experiments with live animals, it is essential to use 3R principles; carrying out a power calculation is an excellent way to produce a robust justification of animal numbers for funding bodies and regulatory authorities.

Important Remarks

5. For a fixed confidence level and treatment effect size, increasing the number of animals increases our statistical power: If our treatment makes a difference, we will detect it with more probability.
6. For a fixed confidence level and statistical power, increasing the number of animals increases our experiment sensitivity (the detectable effect size is smaller).
7. By calculating the sample size before performing the experiment, we can control the type I and II errors at will, assuming that there are not systematic errors causing bias.

The freedom of many researchers to choose the data and the variables that participate in the analysis may inflate the effective false positive rate (type I errors, α) well above the 0.05 level (up to 0.6 as reported by Simmons et al. [24]). The solution suggested by these authors is reporting the specific choices performed, all the data measured, and the analysis with and without any removed data.

Important Remarks

8. Confidence intervals are much more stable than individual tests of significance [8]. There have been recent alarms on the reproducibility of experiments in science [1,3] and its economical impacts [12]. Among many other reasons, experiments with low statistical power and poor (but significant p-values) are behind this recent concern. There has been a recent and very simple proposal to increase the reproducibility in many experiments, simply by lowering the significance threshold from 0.05 to 0.005 and relabeling the experiments with p-values in the range 0.05 to 0.005 as suggestive results [4]. This could be achieved by adequately powering the experiments to a power of 0.9 rather than the power of 0.5 implied by a p-value of 0.05.

6.3 Multiple Testing

In drug screening we can test the effect of thousands of compounds on a cell culture, or microarray experiments give the expression level of thousands of genes. This is going to generate a large number of false positives. A well-known correction is the Bonferroni correction which divides the significance level (typically $p = 0.05$) by the number of tests. While this will maintain the overall significance level to control the generation of false positives, to do so requires us to make the test more stringent, and this will increase the chance of getting false negatives:

$$\alpha = \frac{\alpha_{family}}{K}$$

The Bonferroni test is very conservative, and other corrections have been suggested like Sidak:

$$\alpha = 1 - (1 - \alpha_{family})^{\frac{1}{K}}$$

A very popular approach to control the family type I error is the Benjamini-Hochberg procedure. First, we sort the K p-values of the K tests in ascending order ($p_1, p_2, \ldots, p_K$). Second, we reject the null hypothesis for the k-th test if

$$p_k \leq k\frac{\alpha_{family}}{K}$$

Once we cannot reject the null hypothesis for the test k_0, we cannot reject it for $k > k_0$ and so stop the sequence of comparisons once non-significance is reached.

The best strategy is to minimize the number of tests, restricting it to only those comparisons which are most important. These need to be specified in advance of the experiments being carried out to prevent "data snooping."

7 A Primer in Sample Size Calculations

We can at this point partly understand the logic behind sample size calculation. When we do the experiment, we will reject the null hypothesis if our sample mean is further than a set number of standard errors from the control:

$$\left| \frac{\hat{\mu} - \mu_0}{\frac{\sigma}{\sqrt{N}}} \right| > z_{1-\frac{\alpha}{2}}$$

Treatment effect/standard error has to be greater than the cutoff for statistical significance (for $\alpha = 0.05$, this is 1.96 for a two-tailed test and 1.65 for a one-tailed test). Rewrite the effect size as Δ. We may rearrange the above equation and solve for the sample size:

$$N > \left(\frac{z_{1-\frac{\alpha}{2}}\sigma}{\Delta}\right)^2 = \left(\frac{z_{1-\frac{\alpha}{2}}}{\Delta/\sigma}\right)^2 \quad (1)$$

Our sample size, N, has to be bigger than (cutoff value/standardized effect size)^2. If we want to detect with a confidence of 95% a change of 0.25°C in a thermostat temperature, whose standard deviation is 0.5°C, then we simply need to plug in our specifications into Eq. 1:

$$N > \left(\frac{1.96}{0.25/0.5}\right)^2 = 15.36$$

That is, we need at least 16 samples to detect such changes. Note that this gives us a sample size which will give us a statistically significant result only half of the time. With temperature samples, we may use more if desired, but with animal samples, we run into ethical and economic considerations (why use more animals in an experiment, whose goal has a strong likelihood of being achieved with fewer animals?).

In the graphs we have the distribution of the original control thermostat readings in red and that of the revised thermostat readings with a difference on average of 2.5 degrees in blue. The black line on the graphs is the lower cutoff for a two-tailed significance level p = 0.05. In the upper graph, we have chosen a sample size which is necessary for statistical significance (Fig. 2).

- Including power. If we want to increase our power to detect an effect, then we need to incorporate this into the previous equation:

$$N = \left(\frac{z_{1-\frac{\alpha}{2}} + z_{1-\beta}}{\Delta/\sigma}\right)^2 \quad (2)$$

where the new term is the cutoff for a desired power. A z-value of 0.84 will cut off 80% of the treatment, and a value of 1.28 will cut off 90% of the treatment. Basically we only need four numbers to plug into this equation, 1.96 for a two-tailed test, 1.65 for a one-tailed test, 0.84 for 80% power and 1.28 for 90% power.

For the specifications of the thermostat ($\Delta = 0.25$, $\alpha = 0.05$ and $\beta = 0.2$), we have

$$N = \left(\frac{1.96 + 0.84}{0.25/0.5}\right)^2 = 31.40$$

That is, we need at least 32 samples to detect a departure of 0.25°C from the reference tem-

Parameter	Control	tmt
Mean	20	17.5
SD	5	5
sample size (n)	**15.36**	
Standard Error	1.275775908	
treatment effect	**-2.5**	
Tails	**2**	
Standard Errors to 95% cutoff limit (s)	1.96	
95% Cutoff limit	*17.49947922*	
Power	**0.500**	
Average sig	**0.050**	

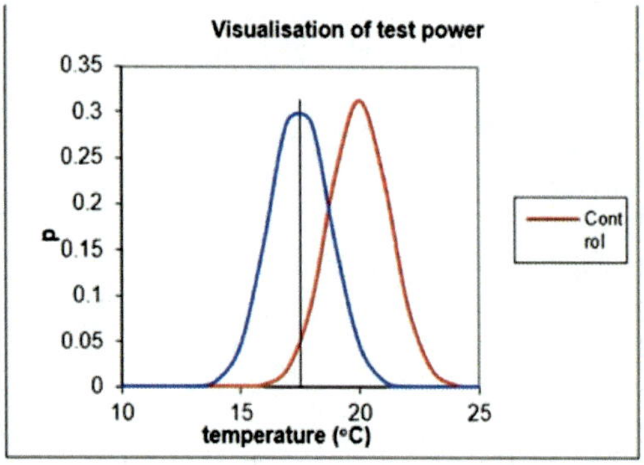

Fig. 2 Significance and power (see text)

Parameter	Control	tmt
Mean	20	17.5
SD	5	5
sample size (n)	**31.4**	
Standard Error	0.892288263	
treatment effect	**-2.5**	
Tails	**2**	
Standard Errors to 95% cutoff limit (s)	1.96	
95% Cutoff limit	*18.251115*	
Power	**0.800**	
Average sig	**0.005**	

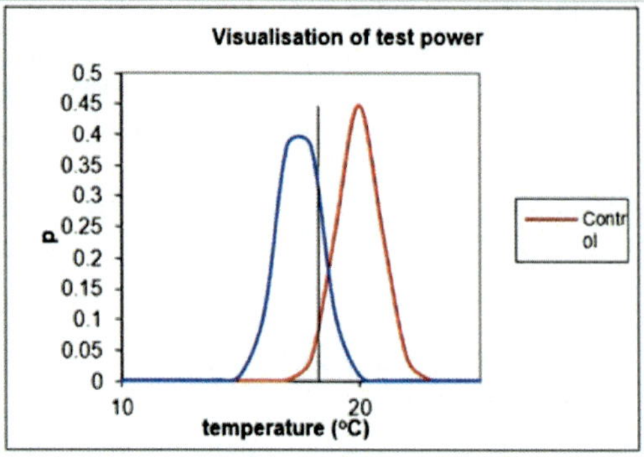

Fig. 3 Power (see text)

perature with a statistical confidence of 95% and a statistical power of 80% (Fig. 3).

7.1 Sample Size Lessons

The main formula for the sample size calculation in the example above was

$$N = \left(\frac{z_{1-\frac{\alpha}{2}} + z_{1-\beta}}{\Delta/\sigma} \right)^2$$

This formula already shows the ideas exposed in Sect. 6:

Important remarks

9. There is no "universal" sample size formula valid for all experiments and situations, but there is a general formula based on the standardized effect size, the significance level chosen, and the power desired.

Non-parametric tests are often used if the experimental data does not fulfill the assumptions of parametric tests. However we can design the sample size based on a parametric test and then correct by some "safety" factor that accounts for the lower efficiency of non-parametric tests. In this way, the sample size is calculated as

$$N_{non-parametric} = \frac{N_{parametric}}{ARE} \quad (3)$$

where ARE is the asymptotic relative efficiency. The following table shows the most common non-parametric tests along with their parametric counterparts and ARE:

Non-parametric	Purpose	Parametric	ARE
Mann-Whitney U test	Compare two independent samples	Student's t-test	$3/\pi =$ 0.955
Wilcoxon signed-rank test	Compare two dependent samples	Paired Student's t-test	$3/\pi =$ 0.955
Spearman correlation test	Correlation between two variables	Pearson's correlation test	0.91
Kruskal-Wallis ANOVA	Compare three or more groups	One-way ANOVA	0.864
If not in this table			0.85

There are a number of situations in which the sample size calculation fails, in particular.

▶ **Important Remarks**

10. If we assume an incorrect variance of the observations. This is a very common error, and we tend to be optimistic about the variability of our experiments.
11. If we violate the assumptions of the hypothesis test, especially the distribution of the observations.
12. If we misunderstand the questions performed by the sample size calculation software. It is advisable, if possible, to use two different software or verify with some easy-to-calculate approximate formula.

Given that we are usually working with an estimate of both the treatment effect and the variability of the data prior to carrying out the experiment, we need to be mindful that the sample size calculations are our best guess as to the sample size required.

The next chapter shows the assumptions and consequences for the most common experimental situations encountered in animal research. It is meant to be a reference chapter, so that we only look up the case in which we are interested at a particular moment. In a first pass over the book, the reader may go over the examples and important remarks to get an idea of the kind of problems he/she may encounter and for which there is already a good statistical solution.

Bibliography

1. Baker M. 1,500 scientists lift the lid on reproducibility. Nature. 2016;533:452–54.
2. Bebarta V, Luyten D, Heard K. Emergency medicine animal research: does use of randomization and blinding affect the results? Acad Emer Med. 2003;10(6):684–7.
3. Begley CG, Ioannidis JPA. Reproducibility in science: improving the standard for basic and preclinical research. Circ Res. 2015;116:116–26.
4. Benjamin DJ, Berger JO, Johannesson M, Nosek BA, Wagenmakers EJ, Berk R, Bollen KA, Brembs B, Brown L, Camerer C, et al. Redefine statistical significance. Nat Hum Behav. 2018;2(1):6.
5. Chia R, Achilli F, Festing MFW, Fisher EMC. The origins and uses of mouse outbred stocks. Nat Genet. 2005;37:1181–6.
6. Chvedoff M, Clarke MR, Faccini JM, Irisarri E, Monro AM. Effects on mice of numbers of animals per cage: an 18-month study (preliminary results). Arch Toxicol Suppl. 1980;4:435–8.
7. Crabbe JC, Wahlsten D, Dudek BC. Genetics of mouse behavior: interactions with laboratory environment. Science (New York, NY). 1999;284:1670–2.
8. Cumming G. Replication and p intervals: p values predict the future only vaguely, but confidence intervals do much better. Perspect Psychol Sci. 2008;3(4):286–300.
9. Ellenberg J. How not to be wrong. The power of mathematical thinking. Penguin Books, USA, 2014.
10. Festing MFW. Principles: The need for better experimental design. Trends Pharmacol Sci. 2003;24:341–5.

11. Festing MFW, Altman DG. Guidelines for the design and statistical analysis of experiments using laboratory animals. ILAR J. 2002;43(4):244–58.
12. Freedman LP, Cockburn IM, Simcoe TS. The economics of reproducibility in preclinical research. PLoS Biol. 2015;13:e1002,165.
13. Higgins JP, Green S. Cochrane handbook for systematic reviews of interventions, vol. 4. John Wiley & Sons, USA, 2011.
14. Hooijmans CR, Rovers MM, de Vries RBM, Leenaars M, Ritskes-Hoitinga M, Langendam MW. Syrcle's risk of bias tool for animal studies. BMC Med Res Methodol. 2014;14:43.
15. Ioannidis JPA. Why most published research findings are false. PLoS Med. 2005;2:e124. https://doi.org/10.1371/journal.pmed.0020124.
16. Jay Jr GE. Variation in response of various mouse strains to hexobarbital (evipal). Proc Soc Exp Biol Med. 1955;90(2):378–80.
17. Johnson WE, Li C, Rabinovic A. Adjusting batch effects in microarray expression data using empirical bayes methods. Biostatistics 2007;8(1):118–27.
18. Kilkenny C, Browne WJ, Cuthill IC, Emerson M, Altman DG. Improving bioscience research reporting: the arrive guidelines for reporting animal research. PLoS Biol. 2010;8:e1000,412.
19. Macleod MR, Fisher M, O'Collins V, Sena ES, Dirnagl U, Bath PMW, Buchan A, Buchan A, van der Worp HB, Traystman RJ, Minematsu K, Donnan GA, Howells DW. Reprint: Good laboratory practice: preventing introduction of bias at the bench. J Cereb Blood Flow Metab. 2009;29:221–3.
20. Macleod MR, Lawson McLean A, Kyriakopoulou A, Serghiou S, de Wilde A, Sherratt N, Hirst T, Hemblade R, Bahor Z, Nunes-Fonseca C, Potluru A, Thomson A, Baginskaite J, Baginskitae J, Egan K, Vesterinen H, Currie GL, Churilov L, Howells DW, Sena ES. Risk of bias in reports of in vivo research: a focus for improvement. PLoS Biol. 2015;13:e1002,273. https://doi.org/10.1371/journal.pbio.1002273
21. Quackenbush J. Microarray data normalization and transformation. Nat Genet. 2002;32(Suppl):496–501.
22. ter Riet G, Korevaar DA, Leenaars M, Sterk PJ, Van Noorden CJF, Bouter LM, Lutter R, Elferink RPO, Hooft L. Publication bias in laboratory animal research: a survey on magnitude, drivers, consequences and potential solutions. PloS One. 2012;7:e43,404. https://doi.org/10.1371/journal.pone.0043404
23. Sackett DL, et al. Bias in analytic research. J Chron Dis. 1979;32:51–63.
24. Simmons JP, Nelson LD, Simonsohn U. False-positive psychology: undisclosed flexibility in data collection and analysis allows presenting anything as significant. Psychol Sci. 2011;22:1359–66.
25. Sorzano COS, Tabas-Madrid D, Núñez F, Fernández-Criado C, Naranjo A. Sample size for pilot studies and precision driven experiments. 2017. arXiv preprint arXiv:170700222.
26. Sullivan LM, Weinberg J, Keaney JF. Common statistical pitfalls in basic science research. J Am Heart Assoc. 2016;5: e004142.
27. Thompson SK. Sampling. John Wiley & Sons, USA, 2012.
28. Zeng X, Zhang Y, Kwong JS, Zhang C, Li S, Sun F, Niu Y, Du L. The methodological quality assessment tools for preclinical and clinical studies, systematic review and meta-analysis, and clinical practice guideline: a systematic review. J Evid Based Med. 2015;8(1):2–10.

Statistical Tests and Sample Size Calculations

Michael Parkinson and Carlos Oscar Sánchez Sorzano

In this chapter we will review the most common cases encountered in animal experiments:

1. Hypothesis test: These studies aim at rejecting a null hypothesis, for example, that our drug has no effect on blood pressure.
2. Confidence intervals: These studies aim at specifying a range of values around the average of a parameter of interest such as the average blood pressure.

Both tests are based on the same statistical inference theory. In fact, the hypothesis test can be calculated by computing a confidence interval on a statistic and checking if this statistic includes the value specified by the null hypothesis.

Calculating the sample size prior to the experiment is vital to scientific success. It is important prior to the experiment to have a reasonable expectation of seeing statistically significant findings out of your research, and power calculations can be a valuable justification for the number of animals used.

M. Parkinson
School of Biotechnology, Dublin City University, Dublin, Ireland
e-mail: michael.parkinson@dcu.ie

C. O. S. Sorzano (✉)
Natl. Center of Biotechnology (CSIC), Madrid, Spain
e-mail: coss@cnb.csic.es

The chapter is written as a reference and there is no need to read it all together. However, in a first reading, we recommend to see the examples to get an idea of the kind of problems that can be successfully solved and that cover a wide spectrum of experimental situations.

1 Sample Size for the Mean

1.1 Hypothesis Test on the Mean of One Sample When the Variance Is Known

The hypothesis test is of the form:

$$\begin{aligned} H_0 &: \mu = \mu_0 \\ H_a &: \mu \neq \mu_0 \end{aligned} \tag{1}$$

The sample size formula was

$$N = \left(\frac{z_{1-\frac{\alpha}{2}} + z_{1-\beta}}{\tilde{\Delta}} \right)^2 \tag{2}$$

Example 3 In the example of the laboratory temperature, the standard deviation of the thermostat is $\sigma = 0.5°$, we wanted to detect a deviation of $\Delta = 0.25°$, with a statistical power of 80% and

© Springer Nature Switzerland AG 2021

J. M. Sánchez Morgado, A. Brønstad (eds.), *Experimental Design and Reproducibility in Preclinical Animal Studies*, Laboratory Animal Science and Medicine 1,
https://doi.org/10.1007/978-3-030-66147-2_7

a statistical confidence of 95%. As we showed above, this requires 32 samples:

$$N = \left(\frac{z_{0.975} + z_{0.8}}{\tilde{\Delta}}\right)^2 = \left(\frac{1.96 + 0.84}{0.25/0.5}\right)^2 = 31.40$$

If we have an additional source of error, for example, if our thermometer also has a measurement error whose standard deviation is 0.2° that adds to the standard deviation of the thermostat and can be factored in as shown below. Independent additive variables (true temperature+thermometer error) add their variances, so that the variance of our observations will be

$$\sigma^2 = \sigma^2_{thermostat} + \sigma^2_{thermometer} = 0.5^2 + 0.2^2 = 0.29$$

The standard deviation of our measurements becomes now

$$\sigma = \sqrt{0.29} = 0.54$$

And the sample size

$$N = \left(\frac{1.96 + 0.84}{0.25/0.54}\right)^2 = 36.57$$

That is, we would need 37 samples to take the decision of stopping the thermostat or not. This is 5h later if we take a sample every hour than in the case of a perfect thermometer due to the extra uncertainty introduced by the measurement process. However, we may reduce the reaction time to the same 32h as in the case of a perfect thermometer by simply taking eight samples every hour of the current temperature and averaging them. The averaging will reduce the uncertainty due to the thermometer, but it cannot reduce the uncertainty due to the thermostat:

$$\sigma^2 = \sigma^2_{thermostat} + \sigma^2_{thermometer}/8 = 0.5^2 + 0.2^2/8 = 0.255$$

and now the required sample size is

$$N = \left(\frac{1.96 + 0.84}{0.25/\sqrt{0.255}}\right)^2 = 31.99$$

That is, $N = 32$.

1.2 Hypothesis Test on the Mean of One Sample When the Variance Is Unknown

This case is much more common than the previous one. If the variance is unknown, we have to estimate it from the samples. Instead of the standard normal distribution, the z-distribution, we have to use the t-distribution instead. The t-value is always bigger than the corresponding z-value, but the larger the sample, the more similar the estimates are between t and z. For sample sizes of 30 or bigger, there is very little difference between t and z, and the estimate is not hugely different for sample sizes of 10 or greater.

Example 4 For the previous example in which the standard deviation of the observations was supposed to be close to 0.54 and we wanted to detect deviations of at least 0.25°C, we would require N = 51.

As expected, this sample size is larger than the one in Example 3, $N = 37$, because we have to estimate the standard deviation from the data, instead of assuming it as known. Less prior information results in larger sample sizes. We are now using t rather than z and t is always larger than the corresponding z value.

1.3 Confidence Interval for the Mean

The sample size design for hypothesis test on a single mean with unknown variance can also be used to calculate the sample size needed to estimate a confidence interval of the mean at t-standard errors.

Example 5 Consider the thermostat Example 4, in which we want to construct a 95% confidence interval whose maximum half-width is 0.25°C. We presume that the standard deviation of the observations will be close to 0.54. The number of samples required for this experiment is

$$N = \left(\frac{t_{0.95,0,N-1}}{0.25/0.54}\right)^2 \Rightarrow N = 21$$

Note that it is much smaller than in the Example 4, the reason being that we only want to construct a confidence interval, rather than testing if the thermostat is malfunctioning with an hypothesis test.

▶ **Important Remarks**

13. Constructing confidence intervals requires much smaller sample sizes than testing a hypothesis because we are essentially working with a power of 0.5 with a confidence interval, whereas we will be powering up for a power of 0.8–0.9 for a statistical test.

1.4 Hypothesis Test on the Mean for Paired Samples

Example 6 Suppose we are interested in the effect of a new compound on eczema. Our model is ear thickening, and since an animal has two ears, we can apply treatment to one ear and have the other as its own control. We could treat each treatment separately and just pool all treatment values and pool all control values, but if we do this, the animal-to-animal variability gets lumped in with error. By using instead the difference in ear thickness between the two ears of the same animal, we remove the variability between subjects, and the effect of the treatment is easier to detect due to the lower variance. We also use half the number of animals since both control and treatment are carried out on the same animal. The statistical analysis is also simpler as we have essentially reduced a hypothesis test on the difference between two samples to a one-sample test.

1.5 Hypothesis Test on the Difference of the Mean of Two Samples

This is, probably, the most common kind of test in biomedical and animal research. We study the difference between the mean of two groups, typically a treatment and a control group. The difference with the case of the previous section is that each subject is not its own control anymore, and the animals in both groups are different. This is, for example, the case of the development of most new drugs. The drug is tested on a treatment group and its effect is compared to a control group. We produce a combined estimate of the standard deviation and test with this. How we calculate this depends upon whether the variances can be considered to be the same or not, and these two different ways of computing the standard deviation will result in a slightly different significance for the test if we assume equal variances than if we assume unequal variances. The decision on whether the variances can be considered equal is made by carrying out an F-test. This may need to be carried out prior to the analysis or may be routinely carried out as part of the computation in the statistical analysis. Apart from the specific details of the formulas, which are irrelevant from a user perspective because these formulas are implemented in software programs that help the researcher to design the experiment, there are some important lessons to learn from the sample size design formulas seen so far:

▶ **Important Remarks**

14. The sample size formula depends on how the data will be analyzed. Specifically, on the test that will be performed (a test on the mean of a sample, on the mean of the difference, on the difference between two means, and also on whether we use a one-tail or two-tail test).
15. If we know the population standard deviation, we use the z-test, and if the variance is unknown and needs to be estimated from the observations, we use Student's t.
16. The normalized effect size plays a crucial role in all designs, and each specific case has its own normalization rules.

1.6 Hypothesis Test on the Mean of Several Groups (ANOVA)

Analysis of variance (ANOVA) is a statistical technique that allows us to test whether the mean of a collection of groups, normally called treatments, is all equal. This is a rather common situation in science, and technically it is called a one-way ANOVA because we have only one variable defining the groups (the different treatment applied to each group).

Example 6 Continuing with the example of the previous section on blood pressure (Example 3), we are simultaneously studying multiple drugs. Each group receives one of the drugs. If at least one of them reduces the blood pressure 5 mm Hg (from 130 of hypertensive mice to 125), then we want to detect this change with a statistical confidence of 95% and a statistical power of 80%?

If there are T treatments, the ANOVA hypotheses are

$$\begin{aligned} H_0 &: \mu_1 = \mu_2 = \ldots = \mu_T \\ H_a &: \mu_i \neq \mu_j \quad \text{foratleasttwoofthetreatments} \end{aligned} \tag{3}$$

For just two groups, ANOVA is equivalent to the hypothesis test on the difference of the mean of two independent samples (see the previous section), in fact F = t-squared. For more than two groups, if the ANOVA test rejects the null hypothesis, then at least one of the groups is different from the rest, but we do not know which one. Thus there are important consequences for interpretation of the results if negative and positive controls are included in your experiment as is usually the case; usually we are interested in the effect of some factor, for example, a drug, but if negative and positive controls are included, then we can expect to see a difference between these, and we will see a significant effect irrespective of what effect your drug is having. It is therefore important to perform *post hoc* tests to identify which groups are different. Multiple t-tests are not the best solution since these will need to be Bonferroni corrected to account for generation of false positives. The *post hoc* tests built into the statistical programs normally explicitly account for the multiple comparisons of inflation of the Type I error (see Sect. 6.3). Among the post hoc procedures, Tukey's honestly significant difference test is one of the most popular, but many other tests exist.

▶ **Important remarks**

17. Sample size designs based on ANOVA are specifically aimed at rejecting the ANOVA null hypothesis (all means are the same), and care needs to be taken in interpreting these if both negative controls and positive controls are included.
18. If post hoc tests are important in our research, we should design the experiment using the two sample designs of the previous section taking into account that we may incur in a Type I error inflation due to multiple testing.

As a simplified design, Mead's resource equation has been proposed. This equation states that the number of samples, N, must fulfill

$$N - 1 = T + B + E \tag{4}$$

where T is the number of treatments, B the number of blocks, and E the number of degrees of freedom available for the residuals, which should be between 10 and 20. This equation is based on the number of degrees of freedom consumed by each one of the different components of the variance (see chapter "Design of Experiments" for a detailed explanation of this decomposition). As can be easily seen, this design does not make any consideration of effect size and power. Although we cannot give an exact number for the effect size addressed by this formula, this can be estimated to be (depending on the number of treatments and blocks) between 1.5 and 2 with a statistical power of 90%. That is, this design is capable of identifying changes in the mean of one of the groups if this change is at least 1.5 times the standard deviation of the observations for each one of the treatments. This may be useful for complicated flavors of ANOVA and as a "rule of thumb" to make sure that the sample size is of the right order, but better is to carry out a power analysis based on expected results.

1.7 Unequal Group Sizes

In the previous section, the variance of our estimate of the difference is

$$\sigma^2_{\hat{\mu}_{\Delta_y}} = \frac{\sigma_1^2}{N_1} + \frac{\sigma_2^2}{N_2}$$

We can minimize total variance while keeping the total number of samples fixed by changing the distribution of samples:

$$\min_{N_1,N_2} \frac{\sigma_1^2}{N_1} + \frac{\sigma_2^2}{N_2} \quad \text{subjectto} N_1 + N_2 = \text{constant}$$

The solution is

$$N_2 = N_1 \frac{\sigma_2}{\sigma_1} \tag{5}$$

▶ **Important Remarks**

19. That is, we should put more samples in the more variable groups, and if the two groups are equally variable, then the number of samples in both groups will be the same $N_1 = N_2$.

Another situation in which we may want to have different group sizes is when the cost of getting samples from Group 1 is different from the cost of getting samples in Group 2.

20. We can put more samples in the less costly group.

Finally, if a number of different treatments are to be compared to a control group, we can minimize the total sample size by using a larger proportion of the total in the comparison group. The solution is

$$N_0 = N_T \sqrt{T} \tag{6}$$

▶ **Important remarks**

21. That is, we should put more samples in the control group, since it will participate in many more comparisons, and diminishing its variance will result into more powerful comparisons.

1.8 Hypothesis Test on the Equivalence of Two Means

Many research experiments respond to the significance test paradigm:

$$H_0 : \mu_1 = \mu_2$$
$$H_a : \mu_1 \neq \mu_2$$

If we reject the null hypothesis, then we presume that the true state of affairs is the alternative hypothesis, and the mean in the group of the new treatment is different from the one in the control.

However, some studies respond to the equivalence test paradigm:

$$H_0 : \mu_1 \neq \mu_2$$
$$H_a : \mu_1 = \mu_2$$

Note that the equal sign has moved from the null hypothesis to the alternative hypothesis. If we reject the null hypothesis, then we presume that the true state of affairs is the alternative hypothesis, and the mean of the treatment and control groups is not different. This is the case, for example, of bioequivalence: we need to show that the effect of our new drug is not different, within limits, from the effect of the reference drug.

Technically, equivalence tests are more expensive in animals than their significance test counterparts. The reason is that the null hypothesis of equivalence tests imply two different tests. To see how this arises, let us first define when two means are considered to be "the same." Normally, it is assumed that two means are the same if their difference, $\Delta\mu = \mu_1 - \mu_2$, is small.

According to the European Medicines Agency Guideline CPMP/EWP/QWP/1401/98, a drug (normally, a new generic coming into the market) is bioequivalent to another (the reference drug) if the effect of the new drug is within a limit from 80% (=0.8) to 125% (=1/0.8) of the effect of the reference (see Fig. 1).

Example 6 We are developing a generic of a drug against hypertension. The reference drug is capable of lowering the mean systolic blood pressure of a mouse model of hypertension from 130 mmHg to 120 mmHg (see Example 3). The effect size of the reference drug is $\Delta = -10$ mmHg. The new drug is a bioequivalent of the reference if its effect size is between 8 and 12.5 mmHg. From this data, we can compute the lower and upper limits for the equivalence tests. $\Delta\mu = \mu_{reference} - \mu_{generic}$, and it must be

$$120 - 122 < \Delta\mu < 120 - 117.5$$

Equivalence tests are therefore usually translated into two one-sided t-tests (TOST) on the upper side of the upper limit and on the lower side of the lower limit (here lower than 117.5 or higher than 122).

Our new drug is bioequivalent to the reference drug if we can reject the two null hypotheses. We will not give at this moment explicit design formulas as the sample size design software implement them and we have already settled the main ideas of sample size calculations.

Example 6 (continued) For our drug bioequivalence problem, we will need $N_{reference} = N_{generic} = 166$ observations (statistical power of 90% and statistical confidence of 95%). If we compare this sample size with the significance test $N = 26$, we see that there is a dramatic increase in required sample size.

Figure 2 shows the statistical distributions of the two null hypotheses and the alternative hypotheses when $\Delta\mu = 0$. For significance tests, the null hypothesis results in a centered distribution of the statistic, and the alternative hypotheses are on each side. However, for equivalence tests, it is just the opposite.

Important Remarks

22. Although equivalence tests use the same "ingredients" as significance tests (statistical confidence and power, one-tail statistical tests), they are used in a different manner. Most importantly, significance tests have a single null hypothesis, while equivalence tests have two.
23. It is much more difficult to show equivalence than significance: the number of samples in equivalence tests is normally much higher.

2 Sample Size for Proportions

Many research studies aim at identifying the proportion of a population that responds to a given treatment that has a certain phenotype or that have a given characteristic. As we did with means, experiments with proportions can be performed with one group (we analyze the proportion within a single group) or two groups (we analyze the difference in proportions between two groups).

2.1 Hypothesis Test on One Small Proportion

Example 7 We are developing a vaccine against a pathogen. We are only interested in vaccines for which the probability of infection when directly exposed to the pathogen is below 1%. How many individuals do we need to show that a given vaccine is useful?

In this example, the hypothesis test we need is

$$H_0 : p \geq 0.01$$
$$H_a : p < 0.01$$

where p is the probability of infection when directly exposed to the pathogen.

We can use the binomial distribution equation to work out the proportion in each class. As with one sample comparison discussed earlier, we are interested in the value of the distribution that cuts off 5% of the value in the lower tail.

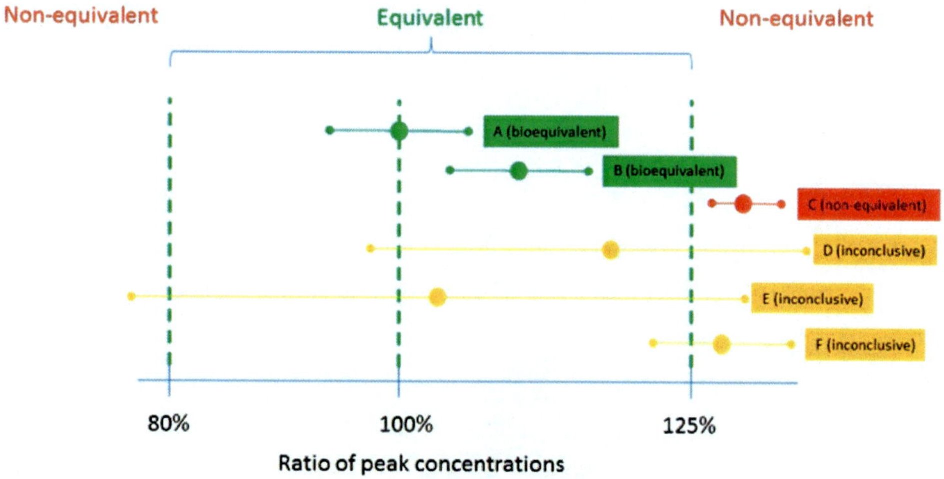

Fig. 1 Two drugs are said to be bioequivalent if the 95% confidence interval of the ratio of variables of relevance (peak concentration, effect, etc.) is inside the bioequivalent area defined between 80% and 125%. The figure shows six different possible confidence intervals and the interpretation of each one of the results

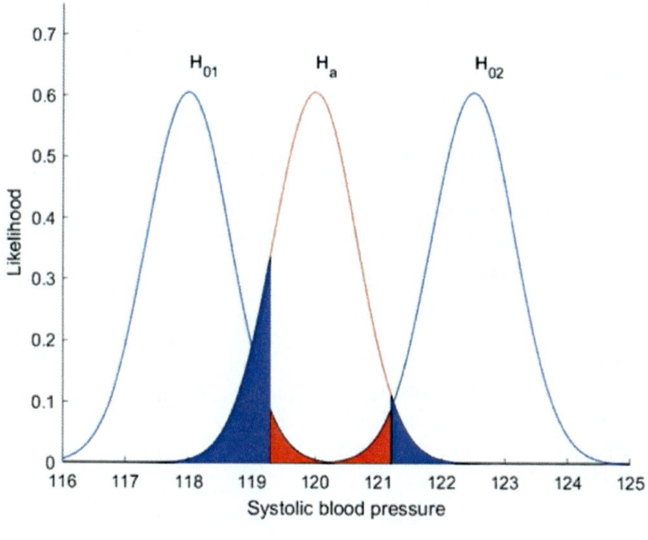

Fig. 2 The red-shaded area is the probability of rejecting any of the null hypotheses if they are true (this area is the complement of the statistical confidence). The blue-shaded area is the probability of not rejecting the null hypotheses when the alternative hypothesis is true (only represented for $\Delta\mu = 0$). The symmetry is broken by the 80% and 125% requirement of the guideline

In the example of the vaccine, the probability of observing x infections among the N mice is

$$\Pr\{X_{\text{infections}} = x\} = \frac{N!}{x!(N-x)!} p^x (1-p)^{N-x}$$

where $x!$ is the factorial of the number x ($x! = x \cdot (x-1) \cdot (x-2) \cdot \ldots \cdot 2 \cdot 1$, for instance, $4! = 4 \cdot 3 \cdot 2 \cdot 1 = 24$). If we use $N = 300$ mice and the true probability of infection is $p = 0.01$, then Fig. 3 shows the probability of observing 0, 1, 2,

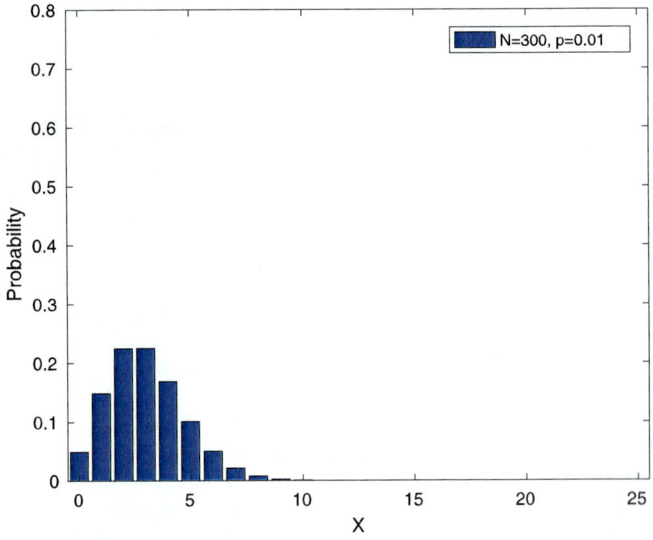

Fig. 3 Probability of observing $x = 0, 1, 2, \ldots$ infections in $N = 300$ animals when the probability of being infected is $p = 0.01$

...infections. The expected number of infections is

$$\mathbb{E}\{X_{\text{infections}}\} = Np$$

That is, in our example we expect to see $300 \cdot 0.01 = 3$ infected animals if the true probability of infection after being vaccinated is $p = 0.01$. In Fig. 3 we can see that $X = 3$ is the most probable result and that observing $X = 0$ infections would happen with probability 4.9% and thus be an unlikely (statistically significant) outcome.

We just happened to choose 300 animals here which magically have given us the exact number that we need to show statistical significance with zero-infected animals. How did we arrive at this sample size? We need to simplify and then rearrange the binomial distribution equation. For $x_0 = 0$, the equation above simplifies to

$$(1 - p_U)^N < \alpha$$

and solving for N

$$N > \frac{\log(\alpha)}{\log(1 - p_U)} \tag{7}$$

for $\alpha = 0.05$ and small p_U (such that $\log(1 - p_U) \approx -p_U$), this equation can be approximated by

$$N > \frac{3}{p_U}$$

that is the famous *rule of 3* used in epidemiology.

Example 7 (continued) In our example we would need

$$N > \frac{\log(0.05)}{\log(0.99)} = 298.07$$

That is, we need $N = 299$ mice.

▶ **Important Remarks**

24. Proving that an event is very rare requires a lot of samples, and the number of samples grows with the inverse of the probability of the event, which can easily grow very quickly as p_U approaches 0.

We can easily turn a problem with a large proportion into a problem of a low proportion by simply changing the event we look for.

Example 8 We want to show that more than 99% of the animals in our animal facility are correctly labeled in their cages. Our test would be of the form:

$$H_0 : p < 0.99$$
$$H_a : p \geq 0.99$$

Instead of having an upper bound of the probability (as in the case of infections), we have a lower bound. In principle, we have not developed the theory for handling these situations, but we can easily do by changing the event we look for. Instead of looking for correctly labeled mice, we may look for mislabeled mice. Then, the test would turn into

$$H_0 : p \geq 0.01$$
$$H_a : p < 0.01$$

▶ **Important Remarks**

25. We can turn superiority tests into inferiority tests or vice versa simply by looking at a different event.

2.2 Confidence Interval for One Proportion

Sometimes we are interested in determining a proportion with a given precision.

Example 9 We are interested in determining the proportion of animals that will develop cancer when they are directly exposed to a given carcinogen. We want to report a confidence interval rather than a point estimate, and we want that our confidence interval is at most 5% wide (for instance, if this proportion is 15%, we want the 95% confidence interval to be between 12.5 and 17.5%). How many animals do we need to expose to achieve this precision?

We could use the binomial distribution equation as we have just done, but this is mathematically very difficult. We saw in the previous graph that the histogram of probability over the number infected approximated to a bell-shaped curve, which is mathematically defined by the normal distribution. An alternative to using the binomial distribution equation is to approximate the distribution of values with the binomial approximation to the normal. Without entering into the mathematical details, the solution of this problem is

$$N > \left(\frac{z_{1-\frac{\alpha}{2}}}{\frac{\Delta_p/2}{\sqrt{p(1-p)}}} \right)^2 \quad (8)$$

▶ **Important Remarks**

26. Designing the sample size for discrete variables can be rather cumbersome mathematically, but in some situations, we may find alternative, approximated, procedures that provide a useful answer for the problem at hand.
27. However, we should not forget that these approximations are just approximations. They provide an order of magnitude and not a precise answer.
28. Additionally, the sample size calculation requires an initial guess of the proportion we are looking for.

Example 9 (continued) Now it is very easy to calculate the sample size with the approximate formula:

$$N > \left(\frac{z_{1-\frac{0.05}{2}}}{\frac{0.05/2}{\sqrt{0.15 \cdot 0.85}}} \right)^2 = \left(\frac{1.96}{\frac{0.025}{0.357}} \right)^2 = 783.7$$

That is, we need to expose 784 animals to the carcinogen to have such a precise confidence interval (the exact samples size provided by the binomial distribution equation is 822 so we see that the approximated solution is in the same order of magnitude).

▶ **Important Remarks**

29. There is a trade-off between sample size and precision of the confidence interval. More precise confidence intervals,

smaller Δ_p, require more samples; conversely, experiments with a low number of samples result in less precise confidence intervals for the proportion.

30. It is easier to be precise in the confidence interval of proportions as they go away from the region of maximum uncertainty, $p = 50\%$. The number of samples for these proportions will be smaller than for proportions close to 50%.

2.3 Hypothesis Test on One Proportion

Example 10 The infection rate of a given pathogen is 5% when adult animals are directly exposed to it. We suspect that the infection rate of newborns is higher. How many newborns do we need to study to test this hypothesis with a 95% confidence level and if we want to have a statistical power of 90% if we anticipate that the infection rate in newborns is above 10%?

Our test is of the form (Fig. 4):

$$H_0 : p \leq 0.05$$
$$H_a : p > 0.05$$

Our cutoff point for statistical significance is the red vertical line to cut off 5

$$N \geq \left(\frac{z_{1-\alpha}\sqrt{p_0(1-p_0)} + z_{1-\beta}\sqrt{p_a(1-p_a)}}{p_a - p_0} \right)^2 \quad (9)$$

Example 10 (continued) The approximated method gives for this case

$$N \geq \left(\frac{z_{0.95}\sqrt{0.05 \cdot 0.95} + z_{0.90}\sqrt{0.1 \cdot 0.9}}{0.1 - 0.05} \right)^2 = 221$$

The exact method gives $N = 233$ and $x_0 = 18$, meaning that when we perform the experiment, if we observe less than 18 infections, we cannot reject the hypothesis that the probability of infection is smaller or equal to 5%.

Important Remarks

31. Hypothesis tests with proportions operate in the same way as with the mean: there are distributions associated with the null hypothesis and with the alternative hypothesis and a cutoff that is used to take the decision to reject the null hypothesis or not.

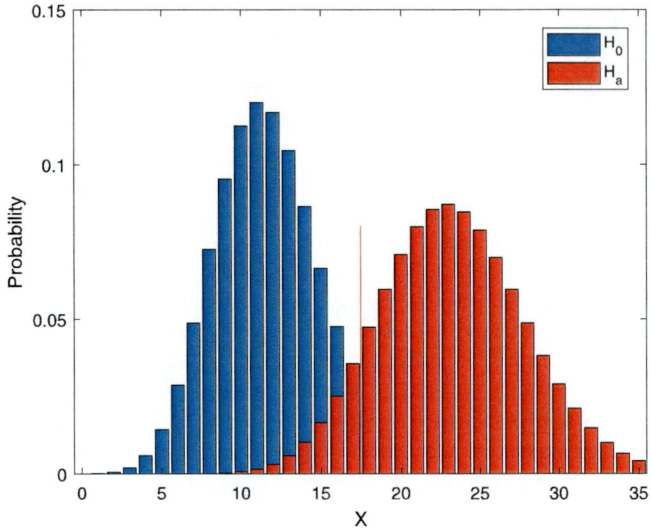

Fig. 4 Probability of observing $x = 0, 1, 2, \ldots$ infections in $N = 233$ animals when the probability of being infected is $p = 5\%$ (blue) and $p = 10\%$ (red)

2.4 Confidence Interval for the Difference of Two Proportions

Example 11 For the example above, let us say that we want to construct a 95% confidence interval on the difference between the two proportions: the proportion of infected adults and the proportion of infected newborns:

$$p_L < p_{newborn} - p_{adults} < p_U$$

For doing so, we will study two groups (adults and newborns) and estimate the proportion of infections in each of the groups. We foresee that $p_{newborn}$ is around 10% and p_{adults} around 5%. Since both proportions are rather close, we want the confidence interval to be very precise such that $p_U - p_L < 5\%$.

In this problem, the statistical variable of interest is

$$\Delta p = p_1 - p_2$$

Let us call the interval width as Δ:

$$\Delta = p_U - p_L$$

Δ is our main design parameter, and it represents how precise we want to be around the observed difference. If the Gaussian approximation of the binomial can be applied ($Np > 5$ and $N(1-p) > 5$), then the sample size design formulas are

$$\begin{aligned} N_1 &= \left(\frac{z_{1-\frac{\alpha}{2}}}{\frac{\Delta/2}{\sqrt{p_1(1-p_1)+p_2(1-p_2)}}}\right)^2 \\ N_2 &= \left(\frac{z_{1-\frac{\alpha}{2}}}{\frac{\Delta/2}{\sqrt{p_1(1-p_1)+p_2(1-p_2)}}}\right)^2 \end{aligned} \qquad (10)$$

Example 11 (continued) Continuing with the example and assuming that we will study the same number of animals on both groups, we require

$$N_1 = N_2 = \left(\frac{z_{0.975}}{\frac{0.05/2}{\sqrt{0.05\cdot 0.95+0.1\cdot 0.9}}}\right)^2 = 846$$

That is, we require 846 animals per group. This large number is due to the inherent inefficiency in testing of binomial data coupled with the small difference.

2.5 Hypothesis Test on the Difference of Two Proportions

Example 12 We are interested in testing if there is a difference in the infection rate of a pathogen in adults and newborns. We expect the infection rate in newborns to be higher than the one in adults (which is expected to be around 5%). If the difference is larger than 5% (i.e., the infection rate in newborns raises above 10%), we want to be able to see it with a statistical power of 90%. The confidence level is set to the standard 95%.

Our statistical test is of the form:

$$\begin{aligned} H_0 &: p_{newborn} \leq p_{adults} \\ H_a &: p_{newborn} > p_{adults} \end{aligned}$$

We may extend the sample design formula for confidence intervals in Eq. 10 to hypothesis tests:

$$N_1 = N_2 = \left(\frac{z_{1-\alpha}+z_{1-\beta}}{\frac{\Delta}{\sqrt{p_1(1-p_1)+p_2(1-p_2)}}}\right)^2 \qquad (11)$$

Note an important difference between the design for the confidence interval and the design for the superiority test: $\Delta/2$ in the confidence interval design (Eq. 10) has turned into Δ for the superiority test (Eq. 11). This results in a large reduction of the sample size.

Example 12 (continued) The required sample size for this example would be

$$N_1 = N_2 = \left(\frac{z_{0.95}+z_{0.9}}{\frac{0.05}{\sqrt{0.05\cdot 0.95+0.1\cdot 0.9}}}\right)^2 = 472$$

Important Remarks

32. In Examples 10, 11, and 12, we have seen three different flavors of the same problem: (1) comparing the proportion of a group to a reference (Example 10), (2) computing a confidence interval for the difference of two groups (Example 11), and (3) showing that the proportion of a group is larger than the proportion in another group (Example 12). The sample size varies widely (N =221, 846, and 472, respectively). This highlights, once again, the need to plan the experiment in advance and decide exactly which is the goal of our experiment.

2.6 Hypothesis Test on the Difference of Two Paired Proportions

Example 13 Does a new treatment reduce the incidence of collapsed lungs (pneumothorax) during lung biopsies? Biopsies using both the conventional and the new procedure are randomly allocated to either lung of pigs. Conventional biopsies lead to about 50% of the animals with collapsed lungs. We want to have a statistical power of 90% if the presence of the symptom drops to 20%. The statistical confidence of the test is set to 95%. How many animals do we need for this test?

After performing the experiment, we can organize the observations in a table depending on whether the animals have the symptom or not before and after treatment:

		New treatment	
		Absent=0	Present=1
Conventional	Absent=0	n_{00}	n_{01}
	Present=1	n_{10}	n_{11}

where the n_{ij} are counts of individuals. The total count of individuals is

$$N = n_{00} + n_{01} + n_{10} + n_{11}$$

There is a fundamental difference between this contingency table and a standard contingency table: the animals with conventional treatment and with new treatment are the same. This is the equivalent of proportions of paired measurements where the same individual serves as its own control. The standard tools for contingency tables (like the χ^2-test) do not apply because those tools are designed for independent samples and not multiple measures on the same individual. The appropriate tool is McNemar's test that determines if the row and column marginal distributions are equal.

The number of animals for the experiment can approximately be calculated with the help of two proxy variables: the total proportion of discordant events (collapsed lung with conventional treatment but not new treatment and collapsed lung with new treatment but not conventional treatment) and the odds ratio between both kinds of discordant events:

$$\begin{aligned} p_D &= p_{10} + p_{01} \\ OR &= p_{10}/p_{01} \end{aligned}$$

Then,

$$N = \left(\frac{z_{1-\frac{\alpha}{2}}(OR+1) + z_{1-\beta}\sqrt{(OR+1)^2 - (OR-1)^2 p_D}}{(OR-1)\sqrt{p_D}} \right)^2 \quad (12)$$

Example 13 (continued) We must translate our previous expectations into proportions in each one of the cells. The following table shows this decomposition:

		After		
		Absent=0	Present=1	
Before	Absent=0	p_{00}=40%	p_{01}=10%	50%
	Present=1	p_{10}=40%	p_{11}=10%	50%
		80%	20%	

For the sample size calculation, we have:

$$p_D = 0.4 + 0.1 = 0.5$$
$$OR = 0.4/0.1 = 4$$
$$N = \left(\frac{z_{0.975}(4+1)+z_{0.9}\sqrt{(4+1)^2-(4-1)^2 0.5}}{(4-1)\sqrt{0.5}}\right)^2 = 55$$

The exact design formula (not shown here) gives $N = 59$.

2.7 Hypothesis Test on the Difference of Multiple Proportions

Example 14 We want to verify if there is a relationship between the incidence of a given pathology and genotype and sex. We will study four genotypes (G_1, G_2, G_3, and G_4) that we will assume equiprobable. If there is no relationship, then we should observe 50% of male and female diseased animals at all genotypes. If there is, then in some of the genotypes, we may observe a deviation from this 50%. We want to have a statistical power of 90% if the deviation is larger than 10%. We want to have a statistical confidence of 95%. How many diseased animals do we need to observe to test this hypothesis?

This kind of studies are addressed through a *contigency table* and subsequent chi-squared analysis, in the example above of diseased animals. When we perform the experiment, we record in this table how many animals we have observed of each kind.

At the moment of experiment design, we cannot input the number of animals observed because the experiment has not started yet. Instead, we will input the expected probabilities at each of the cells. If there is no higher or lower incidence of the disease with sex and/or genotype, all cells should have the same probability as shown below.

		Genotype			
		G_1	G_2	G_3	G_4
Sex	Male=1	$p^0_{11} = 0.125$	$p^0_{12} = 0.125$	$p^0_{13} = 0.125$	$p^0_{14} = 0.125$
	Female=2	$p^0_{21} = 0.125$	$p^0_{22} = 0.125$	$p^0_{23} = 0.125$	$p^0_{24} = 0.125$

If in any of the groups the probability of diseased males and females is unbalanced (*e.g.*, males suffer more frequently the disease than females), then we would observe a different distribution of probabilities. If this happens in Genotype 1, and the deviation is 10%, the expected table of probabilities would be

		Genotype			
		G_1	G_2	G_3	G_4
Sex	Male=1	$p^a_{11} = 0.6 \cdot 0.25 = 0.15$	$p^a_{12} = 0.125$	$p^a_{13} = 0.125$	$p^a_{14} = 0.125$
	Female=2	$p^a_{21} = 0.4 \cdot 0.25 = 0.1$	$p^a_{22} = 0.125$	$p^a_{23} = 0.125$	$p^a_{24} = 0.125$

We may compute the difference between the two distributions (null and alternative) as the square root of the sum of the observed probability in each cell/expected probability squared all divided by the observed probability:

$$w = \sqrt{\sum_{ij} \frac{(p^0_{ij} - p^a_{ij})^2}{p^0_{ij}}}$$

We have named the difference as w, and it is the effect size. In the example above, $w = 0.1$. The test we will do to analyze this data is a χ^2, and the sample size design equation is

$$N = \chi^2 / W^2 \tag{13}$$

Example 14 (continued) The solution is $N = 1,418$. The reason for such a high number is that the effect size is very small.

2.8 Hypothesis Test on the Equivalence of One Proportion

Example 15 We are exploring a new administration route for a drug. Normally, $p = 60\%$ of the animals respond to the drug. How many animals do we need to study to show that the new route is equivalent to the previous one? We want to have a power of 90% when the number of responders is $p_1 = 50\%$ or $p_2 = 70\%$.

As was shown in Sect. 1.8, equivalence tests are translated into two one-sided tests, and they normally require more samples than standard significance tests. In the case of proportions, this is also the case. Again an approximate solution of the number of samples is obtained; if the three binomials can be approximated by the binomial approximation to the normal and $p = \frac{p_{0L}+p_{0U}}{2}$, then we can solve for N as

$$N \geq \left(\frac{z_{1-\alpha} + z_{1-\frac{\beta}{2}}}{\frac{p_{0U}-p_{0L}}{\sqrt{(p_{0L}+p_{0U})(2-p_{0L}-p_{0U})}}} \right)^2 \quad (14)$$

Example 15 (continued) The exact solution requires $N = 255$ samples. We would reject the null hypothesis if the number of respondents is between $x_1 = 142$ and $x_2 = 165$. The approximate solution gives

$$N \geq \left(\frac{z_{0.95} + z_{0.95}}{\frac{0.7-0.5}{\sqrt{(0.5+0.7)(2-0.5-0.7)}}} \right)^2 = 260$$

2.9 Hypothesis Test on the Equivalence of Two Proportions

Example 16 We can solve the same problem as in Example 0 but estimating the proportion from two populations: one with the standard administration route and another one with the alternative route.

As in the previous case, we can solve the problem with two one-sided tests (TOST), for which an exact solution exists based on binomial counting (as in the previous case). In this section we will not give the formulas, which are more complicated than in the previous section, but they have the same flavor.

If we can use the binomial approximation to the normal, then the sample size for a given power $1 - \beta$ is

$$N \geq \left(\frac{z_{1-\alpha} + z_{1-\frac{\beta}{2}}}{\frac{\Delta}{\sqrt{2p(1-p)}}} \right)^2 \quad (15)$$

where Δ is the maximum deviation for which the two proportions are still considered to be equivalent (i.e., $|p_1 - p_2| < \Delta$).

Example 16 The exact solution requires $N = 520$ samples per group. The approximate solution gives

$$N \geq \left(\frac{z_{0.95} + z_{0.95}}{\frac{0.1}{\sqrt{2 \cdot 0.6(1-0.6)}}} \right)^2 = 520$$

Important Remarks

33. If we compare the sample size for an experiment with just one proportion (Example 15) or two proportions (the example above), we see that the size for two proportions is much larger. The reason is that with two proportions, there is much more “uncertainty” involved since we need to estimate the difference in proportion for two groups, instead of just one.

3 Sample Size for the Variance

The following set of procedures aims at designing the sample size for situations in which very little is known about the experiment. Note that in many other sample size designs, the variance of the observations is a key parameter (this is the case of all sample size designs for the mean and for regression). However, there are experimental situations in which even this variance is unknown. The following sample size calculations will allow us to design an experiment by which we will gain some insight into the variability we should expect from our observations.

3.1 Confidence Interval for the Standard Deviation

For instance, let us assume this is the first time, ever in history, that the expression level of a given gene is studied. How many individuals should we study to determine the standard deviation with a confidence interval whose two-sided width is smaller than a given desired precision. When we perform the experiment, we will be able to calculate the sample standard deviation, $\hat{\sigma}$ as

$$\bar{x} = \frac{1}{N}\sum_{i=1}^{N} x_i$$
$$\hat{\sigma} = \sqrt{\frac{1}{N-1}\sum_{i=1}^{N}(x_i - \bar{x})^2}$$

Then, we will construct a two-sided $1-\alpha$ confidence interval (e.g., 95% confidence interval) as

$$\left(\hat{\sigma}\sqrt{\frac{N-1}{\chi^2_{1-\frac{\alpha}{2},N-1}}}, \hat{\sigma}\sqrt{\frac{N-1}{\chi^2_{\frac{\alpha}{2},N-1}}}\right)$$

The confidence interval for the ratio $\frac{\sigma}{\hat{\sigma}}$ is

$$\left(\sqrt{\frac{N-1}{\chi^2_{1-\frac{\alpha}{2},N-1}}}, \sqrt{\frac{N-1}{\chi^2_{\frac{\alpha}{2},N-1}}}\right)$$

whose width is by design to be smaller than δ, so the sample size design equation must be

$$\sqrt{\frac{N-1}{\chi^2_{\frac{\alpha}{2},N-1}}} - \sqrt{\frac{N-1}{\chi^2_{1-\frac{\alpha}{2},N-1}}} \leq \delta \qquad (16)$$

that must be solved numerically.

Example 17 We want to determine a 95% confidence interval for the standard deviation of the gene expression level of a given gene with a two-sided precision less than $\delta = 1$. Then, we need $N = 12$ samples. With this number of samples, the 95% confidence interval for the $\frac{\sigma}{\hat{\sigma}}$ ratio is

$$(0.71, 1.70)$$

That is, the true standard deviation could be as small as $0.71\hat{\sigma}$ or as large as $1.70\hat{\sigma}$. Having more precision in our confidence interval rapidly increases the sample size. For instance, to have only a 10% of two-sided width, the sample size would grow up to $N = 774$ individuals. Then, the confidence interval would be

$$(0.95, 1.05)$$

▶ **Important Remarks**

34. A large precision for the variance or standard deviation rapidly increases the number of samples. For small sample sizes, we need to accept a relatively large uncertainty about the true underlying variability of our population.

3.2 Hypothesis Test for One Variance

Example 18 We regularly monitor the precision of the optical densitometer of our laboratory. Historically, the standard deviation of the measurements has been $\sigma = 0.05$ (arbitrary units). How many samples do we need to detect an increase of variance larger than 50% of the nominal variance with a statistical power of 90% and a confidence of 95%?

In this setting we will perform an hypothesis test (see Fig. 5):

$$H_0 : \sigma^2 \leq 0.05^2$$
$$H_a : \sigma^2 > 0.05^2$$

An approximate solution when N is large is given by the Gaussian approximation:

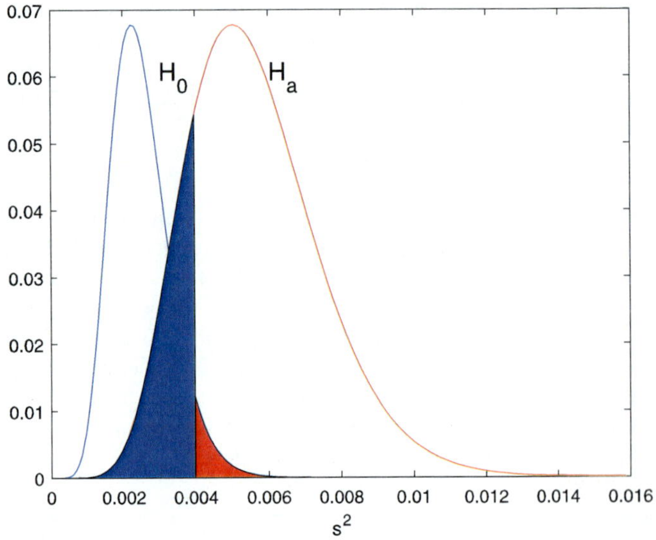

Fig. 5 Example of hypothesis test for a one sample variance. The two distributions show the expected values of the sample variance, $s^2 = \hat{\sigma}^2$, if the null (H_0) or the alternative (H_a) hypotheses are true. The shaded areas represent the probability of Type I (red) and Type II (blue) errors

$$N > \frac{1}{2}\left(\frac{z_{1-\alpha} + z_{1-\beta}}{\log \frac{\sigma_a}{\sigma_0}}\right)^2 \tag{17}$$

3.3 Hypothesis Test for Two Variances

Example 18 We are buying a new optical densitometer that claims to be more precise than our old model. How many samples do we need to take from each densitometer to test if this claim is true? We want to have a statistical power of 90% if the new variance is 50% smaller than the old one.

Now the hypothesis test is given by comparing the variance of both samples. In the following test, we refer to the variance of the old equipment as σ_1^2 and to the variance of the new equipment as σ_2^2

$$H_0 : \sigma_1^2 \leq \sigma_2^2$$
$$H_a : \sigma_1^2 > \sigma_2^2$$

When N is large, this can be approximated by the Gaussian design:

$$N = \left(\frac{z_{1-\alpha} + z_{1-\beta}}{\log \frac{\sigma_1}{\sigma_2}}\right)^2 \tag{18}$$

Example 18 (continued) In this example, we must find N such that

$$\frac{F_{0.95,N-1,N-1}}{F_{0.1,N-1,N-1}} \leq \frac{1}{0.5}$$

whose solution is $N = 74$. The approximate formula gives

$$N = \left(\frac{z_{0.95} + z_{0.9}}{\log \sqrt{\frac{1}{0.5}}}\right)^2 = 72$$

4 Sample Size for Correlations

4.1 Confidence Interval for Correlation

Example 19 We are interested in detecting a weak correlation between aldosterone (an steroid hormone produced by the adrenal gland) concentration in blood plasma and blood pressure.We expect the correlation to be around 0.25. How many individuals do we need to study to determine the correlation with a precision of 0.05 and a level of confidence of 95%.

We are looking for a confidence interval of the form $[\rho_L, \rho_U]$ where L and U refer to the lower and upper bounds, respectively. As with other sample design formulas, for the correlation we need to foresee beforehand which will be approximately the result of the experiment. So that in our case, if we expect the correlation to be around 0.25, the lower and upper bounds will be $[0.2, 0.3]$. With this information we can use Fisher's Z transform that is distributed approximately as a Gaussian:

$$Z = \tanh^{-1}(\hat{\rho}) = \frac{1}{2}\log\frac{1+\hat{\rho}}{1-\hat{\rho}} \sim N\left(\tanh^{-1}(\rho), \frac{1}{N-3}\right)$$

In this way, we transform the confidence interval problem on ρ into a confidence interval problem for Z:

$$\Pr\{\rho_L < \rho < \rho_U\} = 1-\alpha = \Pr\{Z_L < Z < Z_U\}$$

We already know its solution which is

$$\begin{aligned} Z_L &= \tfrac{1}{2}\log\tfrac{1+\rho_L}{1-\rho_L} = \tfrac{1}{2}\log\tfrac{1+\rho}{1-\rho} - z_{1-\frac{\alpha}{2}}\tfrac{1}{\sqrt{N-3}} \\ Z_U &= \tfrac{1}{2}\log\tfrac{1+\rho_U}{1-\rho_U} = \tfrac{1}{2}\log\tfrac{1+\rho}{1-\rho} + z_{1-\frac{\alpha}{2}}\tfrac{1}{\sqrt{N-3}} \end{aligned}$$

If we now subtract the first equation from the second, we have the sample size design formula:

$$Z_U - Z_L = 2z_{1-\frac{\alpha}{2}}\frac{1}{\sqrt{N-3}} \Rightarrow N = \left(\frac{2z_{1-\frac{\alpha}{2}}}{Z_U - Z_L}\right)^2 + 3 \tag{19}$$

Example 19 (continued) In our example

$$\begin{aligned} Z_L &= \tfrac{1}{2}\log\tfrac{1+(0.25-0.05)}{1-(0.25-0.05)} = 0.2027 \\ Z_U &= \tfrac{1}{2}\log\tfrac{1+(0.25+0.05)}{1-(0.25+0.05)} = 0.3095 \\ \Delta Z &= Z_U - Z_L = 0.1068 \\ N &= \left(\tfrac{2z_{0.975}}{0.1068}\right)^2 + 3 = 1,351 \end{aligned}$$

Important Remarks

35. The sample size needed for low correlations is very large precisely because the correlation is so low that it requires many samples to be sure that the detected small correlation is not by chance. For large correlations this is not the case: with relatively few animals, the large correlation quickly becomes apparent.

4.2 Hypothesis Test on One Sample Correlation

Example 20 We suspect that the correlation between the length and weight of an animal is smaller than 0.9. How many individuals do we need to inspect to show so if we want to have a test power of 90% if the correlation is actually 0.8?

We are making a test of the form:

$$\begin{aligned} H_0 &: \rho \geq \rho_0 \\ H_a &: \rho < \rho_0 \end{aligned}$$

This is a test with a single sample (we are not comparing the correlation between length and weight in two groups). Then, we simply have to extend the formula of the previous section to include the statistical power:

$$N = \left(\frac{z_{1-\alpha} + z_{1-\beta}}{Z_0 - Z_a}\right)^2 + 3 \tag{20}$$

where Z_0 is the Fisher's Z transform of ρ_0 and Z_a is the Fisher's Z transform of the correlation for which we already want to have a given statistical power.

Example 20 (continued) In our example

$$\begin{aligned} Z_0 &= \tfrac{1}{2}\log\tfrac{1+0.9}{1-0.9} = 1.4722 \\ Z_a &= \tfrac{1}{2}\log\tfrac{1+0.8}{1-0.8} = 1.0986 \\ N &= \left(\tfrac{z_{0.95}+z_{0.9}}{1.4722-1.0986}\right)^2 + 3 = 65 \end{aligned}$$

4.3 Hypothesis Test for the Correlations in Two Samples

Example 21 The correlation between length and weight in the general population is about 0.8 (Group 1). We wonder if this same correlation holds among diabetes type II animal models

(Group 2) because these animals tend to be fatter. How many control and diseased animals do we need to study to check if the correlation is lower in diabetes type II animals? We want a power of 90% if the correlation drops below 0.7.

We are making a test of the form:

$$\begin{aligned} H_0 &: \rho_1 \leq \rho_2 \\ H_a &: \rho_1 > \rho_2 \end{aligned}$$

We now have two populations (control and diseased animals). After transforming the observed correlations, we will finally compare the difference between both:

$$\Delta Z = Z_1 - Z_2$$

and the test can be reformulated as

$$\begin{aligned} H_0 &: \Delta Z \geq 0 \\ H_a &: \Delta Z < 0 \end{aligned}$$

The variance of ΔZ is

$$\sigma^2_{\Delta Z} = \frac{1}{N_1 - 3} + \frac{1}{N_2 - 3}.$$

If $N_1 = N_2$, then the sample design formula is given by

$$\Delta Z = (z_{1-\alpha} + z_{1-\beta})\sigma_{\Delta Z}$$

that is

$$N = \left(\frac{z_{1-\alpha} + z_{1-\beta}}{\frac{\Delta Z}{\sqrt{2}}}\right)^2 + 3 \tag{21}$$

Example 21 In the example above

$$\begin{aligned} Z_1 &= \tfrac{1}{2}\log\tfrac{1+0.8}{1-0.8} = 1.0986 \\ Z_2 &= \tfrac{1}{2}\log\tfrac{1+0.7}{1-0.7} = 0.8673 \\ \Delta Z &= 0.2313 \\ N &= \left(\frac{z_{0.95}+z_{0.9}}{\frac{0.2313}{\sqrt{2}}}\right)^2 + 3 = 324 \end{aligned}$$

Design of Experiments

Michael Parkinson and Carlos Oscar Sánchez Sorzano

Having an understanding of the factors that can bias or confound our experiments leads us to a consideration of the experimental design.

1 Basic Designs

The main concepts are associated with the most basic designs of experiments.

1.1 Completely Randomized Design (CRD)

The simplest designs of experiment such as t-tests allow us to compare a sample to a standard or to compare two independent samples. What do we do if we have more than two groups to compare? The completely randomized design of analysis of variance (ANOVA) can allow us to determine if there is an effect of treatment.

Example 22 We have two concentrations of drug plus control.

> **Design summary.** We randomly assign animals to treatments to minimize allocation bias. Typically, the same number of animals is analyzed in each group, but this is not essential.
>
> If the treatment is defined by a genetic characteristic (like wild type vs. knockout animals), animals cannot be randomly assigned to the treatment group, but the design is still considered to be completely randomized.
>
> If we anticipate systematic differences in the experiment due to confounding factors, it is better to perform a design with blocks (see Sect. 1.3).

As an example consider an experiment into the effect of two doses of drug plus control on cholesterol levels.

Once we perform the experiment, we may use ANOVA to determine if the drug was effective by comparing the size of the treatment effect against error.

Basically we compare the variability due to treatment with variability due to error. Rather than computing variability directly, we do it in an indirect way by working out the top line of the variability equation first to generate what is

M. Parkinson
School of Biotechnology, Dublin City University, Dublin, Ireland
e-mail: michael.parkinson@dcu.ie

C. O. S. Sorzano (✉)
Natl. Center of Biotechnology (CSIC), Madrid, Spain
e-mail: coss@cnb.csic.es

© Springer Nature Switzerland AG 2021

J. M. Sánchez Morgado, A. Brønstad (eds.), *Experimental Design and Reproducibility in Preclinical Animal Studies*, Laboratory Animal Science and Medicine 1,
https://doi.org/10.1007/978-3-030-66147-2_8

known as a sums of squares. The reason that we do it this way is that the sums of squares are additive so if we know the total sums of squares and the treatment sums of squares, we can work out the error sums of squares by subtraction, and in the days of calculating by hand or on a pocket calculator, this was a useful shortcut. The total sums of squares = the sum of (the difference of each data point from the Grand Mean) squared. For the treatment sums of squares, we essentially do the same thing but use the average of each treatment for every data point rather than its actual value. Error sums of squares can be computed in a very similar way, but this time we use the sum of (the difference of each treatment value from the treatment mean) squared. Each experiment has an associated number of degrees of freedom (the bottom line of the variability equation). Loosely speaking, degrees of freedom are like "tokens of information." If we have an experiment with N animals, then we originally have N tokens. Now, we spend these tokens in estimating different parameters. Every parameter costs a token. We need to estimate the overall mean; then this costs a token, so that the number of degrees of freedom associated with the total sum of squares, SS_T, is no longer N but $N-1$. We need to estimate the treatment effect. In general if we have T treatment groups, we only need $T-1$ degrees of freedom to calculate the main effects of all the groups. We had $N-1$ degrees of freedom to calculate parameters, we have consumed $T-1$, and the remaining $N-T$ are left for the residuals. In this way, we have a decomposition of the degrees of freedom.

We can summarize all this information in the following table, which analyzes the amount of variance explained by each source of information:

Source	Sum of squares	Degrees of freedom	Mean squares ($MS = SS/df$)
Treatments	SS_α	$\#Treatments-1$	$MS_\alpha = SS_\alpha/(df$ Treatment)
Residuals	SS_ϵ	$Difference$	$MS_\epsilon = SS_\epsilon/(df$ Residuals)
Total	SS_T	$N-1$	

Again, the sum of squares decomposition allows the definition of the *coefficient of determination*, normally denoted as R^2, that is, the proportion of the total variance that is explained by the predictions. This value goes from 0 to 1.

The ANOVA table for the data shown in Fig. 1 would be

Source	SS	df	MS	F	p
Treatments	31252	2	15626	13.79	$6.18 \cdot 10^{-5}$
Residuals	30600	27	1133		
Total	61852	29			

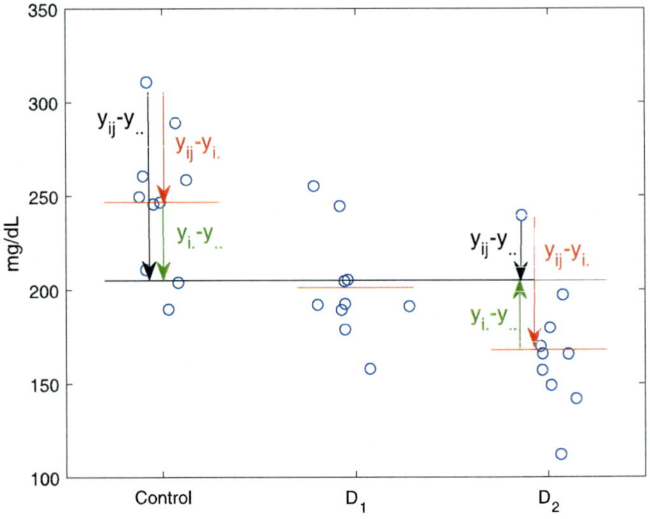

Fig. 1 Example of data analysis by ANOVA. There are three groups (control and two doses) with ten observations each. The horizontal black line is the overall mean. The horizontal red lines are the mean of each of the groups. We can see that within each treatment there is variability and that the three averages are also different

The F-value of MS treatment/MS residuals (15626/1133) = 13.79 gives a very highly significant effect. Consequently, we would reject the null hypothesis and accept that at least two treatments are different to each other. *Post hoc* analysis would now look for the pair or pairs of treatments that are different from each other. Showing this second part of the analysis is out of the scope of this chapter since it would divert us from our main objective, design of experiments. The interested reader is referred to Doncaster and Davey [1]. The R^2 of this ANOVA model (also called eta squared) is $R^2 = 31252/61852 = 0.51$ meaning that it explains a little bit more than 50% of the original variability. If we add additional blocks or factors, these will tend to reduce the error variability, and we are better using partial eta squared instead = treatment SS/(treatment SS + error SS). Eta squared and partial eta squared are very useful in that they can be used directly in power calculations for determination of required sample size.

1.2 Regression Design

In the previous example, we had only 3 levels of drug, but we could design an experiment to test many more levels, for example, 11 levels of a drug from $D = 0$ mg (control), $D = 10$ mg, $D = 20$ mg, ..., $D = 100$ mg. As we saw in the previous section, we could address this design with an ANOVA design of 11 levels for the treatment variable; however this would require 10 degrees of freedom to estimate the 11 levels of the main effects. Given that the dose is continuous, we can turn the linear model above into a regression problem with a generic function, $f(x)$. This model is much cheaper in terms of degrees of freedom (so that we may use fewer individuals for our experiment). It has two other advantages over the ANOVA linear model: (1) the regression can predict the cholesterol level for values in between the doses used in the experiment (for instance, $D = 15$ mg), and (2) regression analysis can check whether any of the regression coefficients is significantly different from 0, meaning that we may simplify the model if we see that we have overparameterized it.

Assuming the regression model has P parameters, and that the model is linear in these parameters (the βs do not participate in a nonlinear way), the data analysis table is given by

Source	Sum of squares	Degrees of freedom
Regression	$SS_\beta = \sum_{ij}(f(D_i) - y_{..})^2$	$P - 1$
Residuals	$SS_\epsilon = \sum_{ij}(y_{ij} - f(D_i))^2$	$N - P$
Total	$SS_T = \sum_{ij}(y_{ij} - y_{..})^2$	$N - 1$

For linear regression (y = a + bx), there are only two parameters (a and b) and only one degree of freedom needed for the treatment effect. The coefficient of determination, R^2, is the proportion of the total variability explained by the model.

Example 22 Figure 2 shows the results of analyzing the effect of 11 dose levels of a new drug on the cholesterol level in blood (see Example 15). There are five individuals per dose level. The data analysis is performed by regression of the results with a polynomial of degree 2. The fitted polynomial is

$$y = 228.2 - 2.567D + 0.0145D^2$$

The following table shows the sum of squares decomposition for this case.

Source	SS	df	MS
Regression	77629	2	38815
Residuals	45967	47	978
Total	123596	49	

We have $f = \frac{38815}{978} = 39.68$, and the associated p-value $p = 8 \cdot 10^{-11}$, which is extremely significant. The model explains $R^2 = 1 - 45967/123596 = 63\%$ of the original variance. Additionally, the confidence intervals for each one of the regression parameters are

$$\beta_0 \in [207.9, 248.5]$$
$$\beta_1 \in [-3.513, -1.621]$$
$$\beta_2 \in [0.005391, 0.02361]$$

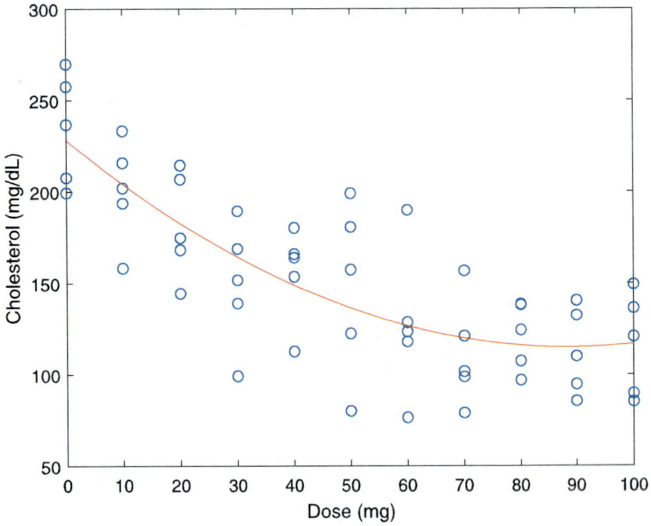

Fig. 2 Experiment in which we are testing the effect of 11 different doses of a new drug on the cholesterol level in blood. The modeling of the response is performed by regression analysis, and the resulting fitted response is shown as a solid, red line

None of these intervals include the zero value; then, all regression coefficients are statistically significant.

Note that we have to be very careful in extrapolating beyond the range explored.

1.3 Randomized Block Design (RBD)

Controlling variability in an experiment by making the experiment more homogeneous will reduce variability but at the expense of scope. A better way to control variability is to block or factor. Which one is used depends upon the reasons for it. Are you going to include the factor in a paper? if so, then it needs to go in as a factor; if not, then as a block. The difference in design is that typically we only put one source of variability into a factor and assume that it may interact with other factors. For blocks we normally do not assume interactions and put as many sources of variability into the blocks as practicable basically keeping the material within a block as homogeneous as possible at the expense of variability between blocks.

In the following experiment, we repeated the earlier experiment but also factored for sex. It is a good practice to keep a balanced design so each level of treatment had the same number of males and females and that there are similar numbers of males and females in each block (Fig. 3).

Sex is now a blocking variable, also called *nuisance factor* in the ANOVA.

Observations have now three indexes: i for the treatment (control, dose 1 or dose 2), j for the block (male or female), and k for the individual within the treatment and block.

Essentially we extend the completely randomized design of ANOVA by computing a block term in exactly the same way that we computed the treatment term but use the average for each block rather than the average of each treatment so the sum of (the Grand Mean – block average) squared for each individual. Again, the degrees of freedom associated with blocks are the number of blocks minus 1.

We can now extend the ANOVA table to include the blocking variable:

Source	Sum of squares	Degrees of freedom
Treatments	$SS_\alpha = \sum_{ijk} \hat{\alpha}_i^2$	$T-1$
Blocks	$SS_\gamma = \sum_{ijk} \hat{\gamma}_j^2$	$B-1$
Residuals	$SS_\epsilon = \sum_{ijk} \hat{\epsilon}_{ijk}^2$	$N-T-B+1$
Total	$SS_T = \sum_{ijk} (y_{ijk} - y_{...})^2$	$N-1$

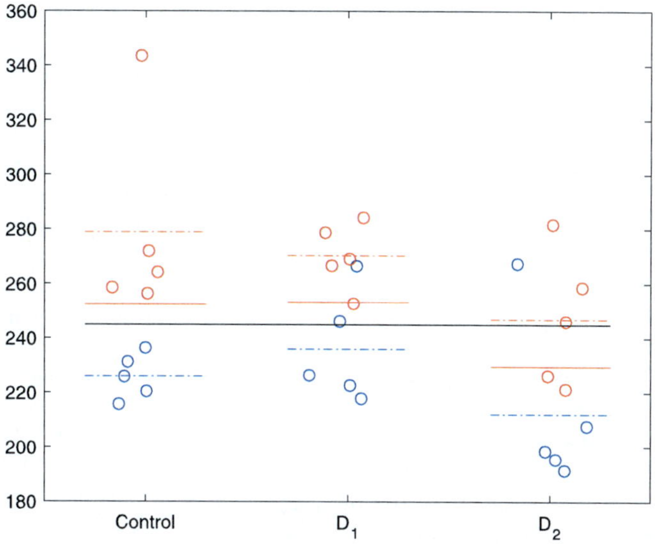

Fig. 3 Data example with sex labels per group (male in red, female in blue). For each group we have drawn the sex average with a dashed line

The p-value is calculated in the same way as before, but the variability explained by the block is taken from the residuals; the sum of squares of the residuals is correspondingly reduced, and it will be easier to show that the treatment is significant (the associated f value will be higher). Before doing an experiment, we cannot know whether blocking will be helpful or not. However, if we suspect that a variable (like sex in our example) could significantly affect the variability of the observations, blocking it and including it in the analysis do not do any harm, and it is a sort of "insurance" just in case we were right about its importance. ANOVA also allows us to analyze the significance of the blocking variables in the same way as we have done for the treatments so we can assess its effect.

We may block the animals according to some continuous variable by splitting it into different cohorts. Suppose we are interested in the effect of four different diets on the growth of pigs and suspect that the initial weight will influence the weight gain. We measure the weight of the animals before the experiment and divide them into three groups: light, medium, and heavy animals. Given four diets it will help balance the experiment if the sample size is a multiple of 4, and we have three weight cohorts so we also ideally would like a multiple of 3 so our experiment will have ideally multiples of 12 animals. Within each block we randomly assign the four different diets.

We can have as many blocks as we want, but do bear in mind that every block will reduce the error degrees of freedom and also make the design of the experiment more complex. The one caveat to blocking is where there is an interaction between block and treatment.

Example 23 We are studying the effect of a hormone on the weight of animals. We will have two groups (control, C, and treatment, T). We have calculated that we need four animals per group, and they will be put in two cages. We are thinking of two designs:

	Cage 1	Cage 2
Design A	CCCC	TTTT
Design B	CCTT	CCTT

From the point of view of eliminating possible cage effects, we would favor Design B over Design A. However, suppose that the hormone does not have an effect on the metabolism of the animals, but on their behavior with animals receiving the hormone being more aggressive or docile. Then, the effect on the animal weight is due to the competition between control and treated animals.

The problem of the interaction of hormone treatment effects with cage effects can be solved by designing the experiment using all possible combinations so that we can then include cage effects as a factor rather than a block and include the cage by treatment interaction.

	Cage 1	Cage 2	Cage 3	Cage 4
Design A+B	CCCC	TTTT	CCTT	CCTT

1.4 Use of Covariates

Blocking addresses discrete variables that might affect our measurements (like sex in the example of the previous section). Covariates can be thought of as blocking for continuous variables. For example, rather than splitting the body weight into different cohorts, we can include it as a variable in the analysis.

The ANOVA table for this model would be

Source	Sum of squares	Degrees of freedom
Covariates	$SS(\beta_w \vert \mu) = RSS(\mu) - RSS(\mu, \beta_w)$	1
Blocks	$SS(\gamma \vert \mu, \beta_w) = RSS(\mu, \beta_w) - RSS(\mu, \beta_w, \gamma)$	$B - 1$
Treatments	$SS(\alpha \vert \mu, \beta_w, \gamma) = RSS(\mu, \beta_w, \gamma) - RSS(\mu, \beta_w, \gamma, \alpha)$	$T - 1$
Residuals	$RSS(\mu, \beta_w, \gamma, \alpha)$	$N - T - B$
Total	$SS_T = RSS(\mu)$	$N - 1$

You may compare these results, with the ones of Example 11. They are different and notably in the estimate of the effect of sex. The ANOVA table is

Source	SS	df	MS	f	p-value
Weight	9866	1	9866	13.8	0.001
Treatments	2626	2	1313	1.84	0.179
Sex	482	1	482	0.68	0.419
Residuals	17837	25	713		
Total	30811	29			

The weight covariate is highly significant, and the sex blocks, which were almost significant in Example 11, have lost most of its significance. The reason is that sex is also correlated with weight. As we have estimated the regression with the weight before sex, then most of the information between sex and cholesterol has been explained by the relationship between weight and cholesterol.

Important Remarks

36. Linear models can be understood as an attempt to progressively explain variance by adding terms that may have an impact in the variability of the observations.
37. When we follow a sequential procedure as the one presented in this section, the parameter estimates, α, β, γ, depend on the order in which the parameters are fitted. They do not depend on the order only if the design is *orthogonal* (orthogonal designs are introduced later in Sect. 1.7).
38. A consequence is that the sum of squares of the ANOVA table must be understood as sum of squares when the variability explained by the previously fitted parameters have been removed. This is highlighted by the notation $SS(\alpha|\mu, \beta_w, \gamma)$; this is the sum of squares explained by the treatments α when the variability explained by the mean, covariates, and blocks has been removed.

1.5 Linear Models, Sample Size, and Replications

Important Remarks

39. Each of the animals in each one of the treatment groups is a replication of the experiment with a given treatment. There is sometimes a confusion between

researchers that they need to replicate the experiment three times in order to have statistically significant results. Experiments that generate a p-value of around 0.05 are under-powered; we would expect to see a statistically significant result only half of the time – you might as well toss a coin. Powering up your experiments to a power of at least 0.8 will give false negatives on average in one fifth of your experiments and an average significance of around 0.01 rather than 0.05. Powering up to a power of 0.9 will give false negatives on average in one tenth of your experiments and an average significance of around 0.001. Rather than repeating an inefficient experiment, it makes more sense to conduct a single experiment which is adequately powered, ideally to a power of around 0.9.

1.6 Factorial Designs (FD)

Blocks assume that there is no interaction with treatments. If you suspect an interaction, or if your factor is interesting from an experimental point of view and its effects need to be teased out, you should include it as a factor in a factorial design rather than as a block.

Design summary. If we study the same number of animals under every possible combination of the levels of all factors, the design is said to be balanced. This is not critical but simplifies the design, analysis, and interpretation of the experiments. In this section we will assume a balanced design, and imbalanced designs will be treated later in Sect. 1.7. As will be shown later, all balanced designs are orthogonal.

Example 24 Following Example 15, we want to know if there are differences in the cholesterol reduction of the second dose (D_2; see Fig. 1), if the drug is taken fasted or fed, and in combination with a special diet rich in fiber. Additionally, we want to know if any of the combinations is particularly useful/useless?

Figure 4 shows the results of two experiments (with and without interactions). If there are no interactions, the two represented lines are parallel to each other. For small interactions, the two lines start to be slightly nonparallel. And for strong interactions, the two lines are clearly nonparallel (in this case, they intersect, but intersection is not a necessary condition for the existence of interactions).

The ANOVA table explains the decomposition of the sum of squares and number of degrees of

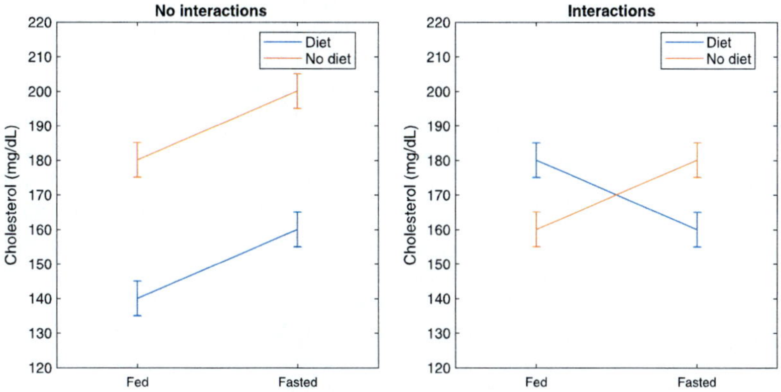

Fig. 4 Example of results with two factors without (left) and with (right) interactions

freedom. We now have two factors, P and Q, and the interaction between them, PQ:

Source	Sum of squares	Degrees of freedom
Treatments P	$SS_{\alpha^{(P)}} = \sum_{ijk} \left(\hat{\alpha}_i^{(P)}\right)^2$	$P-1$
Treatments Q	$SS_{\alpha^{(Q)}} = \sum_{ijk} \left(\hat{\alpha}_j^{(Q)}\right)^2$	$Q-1$
Interactions PQ	$SS_{\alpha^{(PQ)}} = \sum_{ijk} \left(\hat{\alpha}_{ij}^{(PQ)}\right)^2$	(P-1)(Q-1)
Residuals	$SS_{\epsilon} = \sum_{ijk} \hat{\epsilon}_{ijk}^2$	$N-PQ$
Total	$SS_T = \sum_{ijk} (y_{ijk} - y_{...})^2$	$N-1$

In general, there are PQ interactions. However, estimating these many interactions is particularly cheap in terms of degrees of freedom. In this example, it only costs one degree of freedom.

For any of the rows of the ANOVA table, we can test the hypothesis that that row has a statistically significant contribution to the explanation of variability of the observed data. This is done by comparing the corresponding MS to MS_{ϵ}.

Example 24 (continued) Let us assume that we have five individuals per cell and that the ANOVA table is

Source	SS	df	MS	f	p-value
Treatments P	1500	1	1500	1500/900	0.215
Treatments Q	6000	1	6000	6000/900	0.020
Interactions PQ	1500	1	1500	1500/900	0.215
Residuals	14400	16	900		
Total	18900	19			

From this table we see that, with this sample size, only the diet, Q, significantly explains the variability observed in the measurements.

We can easily extend the two-way ANOVA model to multiple factors and include the linear model interactions between pairs of factors (second-order interactions), triples (third-order interactions), etc.

To simplify the table, we can merge all the nonsignificant rows into a single one called *lack of fit*

▶ Important Remarks

40. Our model can include both blocking variables and factors with both treated in a similar way except that we assume that blocks do not interact with factors.
41. Factorial designs are very efficient because we have "hidden" replication where each level of the predictors has been combined with many other predictors and the treatment effects are therefore aggregated over a much larger number of replicates than each individual treatment combination.
42. We should not forget to randomize the animals among the different combinations of factors. The randomization will help avoid the bias induced by uncontrolled factors.

Among all possible designs, factorial designs are most efficient and give the smallest variance in the comparison of any of its components. Consider the following example:

Example 25 We are interested in the effect of a mammalian hormone for water balance in amphibians. We will study two amphibian species (toads and frogs), when animals are dry or wet and with and without hormone. We quantify water balance by measuring the change in weight of the animals after treatment. We thus have 8 treatment combinations and can only manage 24 animals in total. This could yield three animals per treatment combination in a balanced factorial design. Rather than 3 replicates of each treatment, we can see that the effect of species, dryness, and hormone is replicated over 12 animals (24 animals total/2 levels – e.g., toad or frog), the effect of first-order interactions over 6 animals, and only the highest-order interaction of species X wetness X hormone has 3 animals per treatment combination.

– Design 3: We perform a factorial design (we should not forget about the randomization when actually performing the experiment; we only report here the number of animals per group):

Three frogs, dry, no hormone
Three frogs, dry, hormone
Three frogs, Wet, No hormone
Three frogs, wet, hormone
Three toads, dry, no hormone
Three toads, dry, hormone
Three toads, wet, no hormone
Three toads, wet, hormone

The expected variance of the comparison of the effect of the hormone is improved to

$$2\frac{\sigma^2_{\Delta w}}{12}$$

Additionally, the hormone treatment has been tested with many other levels of the other variables (frogs, toads, dry, and wet). Our conclusions from this experiment will be more general than the ones from simpler designs.

Important Remarks

43. In research one way to control confounding is to change one variable at a time holding all the rest fixed. Factorial designs seem to contradict this rule. However, they do not. They propose to hold everything fixed, except those variables of interest. These variables of interest should be combined in all possible ways.
44. Small factorial designs are used when we are interested in estimating possible interactions between factors. For designs with many parameters, we should first determine which factors effectively contribute to the final result. This is done with a fractional (or screening) factorial design.

1.6.1 Single Replicate Factorial Designs

We have just seen how "hidden" replication inherent in factorial designs leads to a very efficient use of animals. In that example we had 24 animals so 23 total degrees of freedom with one for each of the 3 main effects (3), 1 for each of the 3 second-order interactions (3), and 1 for the third-order interaction leaving 16 degrees of freedom for the error. This fits within the 10–20 degrees of freedom suggested by Mead's Resource Equation method for sample size calculation. Note how efficient this design is where we have two levels of each of the factors generating one df for each of the effects. If we had three levels of each factor, then the main effects would each have 2 df (3 treatments $\times$ 2 df = 6 df in total) and each second-order interaction $2 \times 2 = 4$ df (12 in total for the three interactions) and the third-order interaction $2 \times 2 \times 2 = 8$ degrees of freedom. The more levels of each factor, the worse this gets.

It is generally advised to have at least three animals per combination. With a single replicate of every treatment combination, a full analysis partitions all the variability into the factors leaving no variability left for error; this is called a "saturated" design and cannot be used to work out the significance of any of the factors since there is no error variance to work out the F-ratio. However, if we do not expect high-order interactions, we may fit a reduced model in which the high-order interactions are not estimated (they are confounded with the residuals), and we get away with a single animal in each one of the combinations. This strategy is particularly appropriate in large experiments which involve a large number of factors and/or levels and that contain a number of high order interactions.

Example 26 We are interested in maximizing the delivery of a drug so that the exposure is maximum. We have identified a few factors that might influence its absorption: salt form (P, we have identified three different forms of the drug that might have different absorption properties), particle size (Q, by changing the particle size after disintegration of the tablet, the surface area of the microparticles facilitates the absorption; we plan

Table 1 Degrees of freedom associated to a design with multiple factors and their second-order interactions

Source	df
Salt form (P)	2
Particle size (Q)	4
Crystallization form (R)	2
Method of granulation (S)	1
Compression force (T)	3
Interactions PQ	8
Interactions PR	4
Interactions PS	2
Interactions PT	6
Interactions QR	8
Interactions QS	4
Interactions QT	12
Interactions RS	2
Interactions RT	6
Interactions ST	3
Residuals (=3rd, 4th, 5th order interactions)	292
Total	359

to explore five different particle sizes), crystallization form (R, we have identified two polymorphic forms and one amorphous form), method of granulation (S, we may use two different methods of granulation), and compression force (T, we will explore four different forces).

The total number of combinations is $3 \cdot 5 \cdot 3 \cdot 2 \cdot 4 = 360$. If we do not foresee interactions of order higher than 2, we may, then, fit a model only with the main effects and second-order interactions. For every combination we will analyze a single animal. This may seem surprising, but, as we show in Table 1, there are more than enough degrees of freedom for the residuals.

Note that factorial designs very quickly get out of hand in that there is a multiplication of treatment combinations with every added factor.

Important Remarks

45. If we can neglect high-order interactions, we may drastically reduce the number of samples to just one animal per combination, because the high-order interactions act as residuals. However, due to the lack of replication, we cannot construct an unbiased estimate of the noise. That is, if we do not foresee high-order interactions but in reality there are, then our estimate of the noise variance is biased, confounded by the presence of these high-order interactions. Another difficulty of these designs is that we cannot eliminate the effects of blocks, because we need all treatments applied to all block levels, and, therefore, there can only be one block (or at least, as shown in the following section, some of the treatments should be applied to several levels of the blocking variables).
46. Even if we use a single animal per combination, the number of combinations can be very high, 360 in our example above. Fractional factorial designs can even further reduce the number of experiments, but these are out of the scope of these chapters.

1.7 Non-orthogonal, Incomplete, and Imbalanced Designs

1.7.1 Non-orthogonal Designs

In Sect. 1.4, we have seen that one way of estimating linear models is by progressively explaining variance of the observations by adding new terms that might be related to the variability observed in the data. Least squares simultaneously solves all the parameters at once. It is based on trying to solve a linear equation so that the error in each one of the equations is minimized.

Important Remarks

48. A property of orthogonal designs is that the estimates of the parameters do not change whichever sequence we follow. Non-orthogonal designs lose this property, and the model parameters vary depending on the order they are fitted.
49. Designs with covariates are almost never orthogonal because their orthogonality depends on the actual measurements observed in the individuals.

Important Remarks

49. The whole point of experiment design is designing the system matrix X such that the uncertainty associated with the model parameters $\boldsymbol{\theta}$ is minimum. Unfortunately, the uncertainty is given by a matrix, and we cannot "minimize" a matrix. We may minimize its trace (A-optimality), its determinant (D-optimality), its maximum eigenvalue (E-optimality), etc. These different objectives give raise to different designs, with different properties. For some computer programs, the optimality criterion is one of the choices offered to the user.
50. The experiment designs seen in this chapter (completely randomized, randomized block, factorial, etc.) are simple "precooked" designs that guarantee good properties of the covariance matrix of the model parameters.

1.7.2 Incomplete Designs

Incomplete designs are useful when for experimental reasons, we cannot test all treatments in all blocks. For instance, let us consider a factorial design with three factors A, B, and C that can be present (yes) or absent (no). All the possible treatment groups are shown in the table below.

	Factor A	Factor B	Factor C
~~Treatment 0~~	~~No~~	~~No~~	~~No~~
Treatment 1	No	No	Yes
Treatment 2	No	Yes	No
Treatment 3	No	Yes	Yes
Treatment 4	Yes	No	No
Treatment 5	Yes	No	Yes
Treatment 6	Yes	Yes	No
~~Treatment 7~~	~~Yes~~	~~Yes~~	~~Yes~~

However, experimentally it may not make sense to assess the combination (no, no, no) or (yes, yes, yes). We can skip these two treatments and perform only those that make experimental sense. Incomplete designs are a special case of non-orthogonal designs.

We may also use incomplete designs for complicated factorial designs in which not all combinations are to be tested. Additionally, the number of replicates in each one of the combinations may be different.

1.7.3 Imbalanced Designs

Imbalanced designs are useful when we cannot study all possible combinations of treatments and blocks for economical or ethical reasons or any other consideration. Imbalanced designs can also be analyzed by least squares.

Important Remarks

51. There are experimental designs that cannot be analyzed and in which the effects of the treatments and blocks are confounded. Confusion of factors is normal in screening experiments. But they are especially designed to confound in a controlled way.

1.7.4 Balanced Incomplete Block Designs

Having a balanced design helps us keep the estimation equations understandable. Additionally, it does not favor any comparison between treatments. If our blocks cannot hold all treatments, then we may try to find a balanced incomplete block design. A design is *balanced* if:

1. All treatments are applied with the same number of times.
2. All pairs of treatments appear in the same number of blocks.

For instance, the following design is balanced because of the following: (1) each treatment is applied five times, and (2) each pair (AB, AC, AD, AE, AF, BC, BD, BE, BF, CD, CE, CF, DE, DF, EF) appears two times.

	Treatments
Block 1	A B C
Block 2	A B D
Block 3	A C E
Block 4	A D F
Block 5	A E F
Block 6	B C F
Block 7	B D E
Block 8	B E F
Block 9	C D E
Block 10	C D F

Example 27 We want to determine the effect on weight gain of two levels of protein supplement (high or low, represented as P and p, respectively) and vitamin supplement (high or low, represented as V and v). There are four different treatments in total (all possible combinations of protein and vitamin levels that we will represent as A, B, C, and D), and we will use three animals for each of the treatments (12 animals in total). We think that the genetics of the animal may cause a difference, and to account for it, we will use six pairs of siblings. The sibling pair is our block, but we can only test two treatments on each block. The following design is a balanced incomplete design suitable for our needs:

	Treatments
Sibling pair 1	A(pv) B(pV)
Sibling pair 2	A(pv) C(Pv)
Sibling pair 3	A(pv) D(PV)
Sibling pair 4	B(pV) C(Pv)
Sibling pair 5	B(pV) D(PV)
Sibling pair 6	C(Pv) D(PV)

That is, one of the animals of the first sibling pair will receive treatment A (low protein and vitamin supplements), and the other will receive treatment B (low-protein and high-vitamin supplements). It can easily be seen that each treatment is applied to exactly three animals and that all pairs of treatments appear exactly once.

For a comprehensive list of existing solutions, see Zwillinger [2] [Sect. 3.4.2].

An easy way to design experiments is by starting with an initial block (for instance, ABD) and adding 1 to each treatment modulo the number of treatments (i.e., A+1=B; B+1=C; C+1=D; D+1=E; E+1=A). This is called a *cyclic design*. For example, for five blocks of size 3 with five treatments, we would start with the initial block ABD. Then, by adding one to each of the treatments, we would obtain BCE. The rest of blocks are obtained by adding one to the previous block as shown in the following table:

	Treatments
Block 1	A B D
Block 2	B C E
Block 3	C D A
Block 4	D E B
Block 5	E A C

Note that not all initial blocks give raise to a balanced incomplete block design, and you may need to test several initial blocks before finding one that works.

Another easy way to generate balanced incomplete designs is based on lattices. These designs are called *lattice designs*. For example, for seven blocks of size 3 with seven treatments, we construct a Latin square with seven treatments (see Sect. 1.8 and Fig. 5). Then, we take three columns (not any three are valid) and construct the different blocks. These rectangles are called *Youden squares*.

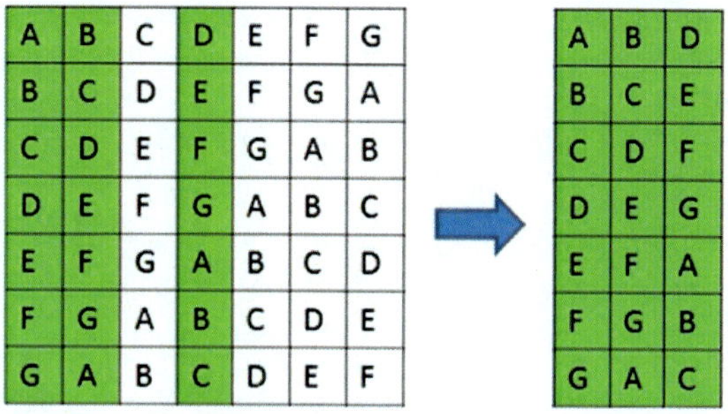

Fig. 5 Example of Youden square. We start from a Latin square of the total number of treatments (left). Then, we select a number of columns equal to the block size (right). If we choose the columns appropriately, the resulting design is balanced

Although outside of the scope of this chapter, for a large number of treatments (a few hundreds), the interested reader may look for cubic lattice designs and alpha lattice designs for large-scale variety trials.

Important Remarks

52. Balanced designs are important to keep estimation equations understandable. If we need to use blocks in which not all treatments fit, balanced incomplete block designs help us keep these two objectives (using blocks and having a balanced design). However, these designs only exist for given combinations of the number of treatments, blocks, and size of the block.

1.8 Latin Squares

Design summary. Latin squares is a special kind of design in which there is a single treatment factor with L levels, and two blocking variables, each one with as many levels as the treatment factor.

Example 28 We want to study the time in hours to recover from a small surgical operation. We can perform it in four different ways (A, B, C, and D), and we will block the researcher performing the operation (four different researchers will be employed). We expect variations depending on the time the operation is performed (9:00, 12:00, 15:00, 18:00) that we also want to block. We may use the design shown below:

Researcher \ Time	9:00	12:00	15:00	18:00
1	A	B	C	D
2	B	C	D	A
3	C	D	A	B
4	D	A	B	C

Each treatment appears only once in all rows and columns (i.e., the property that defines a Latin square). Note that every researcher performs all operations and that all operations are done at a given time. If we perform only one operation per cell in the table, we would have the following table of degrees of freedom:

Source	df
Treatments	3
Researcher	3
Time	3
Residuals	6
Total	15

Having only six degrees of freedom for the residuals has not much statistical power for the standard effect sizes sought in research experiments. After calculating the sample size (see Sect. 1.6), the total number of samples is $N = 25$, we decide to increase it to $N = 32$ in order to have a balanced design and have two samples per combination of blocks and treatments. Instead of repeating twice the same Latin table, we may use a different Latin square as shown below (the upper and lower parts of the table are Latin squares).

Researcher \ Time	9:00	12:00	15:00	18:00
1	A	B	C	D
2	B	C	D	A
3	C	D	A	B
4	D	A	B	C
1	B	D	A	C
2	A	B	C	D
3	D	C	B	A
4	C	A	D	B

We may increase the generalizability of the experiment by studying the treatments with a wider range of researchers and times.

Researcher \ Time	9:00	12:00	15:00	18:00	8:00	11:00	14:00	17:00
1	A	B	C	D				
2	B	C	D	A				
3	C	D	A	B				
4	D	A	B	C				
5					B	D	A	C
6					A	B	C	D
7					D	C	B	A
8					C	A	D	B

The table of degrees of freedom would be

Source	df
Treatments	3
Researcher	7
Time	7
Residuals	14
Total	31

1.9 Graeco-Latin Squares

Design summary. Graeco-Latin squares result from the superposition of two Latin squares, and they allow us to simultaneously perform two different experiments with just one treatment factor and two nuisance factors or to consecutively perform experiments.

Example 29 We are studying the effect of four different cleaning products on the stress of the animals in an animal facility. Four centers participate in the study, and each one of them has four rooms with cages. Simultaneously, we are making a different study, also on the stress of animals, with four different types of cages. Can we perform these two experiments simultaneously without any one of them interfering with the other?

We may use two mutually orthogonal Latin squares: one with the four cleaning products (A, B, C, D) and the other one with the four types of cages (α, β, γ, δ). This kind of designs are called Graeco-Latin squares:

Center \ Room	1	2	3	4
1	Aα	Dδ	Bγ	Cβ
2	Cδ	Bα	Dβ	Aγ
3	Dγ	Aβ	Cα	Bδ
4	Bβ	Cγ	Aδ	Dα

Note that each treatment of one kind (cleaning product or cage) appears exactly once with all treatments of the other kind. The Latin letters form a Latin square, as well as the Greek letters. These two Latin squares are said to be mutually orthogonal, and each combination of pairs of treatments ($A\alpha$, $A\beta$, ..., $D\delta$) appears only once. Each of the cages in the same room would be considered an experimental unit receiving the combined treatment. As we mentioned in the section above, the number of Latin squares of a given size is limited, and the pairs of orthogonal Latin squares are even more limited. For $L = 2$, there is only one pair of mutually orthogonal Latin squares; for $L = 3$, two; for $L = 4$, three; for $L = 5$, four; and for $L = 6$, one.

We have presented Graeco-Latin squares in a context of two simultaneous experiments. But they are also used for consecutive experiments: we first perform the experiment on the cleaning products, and when it is finished, we perform the experiment on the cage types. However, we use a Graeco-Latin design so that there is no carryover effect from the first experiment to the second.

1.10 Crossover Designs

Design summary. In crossover designs we block time and individuals. In this way, we eliminate the intersubject variability from the analysis because an individual is its own control and reduce the number of subjects if we keep fixed the statistical power or increase the statistical power if we keep fixed the number of subjects.

Example 30 We are studying the pain reduction caused by an analgesic. There are two treatments: control (with only the vehicle) and treatment (with the drug). We plan to perform a crossover design in which an animal receives the first one of the treatments, and we perform the measure of pain reduction. Then, we wait for a washout period such that there is no interference between the first and second treatments. Finally, we give the second treatment and measure again. The execution plan is as follows:

Period \ Subject	1	2	3	4	5	6	7	8	9	10	11	12
1	C	T	T	C	C	T	C	T	T	T	C	C
2	T	C	C	T	T	C	T	C	C	C	T	T

Crossover designs can only be used when there is no interference from the first treatment to the second. In a way, the animal seeing the first treatment is not the "same" animal that sees the second, even if it is the same individual. Interferences can be of three kinds:

- Order effects: For instance, if we are using diseased animals and the first treatment cures the disease, we cannot apply the second, or if we apply, its application is useless. The order in which we apply the treatments modifies in an irreversible way the state of the animal.
- Carryover effects: There is still some of the first treatment leftover when we apply the second (for instance, the drug has not been completely eliminated from the body). These negative effects are easily removed by sufficiently long washout periods or by the use of statistical designs aimed at removing first-order, second-order, ...carryover effects, as we will see below.
- Learning effects: Another example is with mice in a maze when one of the rooms has some abuse substance. The study is on the amount of time spent in each of the rooms of the maze. In the second treatment, mice remember which was the configuration of the maze under the first treatment, and this memory modifies the time that naive animals spend in each of the rooms under the second treatment.

A design is *balanced with respect to first-order carryover effects* if each treatment precedes any other treatment the same number of times. For instance, with four treatments (A, B, C, D), a design based on the following sequences is not balanced with respect to first-order carryover effects:

Period			
1	2	3	4
A	B	C	D
B	C	D	A
C	D	A	B
D	A	B	C

The reason is that A precedes B three times, while B never precedes A. However, we can find suitable sequences for four treatments like

Period			
1	2	3	4
A	B	C	D
B	D	A	C
C	A	D	B
D	C	B	A

In this design A precedes B, C, and D only once, and the same happens with all other treatment pairs. Once we have found appropriate sequences of treatments, we must assign the same number of individuals to each of the sequences.

These sequences can be found with the help of Latin squares (see Sect. 1.8), the two previous examples of sequences of four elements were both Latin squares. However, not all Latin squares produce designs balanced with respect to first-order carryover effects. For an even number of treatments, we can find such sequences with the help of a single Latin square. For an odd number of treatments, we require the help of two Latin squares.

Important Remarks

53. In crossover designs, animals are tested more than once reducing the total number of animals needed. Additionally, we can estimate the treatment effects without being affected by the between-animal variability.
54. Thanks to a strongly balanced, uniform within sequences, and period design, we can have estimates of the main effects of the treatments that are unconfounded with the order, period, and carryovers from the immediately previous treatment (first order).
55. If we relax the constraints of the design (strongly balanced, uniform within sequences, and periods), we confound the treatment effects with the order, period, or carryover effects from the previous treatment.

If we repeat this analysis for this design with second-order carryover effects, we see that it is not balanced with respect to them.

1.11 2^k Factorial Designs

Design summary. This is a standard factorial design in which the effect of multiple variables, and their possible interactions, is studied at the same time. The characteristic of this design is that each variable only has two levels. For each combination of the different treatments, we will assume that N animals are studied.

In this section we will study a very common particular case of factorial design in which all factors have only two levels (yes/no, absent/present, ...). If we have k factors, the total number of treatments is 2^k. This kind of designs can be analyzed in the standard way introduced in Sect. 1.

Example 31 We want to know the optimal way of reducing conflicts between animals in cages. For each combination, we will measure the average number of daily conflicts, and we will run our experiment for 10 days. We are interested in the effect of three factors related to the animals in the cage: sex (P), age (Q), and number (R). For each of the factors, we have two levels which we will encode as 0 or 1:

- Sex (P): All animals are of the same sex (0) or different sex (1).
- Age (Q): All animals are within a range of 3 months (0), or the age difference is larger than 3 months (1).
- Number (R): Two animals per cage (0) or four animals per cage (1).

For every treatment we will have two cages of that kind so that we have three observations per treatment. We can arrange the observations as

Sex (P)	Age (Q)	Number (R)	Observations		
0	0	0	y_{0001}	y_{0002}	y_{0003}
0	0	1	y_{0011}	y_{0012}	y_{0013}
0	1	0	y_{0101}	y_{0102}	y_{0103}
0	1	1	y_{0111}	y_{0112}	y_{0113}
1	0	0	y_{1001}	y_{1002}	y_{1003}
1	0	1	y_{1011}	y_{1012}	y_{1013}
1	1	0	y_{1101}	y_{1102}	y_{1103}
1	1	1	y_{1111}	y_{1112}	y_{1113}

We will consider the full factorial model with all interactions:

$$y = \mu+\alpha_P+\alpha_Q+\alpha_R+\alpha_{PQ}+\alpha_{PR}+\alpha_{QR}+\alpha_{PQR}+\epsilon \quad (1)$$

The table of degrees of freedom is

Source	df
P	1
Q	1
R	1
PQ	1
PR	1
QR	1
PQR	1
Residuals	16
Total	23

An interesting feature of 2^k factorial designs (in the example $k = 3$ because we have three factors of interest) is that all model parameters cost only one degree of freedom due to the constraints imposed by linear models. Note that every factor that does not have a significant effect robs the error of degrees of freedom, thereby inflating the error variance (error mean square) and making the whole analysis less significant.

▶ Important Remarks

56. Choosing a model for the observations has important consequences on the statistical power of the analysis. If we foresee second-order, third-order, ...analysis, factorial designs allow estimating all of these interactions. However, if we do not foresee these interactions, choosing an overcomplex model decreases our statistical power, which is our capacity to recognize significant effects.
57. Interactions whose order is larger than two are normally not expected. But, obviously, this depends on the specific system being studied.
58. We should choose the model (main effects, main effects plus second-order interactions, ..., full factorial) before observing the experimental data. We cannot take the decision after seeing the data; this is called *data snooping*, and it constitutes a severe flaw of the analysis.

Bibliography

1. Doncaster CP, Davey A. Analysis of variance and covariance: how to choose and construct models for the life sciences. Cambridge: Cambridge University Press; 2007.
2. Zwillinger D. CRC standard mathematical tables and formulae, 30th edn. Boca Raton: CRC Press; 1996.

Part III

Systematic Reviews and Publishing

Scholarly Publishing and Scientific Reproducibility

Arieh Bomzon and Graham Tobin

Abstract

Poor quality of reporting in published scientific manuscripts has been identified as a major contributor to the low reproducibility of research outcomes. Improved author compliance to a journal's submission guidelines, rigorous editorial vigilance by competent reviewers and journal editors, and revamped research practices and policies by research institutes can raise the reporting quality of submitted manuscripts. In this chapter, we describe the current requirements of scholarly publishing and the responsibilities of authors, peer reviewers, journal editors, scientific journals, and academic institutions. We propose that scientific reproducibility can be improved by (a) upgrading editorial vigilance to assure the quality and accuracy of the scientific record; (b) institutional training in writing in the sciences for research trainees; and (c) institutional adoption of existing standards of quality control in manufacturing and commercial research organizations to develop good publishing and research practices and integrity.

Keywords

Scholarly publishing · Peer review · Writing competency · Editorial competency · Training · Quality control

1 Introduction

Publication in a scholarly journal is probably the most important output of any scientific research, and scholarly journals are a frequently used source of information for scientists [1–4]. A scholarly publication is the culmination of a series of integrated steps, each of which requires unique skills and experience. Additionally, a scholarly publication is often the only tangible evidence that an investigation was done and is used to judge reliability, verifiability, quality, and relevance of the reported research. It is the focus for researchers who want to publish their research findings in prestigious journals: the number and quality of publications are vital to their career because they are used as a measure of a researcher's productivity ("publish or perish") and criteria for recognition and reward ("name and fame") [5].

A. Bomzon (✉)
Laboratory Animals, Pardess Hanna-Karkur, Israel

Consulwrite Editorial Consultancy, Pardess Hanna-Karkur, Israel

Consulvet Consultancy in the Laboratory Animal Sciences, Pardess Hanna-Karkur, Israel
e-mail: arieh@consulwrite.com

G. Tobin
Harlan Teklad, Blackthorn, UK

© Springer Nature Switzerland AG 2021
J. M. Sánchez Morgado, A. Brønstad (eds.), *Experimental Design and Reproducibility in Preclinical Animal Studies*, Laboratory Animal Science and Medicine 1,
https://doi.org/10.1007/978-3-030-66147-2_9

The principles of good reporting encompass accuracy, transparency, and the efficient transfer of knowledge. Good reporting obligates researchers to report their research in journals truthfully [6]. A key component in a scholarly publication is the provision of sufficient information to other researchers in the field to reproduce, replicate, or repeat published findings. An independent and unbiased assessment of a research report is a necessary condition of the scientific process and is typically achieved through a prepublication review of the report by the author's peers [7]. However, the peer-review process is not always infallible in judging the quality of evidence and the clarity of its presentation. Authors of a research report must offer the strongest possible unbiased evidence for their findings in a lucid and coherent manner that convinces the most critical reader and assures the trustworthiness of the report: they should not rely on the peer-review process to improve the report. Authors who intentionally misrepresent data or findings in a publication violate one of the core principles of science, which should serve the public good.

Two of the most important issues in the scientific enterprise are poor quality of reporting in scholarly publishing, which is reflected in (a) the high rejection rate of submitted manuscripts [8–10], which may be about 50% in most journals and up to 90% in prestigious journals [11]; and (b) low reproducibility, which is the variability in outcomes in many studies that purportedly test the same or very similar hypotheses. Of the two, resolving low reproducibility is perhaps seen as the major challenge. For some time, there has been concern that much published research is irreproducible, to such an extent that this low reproducibility has been described by many as a crisis [12–15].

In May 2016, Baker [14] published the results of a global survey of 1576 researchers from a wide range of disciplines, who completed an online questionnaire on reproducibility in research. More than 60% of the participants responded that selective reporting and pressure to publish always or often contributed to irreproducible research while insufficient peer review was listed as a contributor by less than 40%. These responses seem to put the burden for the problem largely with researchers and their institutions. When the respondents were asked to rate 11 different approaches to improve reproducibility, nearly 90% ticked "more robust experimental design" and "better statistics", and 69% ticked "journal checklists".

Understanding the nature and causes of the "reproducibility crisis" has been complicated by the interchangeable use of the terms, "reproducibility", "replicability", and "repeatability" by different authors, yet with apparently different meanings [16–18]. Their meaning in practical speech and writing becomes clear by the context, but much has been written on how they may be precisely defined in respect to scientific data and information. In 2016, the Association for Computing Machinery adopted a set of definitions, which has the merit of simplicity and easy applicability to life sciences: repeatability - same researchers, same experimental setup; replicability - different researchers, same experimental setup; and reproducibility - different researchers, different experimental setup [18]. The definitions of replicability and repeatability are similar to Drummond's definitions [19]. Plesser [18] also added a further dimension to the discussion by arguing that achieving similar results using very different methods (reproducibility) provides better scientific proof than that achieved with classically defined reproducibility.

Beyond this debate on lexicology, there is a genuine concern that experiments that test a common hypothesis commonly produce different outcomes. What are the purported factors that contribute to irreproducible research? Generally, the inability to reproduce the results of published research is increasingly seen as a problem in scientific method and has been attributed to (a) poor experimental design; (b) low statistical power of experiments; (c) measurement error; and (d) poor data analysis [20–24]. The reproducibility crisis has also been attributed to the poor quality of reporting by researchers [14, 25] and constraints in the fostering of responsible research practices and integrity by academic institutions [26, 27].

Accordingly, it has been posited that improving author compliance to submission guidelines and the revamping of research practices and policies by research institutes can substantially raise the acceptance rates of submitted manuscripts. These improvements and revamping, together with better gatekeeping of publications through rigorous editorial vigilance by competent reviewers and journal editors, will assist in resolving the "reproducibility crisis". In this chapter, we describe the existing requirements of scholarly publishing and the responsibilities of authors, peer reviewers, journal editors, and academic institutions. We also provide some suggestions for increasing the likelihood of acceptance of submitted manuscripts, thereby facilitating the reporting of reproducible science.

2 The Process of Scholarly Publishing

Publication in a scholarly journal is the successful outcome of a three-stage information transfer process: submission of information, appraisal of the submitted information, and dissemination of the appraised information. While submission is an assigned responsibility of authors, appraisal is the responsibility of a journal's editorial team, and dissemination is the responsibility of the journal's publisher.

2.1 Submission

2.1.1 The Organization of Information in a Scientific Manuscript

Successful submission dictates that authors submit manuscripts that adhere to existing reporting standards for published research. For this purpose, modern research reports of investigations in most scientific fields are rigidly organized and structured narratives of four sections: an *I*ntroduction, a *M*aterials and Methods section, a *R*esults section, and a *D*iscussion (the IMRaD structure). Authors are also obligated to comply with the target journal's submission guidelines and are recommended to use an appropriate reporting guideline when preparing their manuscript. The IMRaD structure evolved from the letter form in the seventeenth century and was adopted by many journals in the 1940s. It became the standard in the 1980s [28, 29]. The wide use of this format can be attributed to the International Committee of Medical Journal Editors (ICMJE), which published the uniform requirements for manuscripts submitted to biomedical journals in 1978, with the intention of benefitting readers and facilitating peer review of published reports. Since then, the ICMJE has produced multiple editions of these recommendations because problems in publishing were recognized to go well beyond manuscript preparation. The current recommendations are now named the "Recommendations for the Conduct, Reporting, Editing, and Publication of Scholarly Work in Medical Journals" to reflect its broad scope, and more than 3000 journals have stated that they follow these recommendations [30].

The ICMJE recommendations detail the general requirements for reporting of all study designs and manuscript formats. The title page includes the article's title, author information, any disclaimers, sources of support, word count, and sometimes the number of tables and figures. The Introduction provides the context or background of the study (the nature of the problem and its significance). It states the specific purpose, the objective(s), or the hypothesis to be tested.

The Methods section is particularly important for allowing a reader to assess whether the study's protocol and experimental techniques are appropriate to test the hypothesis with sufficient accuracy and precision so that the results are pertinent to the study's objective(s). It should be sufficiently detailed so that another researcher can reproduce the study (methods reproducibility). To this end, authors should unambiguously describe (a) the source of the human or animal population and any inclusion (eligibility) and exclusion criteria; (b) the specific location of the study site; (c) the methods, equipment (details of all apparatus used), and procedures (experimental protocols); (d) all tests performed, including the statistical ones, with enough detail to enable a knowledgeable reader with access to the original data to judge their accuracy and appropriateness for the study and to verify the reported results; and (e) the methods of quantifying and presenting the findings with appropriate indicators of measurement error or uncertainty, such as confidence intervals. For human experimentation, this section should also include statements that the study's protocol was approved by an institutional ethics review board, and the investigation was done according to the principles of the Declaration of Helsinki. For animal-based investigations, this section should also include statements that confirm adherence to national and international guidelines for husbandry, management, and welfare of the animals, and approval of the investigation by an ethics review board.

The Results section presents the key research findings without interpreting their meaning, and its text should draw the reader's attention to what the authors think are the most salient features of the data presented in either the figures or tables. When preparing this section, authors should apply the transformed Newton's third law of motion "For every action, there is an equal and opposite reaction" namely, "For every reported result, there must be a description of the method and for every description of a method, a result must be reported".

The Discussion section is a formal consideration and critical examination of the investigation. The research question should be addressed, and the results considered, in the context of other studies (compare-and-contrast analysis). This section should also emphasize the new and important aspects of the study and its conclusions and imitations. In other words, it should answer the questions posed in the Introduction and explain how the results support the answer(s) and how the answer(s) fit in with existing knowledge on the topic. It should not reiterate a detailed description of the results.

2.1.2 Instructions to Authors or Submission Guidelines

All scientific journals publish a set of instructions to authors (ItAs) to read when preparing a manuscript submission. These instructions or submission guidelines should probably be renamed "information for authors" because they generally include policy statements, as well as a set of instructions: (a) the journal's aims and scope; (b) the article types that the journal publishes, such as a research paper, a short communication, a letter, a commentary, an opinion or perspective, or a review; (c) the journal's policies on peer review, authorship, confidentiality, conflicting interests, research ethics, plagiarism, data manipulation, and prior and duplicate publication; (d) the journal's limits on word count for each article type and requirements for layout, such as font type, line spacing, and margin size, and the format for graphics, in-text citations, and bibliography; and (e) a list of preferred providers of English language editing services because most peer-reviewed scientific articles are published in English and many authors are not native English speakers.

Despite the need for explicit and comprehensible ItAs, the ItAs of many journals are not explicit and comprehensible. Malicki and his colleagues [31] recently reported the results of their analysis of ItAs in 835 health and life sciences journals and arts and humanities journals. Of the 19 topics that they considered to be relevant to transparency in reporting and research integrity, they found that only three topics were addressed in more than one-third of the ItAs namely, conflicts of interest, plagiarism, and the type of peer review used by the journal. Accordingly, they concluded the insufficient attention to transparency could be addressed by more regular updating of their ItAs, thereby ensuring that their requirements match their practices.

2.1.3 Reporting Guidelines

Reporting guidelines were intended to become useful tools for achieving high standards in reporting research and to help authors prepare, and reviewers and journal editors appraise, a scientific manuscript. A reporting guideline comprises statements that provide advice on how to report research methods and findings so that a researcher can present a clear and transparent account of what was done and found in a research study. A reporting guideline is also a checklist that allows assessment of a study and if necessary, reproduction of a study. Some guidelines may request the inclusion of a flow chart to help clarify a complex procedure.

Adherence to a reporting guideline by authors decreases the number of honest reporting errors by taking them through a series of methodical steps so that nothing of importance is omitted, consequently improving the reliability and utility of publications. Reporting guidelines complement a journal's ItAs on the style to be applied to research reports and advice on the basic principles of scientific writing. The inclusion of a completed checklist with a submitted manuscript benefits a journal's editorial team and an article's reviewers by providing clear evidence that the author has met the key basic requirements to justify further effort by them.

Reporting guidelines do not come as a "one-size-fits-all" product because there are many types of investigations and research reports. Accordingly, many reporting guidelines have been developed for reporting each type of investigation. The EQUATOR network (http://www.equator-network.org) is a resource that currently hosts over 400 guidelines for reporting the results of many study types mainly in the health sciences. Irrespective of study type, editorial endorsement on their use requires joint action by the authors, reviewers, and the editorial team of journals [32, 33]. For animal-based investigations, two reporting guidelines were published in 2010: the Gold Standard Publication Checklist (GSPC) [34] and the Animal Research: Reporting of In Vivo Experiments (ARRIVE) reporting guidelines (https://www.nc3rs.org.uk/arrive-guidelines). Of the two, the *ARRIVE* reporting guidelines are the preference of about 1000 biomedical journals. The Meridian Network (https://meridian.cvm.iastate.edu) is a resource that specifically hosts a collection of reporting guidelines, such as ARRIVE, exclusively for animal-based investigations (Meridian–Menagerie of reporting guidelines involving animals). Finally, the Good Publication Practice (GPP) guideline, first published in 2003, updated in 2009 as GPP2, and revised in 2015 as GPP3 [35], was designed to help commercial organizations, such as pharmaceutical, biotechnology, medical device, and diagnostics companies, maintain ethical practices when they report their research findings.

Has the use of reporting guidelines met its objective of improving the quality of reporting? Notwithstanding endorsement of reporting guidelines by scientific journals, their impact on the quality of reporting has not been immense to date. In her inconclusive study of publications in the health sciences, Stevens and her colleagues [36] reported that insufficient evidence existed to determine the relationship between journals' support for reporting guidelines and the completeness of reporting of published reports. The later studies of Bezdjian et al. [37], Leung et al. [38], and Hair et al. [39] were more conclusive: they concluded that journal support for the ARRIVE guidelines has not resulted in a meaningful improvement in reporting quality. In other words, reporting guidelines have not yet arrived because (a) authors do not comply with or use a reporting guideline; (b) reviewers do not always comment on or identify omissions in required information; and (c) the editorial teams of journals do not always insist on submission of a completed checklist at the time of manuscript submission. Lastly, Hair and her colleagues [39] advocated that more stringent editorial policies or a targeted approach to key quality items may promote improvements in reporting and compliance with the ARRIVE guidelines.

2.2 Appraisal

For many journals, a two-step appraisal process is used to select submissions for publishing: an initial internal editorial review, followed by an external peer review of those manuscripts selected. The decision to accept, reject, or revise a manuscript is not an exercise in simple arithmetic where the number of positive and negative points is tallied to generate a final score, which falls above or below a threshold or within a range. Rather, the final editorial decision is based on judicious evaluation of the reviewers' reports, and one major irrecoverable flaw may be sufficient to warrant rejection.

When deciding which papers to publish, the editorial team must remember that the highest priority in publishing an article is to advance science and assure the trustworthiness of the report. The editorial team must also remember that it is accountable for the journal's content and the readers expect that the team will implement procedures to ensure the quality of the published articles in the journal. To these ends, the editorial team (a) must have experience and broad knowledge of the fields covered by the journal; (b) select those manuscripts that reflect the journal's aims and scope and are pertinent for the readership; (c) manage and assure the integrity of the peer review of all manuscripts consistently and impartially; and (d) protect an author's interests during the peer-review process. The editorial team must also be protected from, and be able to resist, any external and internal pressures that could infringe on the integrity of the review process because misconduct can erode a journal's credibility. During the peer-review process, the editorial team should (a) use reliable, competent, and trustworthy reviewers who can meet the journal's timelines; (b) communicate clearly and effectively with the corresponding author and peer reviewers; and (c) coordinate the interaction between the author, peer reviewers, and the journal's publisher. When making the final editorial decision, the team should consider the reviewers' and other editors' comments and synthesize information and opinions from a wide range of resources. Lastly, the editorial team should not suppress the publication of a research report of satisfactory quality.

2.2.1 The Internal Editorial Review ("Triage")

Following its submission, the journal's editorial office first does a technical screen that checks (a) the manuscript's word count and format; (b) whether submission complies with the guidelines; and (c) the submission includes all required documentation. This process is sometimes described as "triage". The manuscript is then assigned to the best-qualified member of the journal's editorial team to (a) establish whether the manuscript falls within the journal's aims and scope; (b) ascertain whether the manuscript would be of interest to the journal's readers in terms of the research question's importance, relevance, and utility; and (c) determine whether the manuscript has the potential for publication in the journal in terms of its methodology, experimental design, statistical analysis, interpretation of the results, and writing style and clarity.

2.2.2 The External Peer Review

Journals use peer review to ensure that the scientific process is robust [7]. Peer review is a process designed to encourage impartiality and typically involves the use of a third party, who is someone neither affiliated directly with the publisher, editorial board, or journal nor too closely associated with the manuscript under review. Additionally, peers submit their reviews without, initially at least, knowledge of other reviewers' comments and recommendations.

Peer review has been a formal part of scientific communication for more than 300 years, and its importance has increased since the 1950s [7, 40]. It is also regarded as the principal mechanism for quality control and ensuring trustworthiness in most scientific disciplines [41]. Nowadays, almost all aspects of the contemporary scientific enterprise, including applications for research funding, rely on quality evaluations by peers. In their study on authors' views of peer review in the digital age, Nicholas et al. [40] reported the findings of a survey of 3650 researchers, who were recruited by six scholarly publishers. The researchers considered peer review to be "a central pillar of trust" in the appraisal of submitted manuscripts and preferred their research findings to be published in journals with robust peer review mechanisms. Peer review has considerable external importance to society: it testifies that researchers take their social responsibility seriously as a self-regulating, normatively driven community. Despite its supposed flaws and critics, such as Richard Smith, a former editor of the British Medical Journal [42–44], the research community views peer review as being synonymous with scientific credibility and the best means for evaluating scientific communications. We discuss the weaknesses of peer review in Subsect. 3.2 "Limitations and Disadvantages of Peer Review".

When done properly, the main outcome of peer review is the selection of the best manuscripts for publication in the journal. In broad terms: it ensures the relevance of the work to the journal; it determines the scientific merit and importance of the research question and the originality of the investigation; it certifies the adherence of scientific standards by appraising the strengths and weaknesses of the investigation's methodology thereby protecting readers from incorrect and flawed research; and it assesses the quality of the presentation, interpretation, and significance of an investigation's finding(s). Specifically, it (a) ensures previous work is acknowledged; (b) checks for factual accuracy of and omissions in a manuscript's content; (c) evaluates the experimental design and the appropriateness and robustness of an investigation's methodology and statistical testing; (d) checks the accuracy of a manuscript's in-text citations and bibliography; and (e) contributes to the detection of fraud and plagiarism. Peer reviewers are not spell, grammar, and punctuation checkers, but they are expected to comment on the quality of a manuscript's language, with examples of inadequacies.

Different degrees of anonymity and openness exist within the peer-review process. The most widely used model is the single-blind review in which the authors' names are known to the reviewers but the reviewers' names are not known to the authors. In the double-blind review, neither the authors' nor the reviewers' names names are known to each other. In the triple-blind review, the authors, the reviewers, and the editors are all unknown to each other. In contrast, in the open and published review, the authors' and reviewers' names are known to each other, and the reviewers' names are published (signed) or not published (blind) with the report. There are also open-identity reviews in which reviewers' reports are published alongside the relevant article (open reports); in open identity and open report reviews, all parties are known to each other and the reviews are published. Finally, there is the post-publication review where readers can comment on a report following its publication (open final-version commenting). For many authors, peer review is an anonymous authority that prolongs publication times. A recent initiative is the introduction of innovative models of peer review in which the process is transparent, rapid, and less onerous for authors: bioRxiv (https://www.biorxiv.org/), PeerJ (https://peerj.com/), F1000Research (https://f1000research.com/), and mSphereDirect (https://msphere.asm.org/content/mspheredirect).

Irrespective of the type of review, two or three reviewers are frequently invited to appraise a submitted manuscript. The selection of a peer reviewer is based on their apparent expertise, which is often gauged in terms of their publication output and impact in the research area. Ensuring an objective review of a scientific report requires peer reviewers to be (a) responsive and timely so that the journal's timelines are satisfied; (b) critical, knowledgeable, and proficient so that the review can improve a report's quality; (c) thorough, impartial, objective, and have no conflicts of interest so that the report's assessment is honest and unbiased; (d) competent and confidential so that the report's assessment is trustworthy and private; and (e) responsible so that the report advances science and contributes to the existing knowledge in the field [45]. Selection of a peer reviewer should depend on the reviewer's ability to fulfill these performance criteria, but in practice, selection is often based on personal acquaintance and experience.

Many researchers do peer review because (a) it is part of their job; (b) it reciprocates for the reviews of their reports; (c) it helps them stay abreast of the latest trends in their field; (d) it ensures the integrity of research published in their field; (e) it is being a good citizen in the scientific community; and (f) it contributes to their personal reputation and career progression.

While the experience of the reviewer and the time spent on a review might be expected to benefit a manuscript's quality, Black and his colleagues [46] found that reviews done by young and less experienced reviewers were generally better than those that were done by old and presumably more experienced reviewers. While the quality of the review did improve with the time spent, they reported that little additional benefit was gained beyond three hours of effort.

2.3 Dissemination

After a manuscript is accepted for publication, the publisher disseminates it in a journal. Scholarly publishing is a profitable business because the costs for creating and appraising the submitted manuscript are minimal. Researchers, whose salaries are paid by their parent institution and whose research is often funded from public money, create and submit the manuscript to their target journal, and the manuscript's appraisers receive no financial reward for their work. Once the manuscript is accepted for publication, the publisher disseminates the article by selling the journal (subscription journals), in which the article is published, to the institutions and organizations that employ and fund the manuscript's creators and appraisers.

In the coming years, the *modus operandi* for disseminating research findings, particularly in Europe, will probably change. Traditionally, publishers locked published manuscripts behind a paywall where readers "pay" to view the article, either via their institutional or personal subscription or on a pay-per-view basis. In the 1990s, individuals began to campaign for open access (OA) to journals because publication paywalls withheld a substantial amount of scientific knowledge from the scientific community and society funded by the public purse. In 2004, the US Congress required the National Institutes of Health (NIH) to develop an OA repository for voluntary submission of published NIH-funded research articles [47]. In 2008, NIH's public access policy became mandatory and directed NIH-funded researchers to "submit or have submitted for them to the National Library of Medicine's PubMed Central an electronic version of their final, peer-reviewed manuscripts upon acceptance for publication, to be made publicly available no later than 12 months after the official date of publication" (http://publicaccess.nih.gov/policy.htm). To comply with NIH's regulations, many journals are now hybrid subscription journals in which some articles are open access after payment of an article-processing charge (APC) and others remain closed access and are unlocked after 12 months. Lastly, many OA journals are legitimate enterprises that contribute to the ever-growing body of scientific knowledge [48]. OA publishers, such as the Public Library of Science (PLoS) and BioMed Central (BMC), maintain peer review to preserve their academic reputations, and many OA journals recover costs by charging an author publication fee [47].

Since 2000, there has been a substantial growth in both the number of journals offering OA publication (18% per annum) and the number of published OA articles (30% per annum) [49] set against the growth of 5% per annum for journals and 4% per annum for articles in overall publishing [50]. Currently, about 15–20% of papers are OA, with a further 10–15% available after a delay following initial publication [50, 51]. In Europe, except for a few countries, such as the UK, the imposition of mandatory OA publishing by funding agencies has been much slower than in the USA. However, OA publishing will soon become mandatory in the Europe Union: the European Commission introduced Plan S, a strategy for accelerating progress toward OA publishing as part of Horizon 2020, its Research and Innovation Programme [52]. In this plan, "After 1 January 2020 scientific publications on the results from research funded by public grants provided by national and European research councils and funding bodies must be published in compliant open access journals or on compliant open access platforms" [53]. It is still too early for us to discuss the implications of a widening of OA in Europe, and we are not qualified to do so, but Richard Horton, the current editor of *The Lancet*, has spelt out some of the consequences to journals that are not compliant or are partially compliant to Plan S [54].

3 Issues Associated with the Publishing Process

3.1 Author Compliance

Many articles on the common errors in rejected manuscripts have been published in numerous life science journals [8, 10, 55–65]. The most frequent reasons for rejection are (a) the topic is outside the journal's aims and scope; (b) the subject matter is not new, does not contribute to the field, has little utility, and is often a false claim of a breakthrough or a discovery; (c) the presence of methodological errors; (d) the experimental design, the data collection process, and the methods of statistical analysis are deficient or suboptimal; and (e) the text lacks clarity and organization. Irrespective of the reasons for rejection, some of these errors originate from non-compliance to the journal's submission guidelines. Other errors can often be avoided by seeking advice from others; for example, common defects in experimental design and statistical analysis can be avoided by consulting a statistician prior to commencement of the study. Lastly, the rejection of a manuscript does not preclude publication. Tracking of rejected papers has perhaps been best studied in medical journals, where publication of previously rejected manuscripts typically ranges between 65 and 75% [66–72]. The delay in publication was about 12–18 months, and publication generally was in less specialized and lower impact journals.

Although improper use of English and poor writing style may make a manuscript's text difficult to follow or understand, it may not necessarily result in outright rejection of a manuscript. However, quality of language does matter because it can influence the reviewers' and editors' overall impression of the work [73] and deficiencies almost certainly need to be corrected before publication. Therefore, authors, whose grasp of English may be weak, will benefit from seeking appropriate support before submission from experienced colleagues with good English writing skills or a professional English-language editing service.

3.2 Limitations and Disadvantages of Peer Review

The UK government (House of Commons Science and Technology Committee) [7] did a broad appraisal of peer review in scholarly publishing after collecting evidence from many eminent individuals in the scientific publishing field. The results of their appraisal are extensive and too detailed to be repeated here, but they provide an extremely valuable oversight of the strengths and weaknesses of the process. The critics of peer review claim that the process is slow, not transparent, nor cost-effective [7, 40, 42, 74–76]. Other declared failings of the process are misjudgment by editors, absence of reviewer impartiality, and submission of inappropriate reviews that are sometimes subjective, intimidating, inconsistent, inadequate, or of variable quality. Additionally, it does not always improve the quality of a report and does not perform well in detecting data manipulation and fraud. Furthermore, peer reviewers often miss errors, especially those in experimental design and statistical analysis.

Editorial decisions on acceptance/rejection of manuscripts are largely influenced by the recommendations of reviewers [77, 78]. Consequently, uniformity of outcome for a manuscript by different reviewers is particularly important. There seems to be no consensus on the inter-rater reliability (IRR) of peer reviews. The majority view is that IRR is poor with recommendations on acceptance or rejection at levels little greater than chance [41, 77, 79–81].

However, contrary views have been expressed. Baethge et al. [78] studied the peer review process at a German general medical journal and reported that their "findings challenge the view that journal peer review, in general, is unreliable". Specifically, they reported that agreement among reviewers was substantial when the recommendation was acceptance or revision of a manuscript, but less so when the recommendation was rejection. They also reported that they considered "concordance among reviewers sufficient for the purposes of editorial decision making". Siler et al. [82] compared the fates of accepted and rejected manuscripts that were eventually published. They examined how many citations each published article eventually garnered, irrespective of whether it was published in the initial target journal or another journal. They reported that peer review added value to manuscripts and generally peer reviewers and editors made good decisions on identifying and promoting quality in scientific manuscripts.

Perhaps it should not be a surprise that sometimes recommendations may differ between reviewers, particularly with respect to rejection, because it is impossible to exclude the human factor and emotion. Some reviewers may consciously or unconsciously balance the inadequacies against the effort that the authors applied in carrying out and producing the manuscript. They may consider the flaws to be correctable rather than necessitating outright rejection. What might be more damning of the peer-review process would be substantial differences in the recognition of factual defects in the manuscript.

The number of submissions to journals is continuously increasing because of relentless and prolonged pressure on researchers to "publish or perish" and the incentives of personal and professional reward ("name and fame"). For all legitimate peer-reviewed journals, the number of submitted manuscripts is far bigger than the number published, and this large number of submissions is overloading the peer-review process. When a manuscript is sent for peer review, initiation of the process automatically places a burden on the scientific community, and this burden is exacerbated when a revision is required or the rejected manuscript is submitted to another journal.

In the 2018 Publons survey "2018 Global State of Peer Review" [83] of 11,800 researchers largely sourced from the Publons community, it was estimated that 13.7 million reviews were required for publishing 2.9 million peer-reviewed articles in 2016. Kovanis et al. [84] investigated the global demand for reviewers in the biomedical sciences over the period 1990–2015, and they reported that the supply of potential reviewers exceeded demand. Although reviewer fatigue is now emerging as a burgeoning problem, Breuning et al. [85] concluded that the process is currently sustainable in terms of volume despite the substantial imbalance in the distribution of peer-review contributions within the scientific community. However, finding competent reviewers for an increasing number of manuscripts will gradually become more and more difficult because of the time required for each review, the reviewer's conflict with other workloads, and the lack of incentives, credit, and recognition for the reviewer. One solution to lessen the burden on expert reviewers is the cascade system. If a manuscript is rejected by the authors' journal of choice, it can be passed on to another journal, crucially, with the reviews from the first journal. This can occur in one of two ways: either within one publishing organization and between its "sister" journals or between journals from different publishers. While publishers are prepared to share reviews with sister journals, sharing outside the "family" is more contentious since "some journals are a bit squeamish about the idea of acknowledging that the paper went somewhere else before it came on to them" [7].

Although peer review is generally highly regarded, there are reviewers who do not act in the best interest of science but rather in their own self-interest [86]. This is most commonly exemplified by manipulating manuscript acceptance to highlight and promote their own work (self-citation). Surprisingly, this is largely achieved through acceptance of low-quality manuscripts rather than rejecting high-quality manuscripts that compete with their own studies. This behavior ensures that approval of their own research will be boosted in an increasing background of poorly conducted studies and low-quality reports and may not always be obvious to editors.

The misconduct of some reviewers should not detract from the substantial contribution made mostly by anonymous volunteers. While reviewers are not always infallible, may not be appropriate for the area of research, or may not be able to give adequate time to the process, the general standard and commitment are high, and overall the process brings about substantial benefits to the quality of a submitted manuscript [87, 88]. If anything, the process should be expanded because "to bypass or diminish peer review may start a process that would undermine the output of research, allow cynics to question its validity, and give free rein to those that prefer their biases to results from well-controlled experimental investigations" [87].

3.3 Reviewer Competence

Most peer reviewers receive neither formal training in reviewing nor training in writing a report, despite a significant proportion of them perceiving that they need one or both. Instead, reviewing is often a skill learnt through the feedback that authors receive on their own submitted manuscripts. Furthermore, many reviewers are not informed on the quality of their reports: they rarely receive any feedback from the journal that requested the review. Given the importance of peer review in scholarly publishing, as well as for grant applications, training in peer review for all early-career researchers should be mandatory [7].

3.4 Editorial Competence

The principal task of a journal's editor is to decide on a journal's content, which includes adjudicating the fate of a submitted manuscript and implementing a journal's internal and external policies. Traditionally, many editors-in-chief of scientific journals are untrained part-time volunteers and discharge their editorial commitments while fulfilling other responsibilities. To improve productivity and decision making and remove the time constraints on a journal's editor-in-chief, numerous scientific journals have an editorial team that can comprise an editor-in-chief, one or more deputy editors, an executive editor, sometimes an executive deputy editor, and an editorial assistant. When a member of the editorial team is not employed by the journal's publisher, the appointment of an individual to the editorial team is usually based on the individual's reputation/stature and expertise in a specific field. The team's reputation is essential for attracting submissions to the journal, and its expertise is essential for proper evaluation of the submissions. Despite these attributes, editors rarely have any formal training in their role, and their scientific expertise does not necessarily imply an ability to be a successful editor. This deficiency has been recognized by Galipeau et al. [89] and Moher et al. [90], who have developed an extensive set of core competencies for editors that can be used to create a training program.

3.5 Publication Practices

Rigorous publication processes help ensure research integrity, and high levels of trust are vital to ensuring that the publication of research results helps to advance research, the global pool of knowledge, and the careers of scientists. Additionally, there are common ethical standards and behaviors to ensure that articles reporting company-sponsored medical research in peer-reviewed journals are of the highest standards [35]. Many publishers are members of organizations that support and facilitate publishing standards and practices. Several such organizations exist, each often with its own focus. The International Association of Scientific, Technical and Medical Publishers (https://www.stm-assoc.org/) is a trade association for academic and professional publishers whose members annually publish nearly 66% of all journal articles and markets itself as the global voice of scholarly publishing. The National Information Standards Organisation (https://groups.niso.org/home) produces information standards for content publishers, libraries, and software developers, while the Committee on Publication Ethics (https://publicationethics.org/) aims to move "the culture of publishing toward one where ethical practices becomes the norm".

Scholarly publishing is not without its weaknesses. In 2008, Young and his colleagues [91] commented that current publishing practices may distort science because (a) they introduce publication bias into the process since only articles that report positive results are generally published, though this is not a consistent finding [92]; (b) the urgency to publish new knowledge often results in false or exaggerated claims that may only be discovered many years after publication; (c) they publish results of an investigation whose real longterm value and utility are largely unpredictable; and (d) publishing in prestigious journals may give a status to a manuscript that is not always justified by its content.

While OA has benefited the science community, it has led to the introduction of OA journals and books in which the author pays for publication without the need for peer review. Some of these publications may be of very low quality and may actively solicit contributions. Sometimes authors will only be notified of a publishing fee after their article is published. In some eyes, the authors are tricked into paying for publication, which has led to the term "predatory" journals or books [93]. However, there is no doubt that some authors are willing to augment their publication output and avoid adequate oversight by paying for publication. A similar process, referred to as "vanity press", is also used for publication of books [48, 94].

A scientific publication has become the prevailing currency of the science community, and scholarly publishing has become an exchange market where there are suppliers (authors) and buyers (journals) of products (scientific manuscripts) [9]. In this market, researchers hawk their manuscripts to those journals with a high impact factor (IF), hoping to add to their personal professional status, and journals seek those manuscripts that will increase their prestige. In other words, good researchers want to publish their research reports in high-ranking journals, which in turn want the good researchers, supposedly with good quality manuscripts, to publish with them. This market is continually expanding and has become dynamic and competitive (see Subsect. 2.3 "Dissemination"). It is expanding because the research community now comprises many non-western researchers, exemplified by China whose researchers are now overtaking US researchers as the dominant source of research publications [50]. It has become dynamic because the Internet has reduced the boundaries between researchers and society and the escalating use of social media and portable Internet devices. For example, Facebook and Twitter are being used to disseminate scientific information, especially from scientific meetings [95–99]. Another example is the "Share this Article" link to various social and professional networks, which enables authors to promote their published article [100]. The market has become more competitive because of a disparity between the increasing size of the research community and the limited availability of printing space in reputable scientific journals. However, it is becoming "ugly" because (a) implementation of existing guidelines for good research practice and publication has not ensured a culture of good research and research integrity in some researchers and research institutions; and (b) publishing in unreliable predatory journals is threatening the integrity of the scientific enterprise.

3.6 Biases

According to Lee and her colleagues [101], bias is "a kind of error in identifying the true quality of the item being rated" and "a deviation from proxy measures for true quality". There are different types of bias in scholarly publishing.

(a) Bias as a function of author characteristics where the evaluation is not based on merit, the excellence of the investigation, or the originality of the finding, but on academic rank, sex, place of work, and social status.
(b) Prestige bias where those individuals who are rich in prestige disproportionately accumulate limited resources, such as grant monies, publication space, and awards, which allows them to garner yet more prestige in a process of cumulative advantage.
(c) Nationality or geographical bias where journals favor reviewers located in the same country as the journal.

(d) Language bias where acceptance rates for authors from English-speaking countries are higher than those for authors from non-English-speaking countries.
(e) Affiliation bias when reviewers and authors have formal or informal relationships.
(f) Content or ego bias or "cognitive cronyism" when reviewers will favorably evaluate the submissions of authors who belong to similar "schools of thought".
(g) Conservatism where there is bias against ground-breaking and innovative research.
(h) Confirmation bias where there is the tendency to gather, interpret, and present evidence in ways that affirm rather than challenge one's existing beliefs.
(i) Bias against interdisciplinary research because disciplinary reviewers prefer mainstream research.
(j) Publication bias where journals prefer to publish research that demonstrates positive rather than negative outcomes [27]. This bias is considered to be a potential major contributor to the lack of reproducibility because "an overworked scientist will struggle to justify investing time and effort into writing up null results, rather than focusing on collecting more data and writing up other, more 'exciting' findings" [102].

In their review, Lee and her colleagues [101] commented that failures in impartiality "threaten the social legitimacy of peer review" lead to outcomes that do not "uphold the meritocratic image of knowledge communities", "protect orthodox theories and approaches", "insulate 'old boy' networks", "encourage authors to chase disputable standards", "mask bad faith efforts by reviewers who are also competitors", and "lead to dissatisfaction among those whose professional success or failure is determined by review outcomes".

While important, bias is not the focus of this chapter, and additional information can be found in Bornmann's report of scientific peer review [41], Gaston and Smart's article on the influences of regional diversity of reviewers [103], and Lerback and Hanson's commentary on gender bias in peer review [104].

3.7 Bibliometric Indices

Bibliometric indices are used to assess the impact and quality of journals and assess and rank a researcher's and institution's research performance. To these ends, at least 2 years of citation data are required. Five indices are used to assess a journal's impact and quality.

(a) The IF, which is derived from the number of citations received in a year by articles published in the preceding 2–5 years.
(b) The source normalized impact per paper (SNIP), which is a ratio of the average number of citations received by articles in a journal (categorized in a particular field) and the citation potential of the field (i.e., the average length of the reference list of articles in that field).
(c) The SCImago Journal Rank (SJR), which is derived from the average number of weighted citations received in a year, divided by the number of articles published in the previous 3 years. The citations received by the journal are weighted according to the subject field, quality, and reputation of the journals citing the articles.
(d) CiteScore, which counts the citations received in a year by articles published in the previous 3 years and divides this by the number of items (articles and other content) published in those 3 years. Contrary to most other journal metrics, CiteScore also includes non-peer-reviewed items, such as editorials, corrigenda, and announcements.
(e) The citation count, which varies widely between fields and depends on the size of the field because it measures the absolute number of citations a journal received in a year.
(f) The Eigenfactor score, which measures a journal's importance to the scientific community.

The IF was originally produced to help the Institute for Scientific Information (ISI) decide whether it should include a journal in its database and librarians to make decisions on the purchase of journal subscriptions [105]. Although researchers use many criteria when selecting a target journal, a journal's bibliometric indices, especially the IF, are widely used because they provide information on journal ranking in their field [106, 107]. Ranking a journal using these indices has long been controversial because their determinants are unrelated to scientific quality [106, 108, 109]. Nevertheless, these indices are being used to rank scientists [106, 110]: they have been repurposed and misused by other researchers and institutions as a proxy for the quality and importance of research publications. Accordingly, researchers are now frequently judged by where their articles are published rather than by the content of their publications.

The "*h* index" (the Hirsch index [111]) and the newer "*g* index" introduced by Egghe in 2006 [112] are bibliometric indices that are designed to measure the importance, significance, and broad impact of a scientist's cumulative research contributions and are often used by institutions to make quantitative comparisons between scientists. Although the *g* index complements the *h* index, it differs by putting more weight on highly cited citations. Elsevier has recently launched and encouraged the use of a new bibliometric tool called SciVal (https://www.scival.com/) for assessing and analyzing the research performance and impact of researchers and institutions.

The use of these two indices to measure a researcher's performance is also controversial. For example, the *h* index has frequently been criticized for the problems of self-citations, field dependency, and multiple authorship [113]. The "h index" and the "g index" have also been criticized because of their damaging effects on the scientific enterprise and the behavior of researchers seeking to boost their rating [114–118]. In the hyper-competitive environment for career development and research funds, scientists have shifted their primary objective from scientific discovery to the adoption of the "least publishable unit" strategy (sometimes referred to as segmented publication, redundant publication, salami slicing, or salami publication). Although a researcher may publish many scientific papers using this strategy, each publication tests a similar hypothesis, uses the same methodology, and presents much the same results without duplicating the text [119, 120]. This change has often been unwittingly and unintentionally supported by institutions that reward scientists according to their publication record, as well as their grant income. Campbell [117], who is the editor-in-chief of the publishing company Springer Nature, wrote that "our own internal research demonstrates how a high journal impact factor can be the skewed result of many citations of a few papers rather than the average level of the majority, reducing its value as an objective measure of an individual paper". Lawrence [115] comments that the use of these indices has "cut a swathe through scientific thinking like a forest fire, turning our thoughts and efforts away from scientific problems and solutions, and toward the process of submission, reviewing and publication". He also comments that "trying to meet the measures involves changing research strategy: risks should not be taken as this can mean long periods trying out new things" and "you risk interesting no one".

It has been claimed that the "publish or perish" mentality has led some researchers, whose submissions have been rejected by traditional subscription journals, to bend the rules or behave unethically [26, 27, 121] and sometimes to publish in "predatory journals" [48, 94]. It is also claimed that such unethical behavior is responsible for increasing cases of academic misconduct, fraud, or sloppiness [26]. These behaviors or transgressions encompass (a) misrepresenting and distorting research data; (b) intentionally spinning a study's findings; (c) problematic statistical techniques; (d) failure to document and preserve research results properly; (e) data and image manipulation; (f) using the same original data in multiple publications; (g) inappropriate authorship; and (h) presenting multiple conference presentations on the same research. Such misconduct damages the public's trust in science and researchers especially when the researcher's profile outside academia is high and the results influence public policy. The response to academic misconduct is frequently not a forensic examination by the researcher's institution to identify the cause(s) or the systemic aspects of their cultures and practices that might have contributed to the misconduct. Wager [122] reported several disappointing institutional attitudes to editors' reports of misconduct: failure to respond to the editor; an unwillingness to take the comment seriously or investigate it; inadequate investigation; and stalling, presumably in the hope that the problem will fizzle out. Worryingly, the failure of UK universities to respond may be consistent with their incomplete adherence to "the Concordat to Support Research Integrity". This policy required those UK universities receiving public funding to deal openly and transparently with research misconduct. Despite being introduced in 2012 by Universities UK, the UK House of Commons Science and Technology Committee on Research Integrity concluded: "Most universities take their research integrity responsibilities seriously, but progress in implementing the Concordat to Support Research Integrity across the whole sector is disappointing. Six years on from the signing of the Concordat, the sector as a whole still falls some way short of full compliance in terms of publishing an annual statement, which risks giving the impression of pockets of complacency. We were surprised by the reasons that some universities gave for not publishing an annual statement on research integrity as recommended by the Concordat" [27]. Furthermore, they noted about 25% of Universities UK members did not even publish an annual report, one of the basic requirements of the Concordat. It would be interesting to know whether this permissiveness to research misconduct applies to academic institutions in other countries.

The first move to document retractions systematically commenced in 2010 with Retraction Watch (https://retractionwatch.com/), which is a blog that was founded by two health journalists, Ivan Oransky and Adam Marcus, and whose aim was to obtain how and why many scientific papers were being withdrawn [123]. In its latest report, Retraction Watch claimed the number of retractions is growing though much of this growth can be attributed to a small number of authors and improved oversight by journals, especially those with low IFs. Retraction does not always mean academic misconduct by the authors or one of the authors [124], and Retraction Watch data suggest that many withdrawn papers were retracted because of unreliability, invalidity, or inadequate interpretation of the data. Unfortunately, a scholarly publication may be withdrawn many years after its original publication by which time much "damage" may have been done.

3.8 English as the Language of Science and Technology

Modern scientific research is a global enterprise whose default language is English. Most of the top journals in any scientific field publish articles in English because they originate from either the USA or the UK, according to SCImago Journal and Country Rank (https://www.scimagojr.com/aboutus.php). This reliance on the English language has had an extraordinary and unprecedented effect on scientific communication, especially for non-native English speakers: they sometimes find it challenging to understand a journal's submission guidelines and convey a coherent message in written English [125]. In the context of the international community of researchers, a journal's submission guidelines should be written in simple, concise, coherent, and precise English because the displacement of English as the default language of science and technology is unlikely to happen in the immediate future.

A researcher's participation in and contribution to the global scientific enterprise is also directly related to his/her ability to write manuscripts in good English [73]. It is also widely accepted that authors of a scientific manuscript that are submitted to journals are responsible for its quality of English [73]. Many non-native English speakers are very capable of writing effective manuscripts despite errors in grammar, syntax, and usage. Unfortunately for authors whose English is not good, reviewers, editors, and journal staff do not have the time or resources to edit manuscripts for the correct use of the English language. Therefore, reviewers of manuscripts that are written by non-native English speakers should focus on the manuscript's science and look beyond errors in grammar, spelling, syntax, and usage because the English can be corrected by others before its publication. When there are language errors or problems in logic and flow of argument in a manuscript, reviewers and editors should provide constructive criticism by identifying examples of the incorrect use of English or problematical text and suggest improvements. Reviewers and editors can also suggest that authors seek the assistance of a professional editing service to assist in preparing a revised version of the manuscript [73].

4 Suggested Improvements to Scholarly Publishing

There is no shortage of suggested improvements to scholarly publishing. Some involve procedural changes and others require changes in attitude and the motivation to engage in inappropriate practices. Begley and Ioannidis [13] summarized 19 proposals made by individual authors and intended to improve research quality. Some of these are very specific, such as quality control of specimens and pathology, while others are wide-ranging suggestions, such as improving editorial standards. They conclude that improvements will not be made by a single entity but require an integrated response from the researchers themselves, their funders, their institutions, and the journals in which they publish. Wicherts [126] considers that among all the possible contributors, the human factor remains of considerable significance. He points out that even "honest people sometimes act slightly dishonestly in particular circumstances" and that other issues such as bias may be ingrained in humans.

A major (if not the greatest) challenge in modern research is the inability to reproduce, replicate, or repeat novel findings. This challenge has inaugurated a surfeit of talkfests (conferences, symposia, and colloquia) and publications to analyze the possible causes of the "reproducibility crisis" and suggest solutions to resolve it. For example, the NIH with the Nature Publishing Group and Science convened a joint workshop on the reproducibility and rigor of research findings in 2014 [127]. The workshop's participants were journal editors from basic/preclinical science journals in which NIH-funded researchers have most often published. The participants agreed on a common set of principles and guidelines to improve the quality of reporting: (a) the journal's submission guidelines should include the journal's policies for statistical analysis; (b) generous limits on the length of the Methods section should be given to authors; (c) authors should complete a checklist to ensure the reporting of key methodological and analytical information to reviewers and readers; and (d) journals should establish best practice guidelines for presenting and analyzing image-based data and describing biological materials and animals.

4.1 Revamping Institutional Research Practices

A university can be viewed as a managed research organization or a professional bureaucracy whose goals are to teach students and to conduct and communicate research [128, 129]. University researchers are highly skilled individuals who sometimes work with considerable autonomy with other individuals or groups external to their university. Increasingly, they have had to share authority over research decisions with those who provide access to funding, thereby influencing their conditions for making a reputation and advancing their careers. Hence, universities and research institutes need to review and overhaul their current policies on research practices because the balance between an individual researcher's authority and that of the institution needs to change.

The ability to express information accurately and succinctly is a basic requirement for any researcher irrespective of whether they remain in academia or not. Many institutions have also replaced traditional essay-based examinations by multiple-choice questions and short-note-based responses further eroding writing skills. Good writing skills are essential throughout research, not only in the submission of manuscripts but in funding requests and teaching. It is also an essential skill if students and postdoctoral researchers are to be the future mentors of others and participate in the scholarly publishing process as reviewers and editors.

Munafo and his colleagues [130] have advocated that institutions should encourage open research practices because they can provide a framework for minimizing academic misconduct in the research community. Individual researchers can protect themselves against their own enthusiasm, and the incentives to discover something by preregistering their study protocols and analysis plans. Making research workflows transparent and subject to potential scrutiny should serve as a quality control measure, including ensuring data are thoroughly checked.

The UK government (House of Commons Science and Technology Committee) has investigated how the current "research culture" could be changed to better support research integrity in UK universities [27]. In this investigation, Professor Dame Ottoline Leyser, from the Nuffield Council on Bioethics, lamented that research is "hypercompetitive and the rules for winning the competition are the wrong rules" and "at some level we have lost sight of what science actually is". The Royal Society also commented that "systems of publishing, assessment and dissemination of work should be adjusted in order to incentivize 'good behavior'".

The sense of these comments is reflected in existing PhD programs, which have changed radically over the last few decades [131]. In most of the twentieth century, it was largely marked by a close relationship between mentor and mentee, and one that is still a highly valued objective in the UK and many other countries. The relationship had the goal of achieving academic skills and competence culminating primarily in the production of the thesis, which was almost entirely developed and written by the mentee and exhibited independent thought on a topic over 3 or more years of study. Publication of papers was desirable but not essential, and certainly, there was no numerical target. The close relationship between mentor and mentee was also expected to include the transfer of good research ethics and practice set by the example of the mentor.

Accentuation of the "publish or perish" maxim has had many undesirable effects on both mentor and mentee. Some mentors may prioritize their need to publish in journals with a high IF beyond the training of the mentee. The mentee is now expected to produce several original papers during the period of training, without which continuation and, in the case of a PhD course of study, even the award of the degree would be at risk. These effects have had unfortunate consequences [132]. In a survey of 467 graduate students and postdoctoral fellows: 25% appeared not to receive adequate mentoring, while 39% had been pressurized to produce "positive" results. Absence of ethical leadership at all levels led to 63% admitting that the pressure to publish influenced the way they reported data, and 24% had omitted results that were inconsistent with their working hypothesis. Perhaps more worryingly, 27% said that they had witnessed extreme research misconduct by others to complete a project or manuscript.

Ultimately setting standards for research ethics and research skills must originate at the top level of institutions. Apparently, a significant minority of academic leaders cannot be relied upon to inculcate a culture of good research integrity and research into an institution's research practices. Hence, a major overhaul is needed, such as implementing a centralized mentoring oversight system to define and maintain standards, as well as a confidential whistleblowing system.

4.2 Competency Training for Researchers, Reviewers, and Journal Editors

i. Researchers
   (a) Authorship training for researchers

One of the key milestones in the training of research mentees is the ability to be the prime author on a research paper. To this end, the mentees need to have developed writing skills to effectively convey their thoughts, ideas, and opinions and to organize experimental data [75], as well as demonstrating an ability to plan and execute experiments. The problem is how best to provide training in writing skills. In principle, it should be achieved through the classic one-to-one relationship between mentor and mentee during doctoral training, and increasingly nowadays during postdoctoral training. While aiming to become successful researchers, mentors have their own pressures on the amount of teaching and supervision they can provide to their mentees. This "publish or perish" mentality creates pressure on the mentor to deliver manuscripts to the best journals and avoid rejection. Moreover, this pressure may cause mentors to assume the primary responsibility for writing to increase the probability of publication and leave the mentee in the role of a highly qualified research assistant. Inconsistency in the amount and quality of training in scientific writing by individual mentors implies a need for universities and other research institutions to provide a "writing for the sciences" course for mentees. Such a course should complement the existing online guidance documents that have been developed by some multinational publishers. Although internal and external training courses in scientific writing are available, some well-trained mentees may participate in such a course in the hope of gaining a "gold nugget" of knowledge.

We all learn by mistakes, but there may be also insufficient time or unwillingness by some mentors to do a thorough failure analysis when a manuscript is rejected. Instead of using rejection as an opportunity for training, the article is too often reformatted for submission to another journal (or even submitted with minimal alteration), and if necessary, the process reiterated until the article is accepted for publication. This hawking of papers around journals not only provides poor training, but places an unnecessary burden on journals and peer reviewers. Since we support the cascade system for lessening the burden on the peer-review process, we would like to see editors or journals require authors to declare whether the manuscript has been previously rejected and the basis for that rejection. Such rejection should not preclude publication because initial rejection may have been based on non-quality issues, such as one of the biases described previously. Nonetheless, it should pressure authors to re-examine their paper thoroughly in the light of justifiable peer reviewer comments. Authors might also consider preregistering the report with the Center for Open Science (https://cos.io/our-services/top-guidelines/) whose aim is to promote an open research culture which comprises a set of guidelines with eight standards to align scientific ideals with practices [133].

(b) Measuring researcher competence

It is somewhat paradoxical that many training organizations, such as universities, have neither documented training requirements for individual graduate students or postdoctoral fellows nor a detailed assessment of competencies. This contrasts with many non-academic environments, particularly those with quality accreditations (see Sect. 5 "Institutional Responsibilities: Can Research Quality be Improved by Formal Quality Systems?").

Authorship of papers is often presumed to be a measure of competence. The ICMJE recommends that authorship be based on (a) substantial contributions to the conception or design of the work or the acquisition, analysis, or interpretation of data for the work; (b) drafting the work or revising it critically for important intellectual content; (c) final approval of the version to be published; and (d) agreement to be accountable for all aspects of the work in ensuring that questions related to the accuracy or integrity of any part of the work are appropriately investigated and resolved [30]. The presumption that competence of mentees is reflected in the authorship of a paper may not be valid because the number of authors on individual papers is growing (author inflation) due to collaborations, specialization of research expertise, and honorary authorships (gift authorships) [134]. It is becoming increasingly difficult to recognize the competencies of individual investigators [135] and ascertain the contribution of each author in multi-authored papers from the order in which they appear on a manuscript [136, 137]. To these ends, McNutt and her colleagues [135] recommended that journals adopt the Contributor Roles Taxonomy (CRediT) methodology (https://casrai.org/credit/) for attributing contributions and require authors to identify themselves in research, scholarship, and innovation activities using ORCID's digital identifier (https://orcid.org). They also recommended that universities and research institutions articulate their expectations about author roles and responsibilities. This inability to determine an individual's competence from their publication record is also evidence for an alternative method for determining competence, such as maintenance of training records of each trainee, which are commonly used in non-academic environments.

ii. Reviewers

There is no body of literature that has systematically identified the roles and tasks of peer reviewers of biomedical journals. To address this deficiency, Glonti et al. [138] announced the establishment of a scoping review whose purpose is to determine the competency requirements for peer reviewers. Despite this deficiency, training programs and online guidance documents to foster standards so that reviewers can acquire a set of core competencies have been developed by some multinational publishers (Wiley-Blackwell, Elsevier, BioMed Central, BMJ Publishing Group, Springer), Publons (Publons Academy), the European Peer Review Association (http://www.peere.org/school/), and the Peer Review European Network (http://www.peer-review-network.eu/pages/training.php). Collectively, it is envisaged that these programs and guidance documents will educate new reviewers and provide a repository of tools and innovations for experienced reviewers. It is also envisaged that the certification of reviewers will identify skilled reviewers and increase trust and transparency in the peer-review process. Finally in 2018, Pinto da Costa et al. [139] published a list of organizations where researchers can learn how to peer-review a research report, and Tokalic and Marusic [140] have developed a card exchange game for teaching integrity and ethics in peer-review training.

iii. Journal Editors

Journal editors are crucial to scholarly publishing because they are responsible for ensuring that the articles that are published in their journals are clear, complete, transparent, and as free as possible from bias. In an effort to improve the quality of scientific reports, some scholarly journals in the health and life sciences have revised their submission guidelines [141], as well as endorsing reporting guidelines to improve the quality of reporting.

Moher et al. [90] assert that no documentation on the required knowledge, skills, and characteristics of journal editors exists and no core competencies for the tasks of journal editors have been developed. Accordingly, they have created a set of 14 core competencies for scientific editors so that a scientific editor can proficiently fulfill his/her duties at a biomedical journal. By developing these core competencies, Moher and his colleagues envisage "endorsement across a broad spectrum of journals and editorial groups". This will lead to the development of "a core competency-based curriculum with which to train scientific editors of biomedical journals" and "a certification process whereby journal editors can obtain official recognition for demonstrating that they possess all of the core competencies". They concluded that "the downstream consequences of these efforts might include an increase in the research value of science and a higher quality of scientific publications". In other words, revising submission guidelines, advocating the use of a reporting guideline, and training can collectively contribute to the upgrading of editorial vigilance.

5 Institutional Responsibilities: Can Research Quality Be Improved by Formal Quality Systems?

Currently, about 50% of the manuscripts produced by academic research are rejected on the grounds of poor quality [9] due mainly to defects in study formulation, design, execution, and accuracy and comprehensiveness of reporting. High rejection rates have been occurring for a considerable period with little evidence of a strong desire to rectify the situation. The economic cost of failure is extremely high and is a major contributor to the estimated $100 billion "waste" in biomedical research each year [89]. Irreproducible research in preclinical studies in the USA alone is estimated to waste $28 billion annually [142]. Since these costs are met largely directly or indirectly from the public purse, it is only a matter of time before the acceptance of such waste is challenged. If the research enterprise is to remain intact, the issues of study and data quality need to be addressed urgently. There are also ethical questions, not least the waste of animals in animal-based research.

The problems of study design and execution, data reliability, and research quality began to be addressed in commercial life science research and in manufacturing over 40 years ago. The primary means by which these issues have been successfully addressed in these areas is the introduction of quality standards and systems that result in transparent and independently checked data; documented, appropriate, and validated methods and processes; and a mechanism of learning from mistakes or potential mistakes. In the case of life science contract research organizations (CROs) and pharmaceutical companies (Pharmas), a system referred to as Good Laboratory Practice (GLP) was introduced in regulatory studies. Its introduction was initially driven by the US Food and Drug Administration in the late 1970s as a result of systemic failures in some CROs and Pharmas [143, 144] and then quickly adopted by countries within the Organisation for Economic Co-operation and Development (OECD). A detailed description of GLP is outside the scope of this chapter but is given by Cooper-Hannan [145] and Seiler [146].

The benefits of applying the principles of GLP and its clinical research equivalent, Good Clinical Practice (GCP), to academic research through the concept of Good Research Practice (GRP) have been recognized for many years [147–150]. However, it is important to note that GLP is narrow in the range of activities to which it applies, is enforced at a government level, and would be difficult to apply to all academic research activities.

Individual manufacturing entities also adopted various quality systems in the 1970s to tackle perceived deficiencies in product quality. One of the main systems was the British Standard BS5750, which subsequently metamorphosed into ISO 9000, a family of international standards on quality management and quality assurance. Subsequently, this family became a single standard, ISO 9001. The standard is used not only in manufacturing environments but in many technology laboratories and consultancies that are perhaps at first sight more similar to academic research environments. We believe that much can be learnt from those using a quality assurance system to deliver a high-quality product and good commercial research. Perhaps surprisingly, academic research has much in common with manufacturing: it results in a product, such as a scholarly publication or a thesis whose intrinsic value is the knowledge it conveys, and has customers, namely, the researchers' peers, funding bodies, and society.

The ISO 9001 standard might form a good basis for developing good practices in academic research, and many of its principles would be recognizable to academic researchers, who should already be familiar with the benefits of standards which can be basically described as "processes, actions, or procedures that are deemed essential by authority, custom, or general consent" [151]. At their simplest, they may represent uniform ways of measurement to ensure consistency and help scientific cooperation, for example, the use of the SI system of measurement units.

One of the benefits of the ISO 9001 standard is that it has been designed to apply to a wide range of manufacturing and service activities and its principles would encompass all the academic disciplines and their activities, for example, from the interpretation of metadata through to practical laboratory and field experiments. It has a focus on continuing improvement, includes an emphasis on design and development that would fit that of experimental studies, is a global and well-recognized system, and is managed by commercial bodies rather than government. It can also be applied to parts of an organization rather than requiring compliance by the whole: individual research departments can progressively claim compliance as they demonstrate adherence to its principles. Some non-academic research organizations have adopted both GLP (for their regulatory work) and the ISO 9001 standards as an overall quality system. Hence, it would be possible for academic organizations in the life sciences to adopt a similar policy, taking the best of GLP and integrating it into an ISO 9001-based quality system.

The ISO 9001 standard also recognizes the importance of the human factor to product quality and requires identification of appropriate training to ensure quality and measurement of the competence of individuals in the required skills. Both must be documented and signed off by mentor and mentee. Working in such an environment not only improves the training of mentees and junior researchers, but prepares them for the practical environment that they are likely to meet outside of academia. It is perhaps paradoxical that focus on training and training procedures and measurement and documentation of competence in academia are often weaker than that in industry.

The ISO 9001 standard also includes an independent internal auditing system by which peers can ensure that the desired research standards and data quality are being maintained. Thus, journal reviewers can be satisfied that unseen material underpinning the manuscript is almost certainly of an appropriate standard and has been independently and internally audited. The organization also regularly assesses to what extent its customers are satisfied with its product: in the case of research, feedback from journals on the quality of submitted manuscripts would be high on that assessment. From both the auditing procedure and measurement of customer satisfaction, the organization can correct, and prevent in the future, any deficiencies, ensure that it does not release substandard "product", and can engage in a process of continuous improvement.

Quality systems, such as ISO 9001, GLP, and GCP, also formally address the issue of data retention and its transparency, and one of the functions of the auditing system is to ensure that data do not go "missing". Poor availability of underlying original data is often seen as one of the key factors in scientific irreproducibility [152]. For some journals, such as the PLoS family of journals, authors are strongly recommended to deposit their research data in a cloud-based data retention system, such as Dryad [153, 154] and others listed in the registry of research data repositories (https://www.re3data.org/), and make the data available to all interested researchers upon request (https://journals.plos.org/plosbiology/s/data-availability). However, the storage of data alone and its open access are not a complete solution: investigators may be selective in the data that they choose to use in an article to support their hypothesis. In regulatory systems, such as GLP and GCP, all data must be archived, be complete, and include any data excluded from consideration in the study outcome, irrespective of the reason. No data may be eliminated on the whim of the investigator, and any data changes (deletions or amendments) must be fully explained.

Formal quality systems are sometimes mistakenly criticized because they do not necessarily equate to good science. However, irreproducibility in the research enterprise reveals an existing failure to always yield good science. The ISO 9001 standard does address absolute quality: for example, not every car has to be of the standard of a Rolls-Royce for the ISO 9001 standard to be relevant in its manufacture. However, the manufacturer must define the specification (quality) of the product and show its ability to meet that specification consistently. That specification is driven by the needs of the customer, which in academia would be the funding organizations and the researchers' peers. For example, the best methodology for measuring plasma glucose levels with a required accuracy and sensitivity is determined by the research community: the ISO 9001 standard would not dictate the methodology, but would ensure that the organization has assessed and used correctly what is appropriate to meet the required quality of measurement. This process would include validation and documentation of the method; regular calibration and maintenance of any equipment according to the supplier's specification; training and assessment of competence of those using the equipment; and documentation of these activities. All these components of the process are good scientific practice.

It is hard to believe that individual researchers or research groups will voluntarily incur the additional cost of independent quality assessment. Implementation of such practices can only be achieved at an institutional level where balancing the cost of quality assessment and management versus additional teaching or research staff can be appropriately judged. Many investigators may consider that formal quality systems may negatively impinge on research creativity. We consider this to be a short-term view, and not necessarily valid. In the long term, the introduction of such practices will strengthen the position of life sciences in society. If the economic scale of waste through poor research quality is fully recognized, change will be externally imposed, probably through the level of funding. If we consider research as a product, how many manufacturers (or their stakeholders) would accept a product failure rate of 50% without taking effective action?

6 Conclusions

In this chapter, we have discussed the relationship between the quality of reporting in scholarly publishing and scientific reproducibility. We have also described some of the innovations that could change the current face and dynamics of scholarly publishing. We have also focused on how improvements in scholarly publishing from the author's submission of research findings in well-written, accurate, and honest publications through to their dissemination by a publisher might help the quality of what is published and improve reproducibility. Additionally, we have identified many inadequacies in scholarly publishing, as well as many adequacies, such as the contribution of peer review.

Against this background, several inadequacies in need of solution are high on our list of priorities. We believe that the quality of scientific writing is declining. The importance of concise, precise, coherent, and lucid scientific writing is perhaps best summarized in Gopen's statement that "The perfect piece of literature, when read by 1000 readers, should result in at least 1000 interpretations. The perfect piece of writing in the professional world, when read by 1000 readers, should produce one and only one interpretation" [155]. Hence, improvement in scientific writing needs to be addressed centrally through the institutional provision of "writing in the sciences" courses. This idea is also echoed by postgraduate students and postdoctoral fellows. Training may be even more important in the future where "short-hand" writing, such as texting, is becoming the dominant method of writing.

Reviewer competence and editorial vigilance are crucial to assuring the quality and accuracy of the scientific record. Accordingly, we advocate that peer reviewers and journal editors must become more circumspect when appraising submissions than they currently are. There is little point in attempting to improve the quality of reporting in scientific manuscripts when those who assess them are limited due to inadequate training and/or competence in the process. Since most reviewers and editors acquire the necessary skills to perform their respective tasks by on-the-job training, we believe that this should be complemented with institutionally based training. We also see the definition of required competencies and provision of training as being important not only for those involved in peer review and editing, but also for authors. While the peer-review process is valuable in not only acting as a gatekeeper for granting passage to authors into scholarly publishing, it also provides authors with independent and continuing development in research and writing skills. If authors are to gain anything from the rejection or referral of a manuscript, the peer review should be sufficiently constructed, objective, and explanatory so as to provide the basis for an author's advancement, development, and improvement. Lastly, the training to be given to postgraduate students and postdoctoral fellows needs defining, and the documentation of such training and the acquisition of competencies need recording. At the end of their training, each should leave with a record that can accompany them throughout their career and can be regularly updated.

When process and product failures occurred, manufacturers and non-academic research institutes responded by introducing formal quality systems, such as GLP, GCP, and/or ISO 9001. Hence, we advocate the adoption of the existing standards of quality control in manufacturing by academic institutions to encourage open and good research practices and develop good publishing practices. We recognize that the introduction of a robust quality system is a challenge for academic institutions and will not be quickly adopted. Nevertheless, quality systems have been introduced in a wide range of disciplines with highly successful outcomes. In the short term, these may be seen as an inconvenient burden on a research environment already underfunded. In the long term, academic researchers and institutions need to realize that acceptance of high failure rates and substantial financial waste is and will not be acceptable to society.

We have also highlighted the opinions of some individuals in the field of scholarly publishing that academic institutions are often slow to address instances of research misconduct and failure to do so inevitably adversely impacts society's view of science. Accordingly, we believe that institutions need to be more active in managing the quality of research and research publications than they currently are. This pro-activity can be implemented and achieved through both preventive and corrective steps, such as revamping existing institutional policies of research practices and integrity and responding rapidly to allegations of academic misconduct. Institutions also need to take preventive and corrective actions to improve the behavior of researchers and the quality and reproducibility of scientific research.

Disclosures The authors have no conflicts of interest to disclose.

Acknowledgements The authors thank Dr. Eoghan McAlpine and Dr. Ze'ev Bomzon for their constructive criticisms and helpful suggestions. The authors also thank Statler and Waldorf for encouraging and inspiring us to write this chapter.

References

1. Levitan KB. Scientific societies and their journals: biomedical scientists assess the relationship. Soc Stud Sci. 1979;9:393–400.
2. Tenopir C, King DW, Boyce P, et al. Patterns of journal use by scientists through three evolutionary phases. D-Lib Mag. 2003;9:1082.
3. Niu X, Hemminger BM. A study of factors that affect the information-seeking behavior of academic scientists. J Am Soc Inf Sci Technol. 2011;63:336–53.
4. Nicholas D, Watkinson A, Volentine R, et al. Trust and authority in scholarly communications in the light of the digital transition: setting the scene for a major study. Learn Publ. 2014;27:121–34.
5. Jubb M. Communication or competition: what motivates researchers to write articles for journals? Learn Publ. 2014;27:251–2.
6. Shamseer L, Moher D, Maduekwe O, et al. Potential predatory and legitimate biomedical journals: can you tell the difference? a cross-sectional comparison. BMC Med. 2017;15:28.
7. Peer review in scientific publications. London: Science and Technology Committee, House of Commons; 2011.
8. Byrne DW. Common reasons for rejecting manuscripts at medical journals: a survey of editors and peer reviewers. Science. 2000;23:39–44.
9. Sugimoto CR, Lariviere V, Ni C, Cronin B. Journal acceptance rates: a cross-disciplinary analysis of variability and relationships with journal measures. J Informetr. 2013;7:897–906.
10. Lamb CR, Mai W. Acceptance rate and reasons for rejection of manuscripts submitted to Veterinary Radiology & Ultrasound during 2012. Vet Radiol Ultrasound. 2014;56:103–8.
11. Reich ES. The golden club. Nature. 2013;502:291–3.
12. Casadevall A, Fang FC. Reproducible science. Infect Immun. 2010;78:4972–5.
13. Begley CG, Ioannidis JPA. Reproducibility in science. Circ Res. 2015;116:116–26.
14. Baker M. Is there a reproducibility crisis? Nature. 2016;533:452–4.
15. Fanelli D. Opinion: Is science really facing a reproducibility crisis, and do we need it to? Proc Natl Acad Sci USA. 2008;115:2628–31
16. Goodman SN, Fanelli D, Ioannidis JPA. What does research reproducibility mean? Sci Transl Med. 2016;8:341ps12.
17. Barba LA. Terminologies for reproducible research. arXiv. 2018;1802 03311v1 [cs DL].

18. Plesser HE. Reproducibility vs. replicability: a brief history of a confused terminology. Front Neuroinform. 2018;11:76.
19. Drummond C. Replicability is not reproducibility: nor is it good science. In: Proceedings of the Evaluation Methods for Machine Learning Workshop at the 26th ICML. Montreal, Canada: National Research Council of Canada; 2009.
20. Ioannidis JPA. Why most published research findings are false. PLoS Med. 2005;2:e124.
21. Prinz F, Schlange T, Asadullah K. Believe it or not: how much can we rely on published data on potential drug targets? Nat Rev Drug Discov. 2011;10:712.
22. Peng R. The reproducibility crisis in science: a statistical counterattack. Significance. 2015;12:30–2.
23. Loken E, Gelman A. Measurement error and the replication crisis. Science. 2017;355:584–5.
24. Munafo MR, Nosek BA, Bishop DVM, et al. A manifesto for reproducible science. Nat Hum Behav. 2017;1:0021.
25. Enserink M. Sloppy reporting on animal studies proves hard to change. Science. 2017;357:1337–8.
26. Nuffield Council of Bioethics. The culture of scientific research in the UK. London: Nuffield Council of Bioethics; 2014.
27. Research integrity. London: Science and Technology Commitee, House of Commons; 2018
28. Day RA. The origins of the scientific paper: the IMRAD format. J Am Med Writ Assoc. 1989;4:16–8.
29. Sollaci LB, Pereira MG. The introduction, methods, results, and discussion (IMRAD) structure: a fifty-year survey. J Med Libr Assoc. 2004;92:364–71.
30. International Committee of Medical Journal Editors. Recommendations for the conduct, reporting, editing, and publication of scholarly work in medical journals. 2018. http://www.icmje.org/icmje-recommendations.pdf.
31. Malicki M, Aalbersberg IJ, Bouter L, ter Riet G. Journals' instructions to authors: A cross-sectional study across scientific disciplines. PLoS One. 2019;14:e0222157.
32. Baker D, Lidster K, Sottomayor A, Amor S. Two years later: journals are not yet enforcing the ARRIVE guidelines on reporting standards for pre-clinical animal studies. PLoS Biol. 2014;12:e1001756.
33. McGrath JC, Lilley E. Implementing guidelines on reporting research using animals (ARRIVE etc.): new requirements for publication in BJP. Br J Pharmacol. 2015;172:3189–93.
34. Hooijmans CR, Leenaars M, Ritskes-Hoitinga M. A gold standard publication checklist to improve the quality of animal studies, to fully integrate the three Rs, and to make systematic reviews more feasible. Alt Lab Anim. 2010;38:167–82.
35. Battisti WP, Wager E, Baltzer L. Good publication practice for communicating company-sponsored medical research: GPP3. Ann Intern Med. 2015;163:461–4.
36. Stevens A, Shamseer L, Weinstein E, et al. Relation of completeness of reporting of health research to journals' endorsement of reporting guidelines: systematic review. Br Med J. 2014;348:g3804.
37. Bezdjian A, Klis SFL, Peters JPM, et al. Quality of reporting of otorhinolaryngology articles using animal models with the ARRIVE statement. Lab Anim. 2017;52:79–87.
38. Leung V, Rousseau-Blass F, Beauchamp G, Pang DSJ. ARRIVE has not ARRIVEd: support for the ARRIVE (Animal Research: reporting of in vivo Experiments) guidelines does not improve the reporting quality of papers in animal welfare, analgesia or anesthesia. PLoS One. 2018;13:e0197882.
39. Hair K, Macleod MR, Sena ES, et al. A randomised controlled trial of an intervention to improve compliance with the ARRIVE guidelines (IICARus). Res Integr Peer Rev. 2019;4:12.
40. Nicholas D, Watkinson A, Jamali HR, et al. Peer review: still king in the digital age. Learn Publ. 2015;28:15–21.
41. Bornmann L. Scientific peer review. Ann Rev Info Sci Technol. 2011;45:197–245.
42. Smith R. Peer review: a flawed process at the heart of science and journals. J R Soc Med. 2006;99:178–82.
43. Smith R. Classical peer review: an empty gun. Breast Cancer Res. 2010;12:S13.
44. Smith R. Roger Bacon on ignorance and peer review. 2017. https://blogs.bmj.com/bmj/2017/05/04/richard-smith-roger-bacon-on-ignorance-and-peer-review/.
45. Wagner PD, Bates JHT. Maintaining the integrity of peer review. J Appl Physiol. 2016;120:479–80.
46. Black N, van RS, Godlee F, et al. What makes a good reviewer and a good review for a general medical journal? JAMA. 1998;280:231–3.
47. Albert KM. Open access: implications for scholarly publishing and medical libraries. J Med Libr Assoc. 2006;94:253–62.
48. Bartholomew RE. Science for sale: the rise of predatory journals. J R Soc Med. 2014;107:384–5.
49. Laakso M, Welling P, Bukvova H, et al. The development of open access journal publishing from 1993 to 2009. PLoS One. 2011;6:e20961.
50. Johnson R, Watkinson A, Mabe M. An overview of scientific and scholarly publishing. 5th ed. The Hague: International Association of Scientific, Technical and Medical Publishers; 2018. https://www.stm-assoc.org/2018_10_04_STM_Report_2018.pdf.
51. Bjork BC, Welling P, Laakso M, et al. Open access to the scientific journal literature: situation 2009. PLoS One. 2010;5:e11273.
52. Guedj D, Ramjoue C. European Commission policy on open-access to scientific publications and research data in Horizon 2020. Biomed Data J. 2015;1:11–4.

53. Schiltz M. Science without publication paywalls: cOAlition S for the realisation of full and immediate open access. PLoS Med. 2018;15:e1002663.
54. Horton R. The future of scientific knowledge. Lancet. 2018;392:2337.
55. Bordage G. Reasons reviewers reject and accept manuscripts: the strengths and weaknesses in medical education reports. Acad Med. 2001;76:889–96
56. Pierson DJ. The top 10 reasons why manuscripts are not accepted for publication. Respir Care. 2004;49:1246–52.
57. Ehara S, Takahashi K. Reasons for rejection of manuscripts submitted to AJR by international authors. Am J Roentgenol. 2007;188:W113–6.
58. Harris AHS, Reeder R, Hyun JK. Common statistical and research design problems in manuscripts submitted to high-impact psychiatry journals: what editors and reviewers want authors to know. J Psychiatr Res. 2009;43:1231–4.
59. Johnson C, Green B. Submitting manuscripts to biomedical journals: common errors and helpful solutions. J Manip Physiol Ther. 2009;32:1–12.
60. Wyness T, McGhee CN, Patel DV. Manuscript rejection in ophthalmology and visual science journals: identifying and avoiding the common pitfalls. Clin Exp Ophthalmol. 2009;37:864–7.
61. Ali J. Manuscript rejection: causes and remedies. J Young Pharm. 2010;2:3–6.
62. Harris AHS, Reeder RN, Hyun JK. Survey of editors and reviewers of high-impact psychology journals: statistical and research design problems in submitted manuscripts. J Psychol. 2011;145:195–209.
63. Pimm J. Dear editor, why have you rejected my article? Psychiatrist. 2013;37:313–4.
64. Garg A, Das S, Jain H. Why we say no! A look through the editor's eye. J Clin Diagn Res. 2015;9:JB01–5.
65. Meyer HS, Durning SJ, Sklar DP, Maggio LA. Making the first cut: an analysis of academic medicine editors' reasons for not sending manuscripts out for external peer review. Acad Med. 2018;93:464–70.
66. Chew FS. Fate of manuscripts rejected for publication in the AJR. Am J Roentgenol. 1991;156:627–32.
67. Ray J, Berkwits M, Davidoff F. The fate of manuscripts rejected by a general medical journal. Am J Med. 2000;109:131–5.
68. Wijnhoven BPL, Dejong CHC. Fate of manuscripts declined by the British Journal of Surgery. Br J Surg. 2010;97:450–4.
69. Khosla A, McDonald RJ, Bornmann L, Kallmes DF. Getting to yes: the fate of neuroradiology manuscripts rejected by Radiology over a 2-year period. Radiology. 2011;260:3–5.
70. Okike K, Kocher MS, Nwachukwu BU, et al. The fate of manuscripts rejected by the Journal of Bone and Joint Surgery (American Volume). J Bone Joint Surg AM. 2012;94:e130
71. Grant WD, Cone DC. If at first you don't succeed: the fate of manuscripts rejected by Academic Emergency Medicine. Acad Emerg Med. 2015;22:1213–7.
72. Docherty AB, Klein AA. The fate of manuscripts rejected from Anaesthesia. Anaesthesia. 2017;72:427–30.
73. Cronin B. Language matters. J Am Soc Inf Sci Technol. 2011;63:217.
74. Wager E, Jefferson T. Shortcomings of peer review in biomedical journals. Learn Publ. 2001;14:257–63.
75. Vale RD. Accelerating scientific publication in biology. Proc Natl Acad Sci USA. 2015;112:13439–46.
76. Allison DB, Brown AW, George BJ, Kaiser KA. A tragedy of errors. Nature. 2016;530:27–9.
77. Kravitz RL, Franks P, Feldman MD, et al. Editorial peer reviewers' recommendations at a general medical journal: are they reliable and do editors care? PLoS One. 2010;5:e10072.
78. Baethge C, Franklin J, Mertens S. Substantial agreement of referee recommendations at a general medical journal – a peer review evaluation at Deutsches Arzteblatt International. PLoS One. 2013;8:e61401.
79. Rothwell PM, Martyn CN. Reproducibility of peer review in clinical neuroscienceIs agreement between reviewers any greater than would be expected by chance alone? Brain. 2000;123:1964–9.
80. Bornmann L, Mutz R, Daniel H-D. A reliability-generalization study of journal peer reviews: a multilevel meta-analysis of inter-rater reliability and its determinants. PLoS One. 2010;5:e14331.
81. Jirschitzka J, Oeberst A, Gollner R, Cress U. Inter-rater reliability and validity of peer reviews in an interdisciplinary field. Scientometrics. 2017;113:1059–92.
82. Siler K, Lee K, Bero L. Measuring the effectiveness of scientific gatekeeping. Proc Natl Acad Sci USA. 2015;112:360–5.
83. Publons. Global State of Peer Review. 2018.
84. Kovanis M, Porcher R, Ravaud P, Trinquart L. The global burden of journal peer review in the biomedical literature: strong imbalance in the collective enterprise. PLoS One. 2016;11:e0166387.
85. Breuning M, Backstrom J, Brannon J, et al. Reviewer fatigue? Why scholars decline to review their peers' work. PS: Polit Sci Polit. 2015;48:595–600.
86. D'Andrea R, O'Dwyer JP. Can editors save peer review from peer reviewers? PLoS One. 2017;12:e0186111.
87. Gannon F. The essential role of peer review. EMBO Rep. 2001;2:743.
88. Jackson JL, Srinivasan M, Rea J, et al. The validity of peer review in a general medicine journal. PLoS One. 2011;6:e22475.
89. Galipeau J, Barbour V, Baskin P, et al. A scoping review of competencies for scientific editors of biomedical journals. BMC Med. 2016;14:16.

90. Moher D, Galipeau J, Alam S, et al. Core competencies for scientific editors of biomedical journals: consensus statement. BMC Med. 2017;15:167.
91. Young NS, Ioannidis JPA, Al-Ubaydli O. Why current publication practices may distort science. PLoS Med. 2008;5:e201.
92. van Lent M, Overbeke J, Out HJ. Role of editorial and peer review processes in publication bias: analysis of drug trials submitted to eight medical journals. PLoS One. 2014;9:e104846.
93. Beall J. Predatory publishers are corrupting open access. Nature. 2012;489:179.
94. Butler D. Investigating journal: the dark side of publishing. Nature. 2013;495:433–5.
95. Bert F, Paget DZ. Scaioli G. A social way to experience a scientific event: Twitter use at the 7th European Public Health Conference. Scand J Public Health. 1999;44:130–3.
96. Kiernan M, Wigglesworth N. The use of social media in the dissemination of information from scientific meetings. J Infect Prev. 2011;12:224–5.
97. Kapp JM, Hensel B, Schnoring KT. Is Twitter a forum for disseminating research to health policy makers? Ann Epidemiol. 2015;25:883–7.
98. Allen CG, Andersen B, Chambers DA, et al. Twitter use at the 2016 conference on the science of dissemination and implementation in health: analyzing #DIScience16. Implement Sci. 2018;13:34.
99. McClain CR. Practices and promises of Facebook for science outreach: becoming a "Nerd of Trust". PLoS Biol. 2017;15:e2002020.
100. Science is social. Nat Genet. 2018;50:1619.
101. Lee CJ, Sugimoto CR, Zhang G, Cronin B. Bias in peer review. J Am Soc Inf Sci Technol. 2012;64:2–17.
102. Munafo M, Neill J. Null is beautiful: on the importance of publishing null results. J Psychopharmacol. 2016;30:585.
103. Gaston T, Smart P. What influences the regional diversity of reviewers: a study of medical and agricultural/biological sciences journals. Learn Publ. 2018;31:189–97.
104. Lerback J, Hanson B. Journals invite too few women to referee. Nature. 2017;541:455–7.
105. Garfield E. Citation analysis as a tool in journal evaluation. Science. 1972;178:471–9.
106. Rogers LF. Impact factor; the numbers game. Am J Roentgenol. 2002;178:541–2.
107. Tsikliras AC. Chasing after the high impact. ESEP. 2008;8:45–7.
108. Seglen PO. Why the impact factor of journals should not be used for evaluating research. Br Med J. 1997;314:498–502.
109. Hecht F, Hecht BK, Sandberg AA. The journal "Impact Factor": A misnamed, misleading, misused measure. Cancer Genet Cytogenet. 1998;104:77–81.
110. Bertuzzi S, Drubin DG. No shortcuts for research assessment. Mol Biol Cell. 2013;24:1505–6.
111. Hirsch JE. An index to quantify an individual's scientific research output. Proc Natl Acad Sci USA. 2005;102:16569–72.
112. Egghe L. Theory and practise of the g-index. Scientometrics. 2006;69:131–52.
113. Patel VM, Ashrafian H, Bornmann L, et al. Enhancing the h index for the objective assessment of healthcare researcher performance and impact. J R Soc Med. 2013;106:19–29.
114. Lawrence PA. The politics of publication. Nature. 2003;422:259–61.
115. Lawrence PA. The mismeasurement of science. Curr Biol. 2007;17:R583–5.
116. Lawrence PA. Lost in publication: how measurement harms science. Ethics Sci Environ Polit. 2008;8:9–11.
117. Campbell P. Escape from the impact factor. Ethics Sci Environ Polit. 2008;8:5–7.
118. Boutron I, Ravaud P. Misrepresentation and distortion of research in biomedical literature. Proc Natl Acad Sci USA. 2018;115:2613–9.
119. Angell M, Relman AS. Redundant publication. N Engl J Med. 1989;320:1212–4.
120. Budd JM. Stewart KN. Is there such a thing as "least publishable unit"? an empirical investigation. LIBRES 2015;25:78–85.
121. Day NE. The silent majority: manuscript rejection and its impact on scholars. Acad Man Learn Edu. 2011;10:704–18.
122. Wager E. Coping with scientific misconduct. Br Med J. 2011;343:d6586.
123. Brainard J. Rethinking retractions. Science. 2018;362:390–3.
124. Grieneisen ML, Zhang M. A comprehensive survey of retracted articles from the scholarly literature. PLoS One. 2012;7:e44118.
125. Drubin DG, Kellogg DR. English as the universal language of science: opportunities and challenges. Mol Biol Cell. 2012;23:1399.
126. Wicherts MJ. The weak spots in contemporary science (and how to fix them). Animals. 2017;7:90.
127. McNutt M. Journals unite for reproducibility. Science. 2014;346:679.
128. Cruz-Castro L, Sanz-Menendez L. Autonomy and authority in public research organisations: structure and funding factors. Minerva. 2018;56:135–60.
129. Tartari V, Perkmann M, Salter A. In good company: the influence of peers on industry engagement by academic scientists. Res Policy. 2014;43:1189–203.
130. Munafo MR, Hollands GJ, Marteau TM. Open science prevents mindless science. Br Med J. 2018;363:k4309.
131. Review of Wellcome Trust PhD research training: the supervisor perspective. London: Wellcome Trust; 2001.
132. Boulbes DR, Costello TJ, Baggerly KA, et al. A survey on data reproducibility and the effect of publication process on the ethical reporting of laboratory research. Clin Cancer Res. 2018;24:3447–55.

133. Nosek BA, Alter G, Banks GC, et al. Promoting an open research culture. Science. 2015;348:1422–5.
134. Wren JD, Kozak KZ, Johnson KR, et al. The write position. A survey of perceived contributions to papers based on byline position and number of authors. EMBO Rep. 2007;8:988–91.
135. McNutt MK, Bradford M, Drazen JM, et al. Transparency in authors' contributions and responsibilities to promote integrity in scientific publication. Proc Natl Acad Sci USA. 2018;115:2557–60.
136. Laurance WF. Second thoughts on who goes where in author lists. Nature. 2006;442:26.
137. Greene M. The demise of the lone author. Nature. 2007;450:1165.
138. Glonti K, Cauchi D, Cobo E, et al. A scoping review protocol on the roles and tasks of peer reviewers in the manuscript review process in biomedical journals. BMJ Open. 2017;7:e017468
139. Pinto da Costa M, Oliveira J, Abdulmalik J. Where can early career researchers learn how to peer review a scientific paper? Eur Sci Editing. 2018;44:4–7, 18.
140. Tokalic R, Marusic A. A peer review card exchange game. Eur Sci Editing. 2018;44:52–5.
141. Yosten GLC, Adams JC, Bennett CN, et al. Editorial: revised guidelines to enhance the rigor and reproducibility of research published in American Physiological Society Journals. Am J Physiol Regul Integr Comp Physiol. 2018;315:R1251–R1253
142. Freedman LP, Cockburn IM, Simcoe TS. The economics of reproducibility in preclinical research. PLoS Biol. 2015;13:e1002165.
143. Schneider K. Faking it: the case against industrial bio-test laboratories. Amicus J. 1983;Spring edition:14–26.
144. Baldeshwiler AM. History of FDA good laboratory practices. Qual Assur J. 2003;7:157–61.
145. Cooper-Hannan R, Harbell JW, Coecke S, et al. The principles of good laboratory practice: application to in vitro toxicology studies. Alt Lab Anim. 1999;27:539–77.
146. Seiler JP. Good laboratory practice: the why and the how. Berlin: Springer; 2006.
147. Glick JL, Shamoo AE. A call for the development of "good research practices" (GRP) guidelines. Account Res. 1993;2:231–5.
148. Murray GD. Promoting good research practice. Stat Methods Med Res. 2000;9:17–24.
149. Davies R. Good research practice: it is time to do what others think we do. Quasar. 2013;124:21–3.
150. Pedro-Roig L, Emmerich CH. The reproducibility crisis in preclinical research – lessons to be learnt from clinical research. Med Writ. 2017;26:28–32.
151. Dickersin K, Mayo-Wilson E. Standards for design and measurement would make clinical research reproducible and usable. Proc Natl Acad Sci USA. 2018;115:2590–4.
152. Whitlock MC, McPeek MA, Rausher MD, et al. Data archiving. Am Nat. 2010;175:145–6.
153. Mannheimer S, Yoon A, Greenberg J, et al. A balancing act: the ideal and the realistic in developing Dryad's preservation policy. First Monday. 2014;19
154. Vines TH, Albert AYK, Andrew RL, et al. The availability of research data declines rapidly with article age. Curr Biol. 2014;24:94–7.
155. Gopen GD. Expectations: teaching writing from the reader's perspective. London: Pearson Longman; 2004.

Systematic Reviews

Janet Becker Rodgers and Merel Ritskes-Hoitinga

Abstract

Systematic reviews are a firmly established method of ensuring that proposed research is based upon the best available scientific evidence. In this chapter, we provide a brief history of systematic reviews and discuss their adaptation to preclinical studies. The steps in conducting a systematic review are explained, with examples of best practice. Readers will learn how to critically evaluate the quality of systematic reviews in their own fields. Basic guidance on the parts of a systematic review and meta-analysis are explained. Critically appraised topics (or knowledge summaries) are also described, and their relevance for preclinical research is explained, including a worked example.

Keywords

Systematic review · Meta-analysis · Critically appraised topic · Evidence-based medicine · Evidence-based veterinary medicine · Risk of bias

J. B. Rodgers (✉) · M. Ritskes-Hoitinga
Professor in Evidence-Based Laboratory Animal Science, RadboudUMC, Nijmegen, The Netherlands
e-mail: janet.rodgers@retired.ox.ac.uk; Merel.Ritskes-Hoitinga@radboudumc.nl

Glossary

AMSTAR Assessment of multiple systematic reviews, a tool, designed for health professionals and policy makers who do not necessarily have epidemiological expertise, to assess the quality of systematic reviews and meta-analyses [1], updated to AMSTAR 2 in 2017 [2]. Note that PRISMA is a list of guidelines for producing a systematic review, whereas AMSTAR is a method of assessing the quality of the published review.

ARRIVE Animal Research: Reporting of In Vivo Experiments, checklist covering key information to be described in scientific publications [3].

Bias Systematic deviation from the effect of intervention that would be observed in a large randomised trial without any flaws [4].

CAMARADES Collaborative Approach to Meta-Analysis and Review of Animal Data from Experimental Studies (research).

CONSORT Consolidated Standards of Reporting Trials, used to improve reporting of human randomised controlled trials (group).

EQUATOR Enhancing the Quality and Transparency of Health Research (medicine).

GRADE Grading of Recommendations Assessment, Development and Evaluation,

© Springer Nature Switzerland AG 2021

J. M. Sánchez Morgado, A. Brønstad (eds.), *Experimental Design and Reproducibility in Preclinical Animal Studies*, Laboratory Animal Science and Medicine 1,
https://doi.org/10.1007/978-3-030-66147-2_10

a system for grading evidence for clinical guidelines [8–10].

Grey literature Reports, theses, dissertations, conference proceedings, technical specifications or standards, bibliography collections, and other documents not usually incorporated into standard science publication databases. Slide presentations and unpublished data are also considered in this category.

HARRP guidelines Harmonised Animal Research Reporting Principles, a list of guidelines for reporting primary animal research [11].

PICO(T) The accepted format for the research question in a systematic review. P = patients or population (or animal subjects), I = intervention, C = comparator, O = outcome measured, and T = time of follow-up if this is important.

PRISMA Preferred Reporting Items for Systematic Reviews and Meta-analyses, a minimum set of items for reporting in systematic reviews and meta-analyses, consisting of a checklist (containing the subheadings Title, Abstract, Introduction, Methods, Results, Discussion, and Funding) and a flow diagram (used to depict numbers of retrieved items and how they are modified during screening, eligibility assessment, and finally inclusion in the systematic review) [12].

PROSPERO International prospective register of systematic reviews with health-related outcomes, which also publishes protocols of animal intervention studies. It is funded by the National Institute for Health Research in the UK and prioritises UK submissions. Animal intervention study protocols are accepted. Approximately 350 were registered at the time of writing (research).

Qualitative systematic review A means of analysing and summarising qualitative information derived, e.g. from interviews, surveys, focus groups, and patient-reported outcome measures.

RCT Randomised controlled trial.

SYRCLE Systematic Review Center for Laboratory Animal Experimentation. Systematic review protocols on laboratory animal science topics are published on this website (RadboudUMC).

SyRF A free platform for conducting systematic reviews and meta-analyses of animal studies (research).

1 Introduction

> [The meaning of 'experiment,'] according to the OED and normal scientific use, is 'to test a hypothesis.' It has been taken over by journalists and debased from its usual meaning and is now being used in its archaic sense of 'action of trying anything . . . '
>
> – Archibald Cochrane, *Effectiveness and Efficiency: Random Reflections on Health Services* (1972)

1.1 Objectives of This Chapter

This chapter has two objectives: to aid the reader in understanding what a properly written systematic review is and to describe a simpler project, the critically appraised topic, as a useful aid in designing and conducting experiments.

1.2 Brief History of Research Synthesis

Archie Cochrane (1909–1988) (Fig. 1), the British medic who advocated the current movement of clinical medicine towards evidence-based decision-making, focused attention on the idea that physicians needed to rely more on scientific evidence when making judgements about patient care. According to Cochrane, the critical step in changing medical research from its reliance on expert opinion and observation into one of experimentation was initiated by the 1952 analysis of a trio of randomised controlled trials (RCTs) by Daniels and Hill [16]. They integrated three separate RCTs of the anti-tubercular drugs streptomycin and para-aminosalicylic acid, producing new evidence that a combination of the two drugs worked better than either drug alone. They also showed that streptomycin-

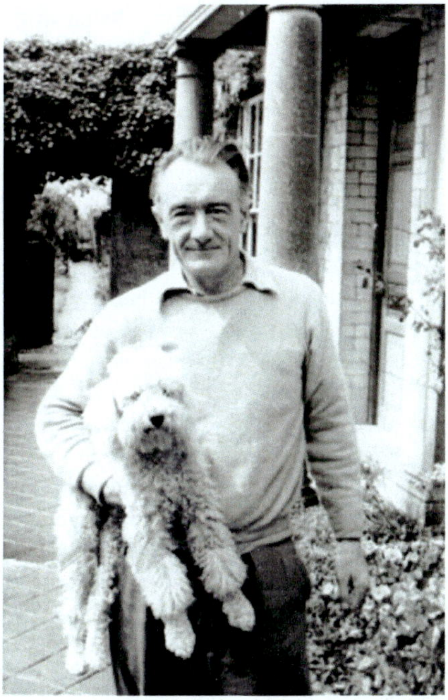

Fig. 1 Archie Cochrane at his home, ca 1956 [18]

resistant strains emerged much more frequently in patients treated with streptomycin only. Great care was taken to show that treatment groups in the three trials were similar in terms of the measured outcomes. This work was possible, the authors wrote, because of the strict adherence to a centrally devised plan and to the remarkable team spirit of all involved in the experiments.

Cochrane also wrote that although the randomised controlled trial process had 'snags', it was nonetheless a widely applicable and elegant technique. After devising the concept of *randomising* patients to treatment groups in the RCT, the *double-blind* RCT was invented because:

> When humans have to make observations there is always a possibility of bias. [15]

Earlier scientists had emphasised the need to combine previous observations, opinions, and experiments into a cogent theory [19]:

- James Lind, a Scottish naval surgeon, noted the importance of conducting a full critical appraisal of previous publications about scurvy in the eighteenth century, after 'removing a great deal of rubbish'.
- Adrien-Marie Legendre developed the least squares technique for regression analysis of astronomical observations in the early nineteenth century.
- Karl Pearson combined correlation coefficients of studies on the effectiveness of typhoid vaccines in 1904.
- Joseph Goldberger analysed bacteriuria in typhoid fever using a strategy now used in systematic reviews: review the literature; select studies for analysis using pre-specified criteria; tabulate data from those studies; and analyse the abstracted data to derive a more meaningful result than any of the studies alone. His results were published in 1907.
- Ronald Fisher, working largely with data from crops grown at the Rothamsted Experiment Station in England, devised numerous important statistical methods including the p value and ANOVA and published 14 editions of *Statistical Methods for Research Workers* beginning in 1925. Of his work, Pearce (1992) [20] wrote:

> At the heart of his approach were the twin ideas of randomisation and significance... Significance was received with delight because it met a psychological need... Randomisation, on the other hand, was rejected from the first. It led to many difficulties in the field and was therefore rejected as unpractical.

After social scientists established that narrative reviews could be biased, for example, in the selection of papers for the review, biomedical scientists began to adopt similar strategies. A seminal work was a 1987 analysis of 50 medical review papers conducted by Mulrow [21]. Measured against a set of quality criteria, she demonstrated that while the majority incorporated qualitative synthesis, only three attempted quantitative methods, and none measured interactions or small effects in the combined data. She suggested six steps to improve reviews, including formulation of a precise question to be addressed, efficient search strategies, inclusion criteria, appraisal methodology, multiple reviewers from different disciplines, and systematic synthesis of the results with weighted evidence.

In the late 1980s, syntheses of research, particularly in cardiovascular medicine and cancer, made their debut in the literature. The landmark publication of the two-volume book *Effective Care in Pregnancy and Childbirth* (Chalmers et al. [22]) added this discipline to the burgeoning list of biomedical research areas which were applying systematic methods to review previous studies. Sir Ian Chalmers formed a group in Oxford in 1993 which ultimately became the behemoth Cochrane, named in honour of Archie Cochrane's call for useful up-to-date information for medical practitioners.

1.3 What Is a Systematic Review?

One definition of a systematic review [23] rephrases Egger [24] is:

> A systematic review is a protocol-driven literature review that addresses a specific research question by collecting all relevant papers on the topic and extracting and analysing their data in a transparent and objective manner. The systematic review results in a qualitative data analysis and may result in a quantitative meta-analysis.

Systematic review is based upon both transparency of the methods and reproducibility of the review. It follows scientific methodology, including an initial protocol to define the scope of the review, as well as transparency in the selection of publications to be included and excluded. Another key feature of systematic reviews is that they assess the quality of the evidence in the studies selected for inclusion, which is not part of narrative reviews.

Narrative reviews, the long-standing mainstay of publications used to guide future direction of a particular research area, are often subjective and prone to bias and error. A somewhat pejorative description of a narrative review is *a summary of the information available to the author from the point of view of the author* [25, 154]. Authors may be eager to promote expertise in a specific area, such as a pathophysiological theory or treatment, resulting in biased selection of publications covered in the review.

Systematic reviews as well as narrative reviews, original research, and opinion pieces contribute to the advancement of science, but scientists must be cognisant of how accepted truths develop in society. Citation networks are used to analyse *the path from data to belief across a network of all papers* [26, 27]. Mathematical analysis of how authors cite other papers in their own work reveals that, as with other forms of social communication, accepted beliefs achieve undeserved authority by a process of 'citation votes'. Numerous forms of bias and error occur in the process of citing papers. Claims may be amplified without any data to support them, papers containing negative results may be ignored while those with positive results are over-cited, and facts may even be invented through distortion. As an example, a systematic review of tissue plasminogen activator (tPA) in a mouse stroke model resulted in a visually compelling tornado-shaped cumulative funnel plot showing how 104 animal studies, conducted between 1990 and 2008, converged on a clearly beneficial outcome by the year 2001 (Fig. 3 in [28]). In the Discussion, the authors stated that the efficacy estimates were stable after data had been obtained from 1500 mice, but experiments continued in subsequent years with nearly 2000 more mice. After a sentence declaring that systematic reviews are an important tool to reduce unnecessary animal usage, the authors then admitted that most of the later studies used the drug as either a positive control, a comparator to other candidate drugs, or in combination with other drugs to examine risk modification. Later authors failed to note this important clarification. Chalmers et al., in a scathing series published in the *Lancet* decrying the waste of funds in research, stated that the Sena review was an example of how animal experiments are unnecessarily replicated: *the efficacy of tPA would not have continued for almost a decade after its benefit had been shown in stroke models* (Panel 2 in [29]). tPA experiments in humans and animals had proceeded in parallel, yet Chalmers and others continue to reproduce the famous funnel plot to advocate for reducing animal research funding.

While narrative reviews may be important in offering expert perspective on a topic, a well-conducted systematic review offers much more to the reader. Along with expert opinion provided by the narrative reviewer, a systematic review provides specific direction for future research based on scientific evidence, in order to produce useful data which can be folded in with previous work. In order to write meaningful systematic reviews, it is important to assemble a multidisciplinary team of specialists, including methodological and subject matter experts.

Not all systematic reviews lend themselves to a combination of statistical data in a meta-analysis, because they set out to do something entirely different. Questions amenable to systematic review but not meta-analysis might include, for example:

- What animal models are most relevant to a particular aspect of a human condition?
- Which procedure is best for administering my drug, collecting my samples, breeding my mice, or affixing a head cap to a cranium?
- How do anaesthesia or analgesia affect animals, and for how long?
- Do I have to wait a week for my animals to become acclimated to their new housing?
- Do I have to wear sterile gloves to do rodent surgery?

Conducting a systematic, rather than a narrative, review of questions such as these will provide a better and more scientifically reliable answer, with a comprehensive and thorough search of the options and a less biased assessment of the procedures. In essence, they provide tables of studies, grouped in various ways, to provide others with a complete, up-to-date summary of relevant studies, which can be updated as new information comes to light without having to undergo the entire systematic review process all over again.

If the results of the studies included in the systematic review lend themselves to statistical analysis, such as numerical measures of treatment effects, meta-analysis can be used to summarise the results and take advantage of the larger sample size and multisite replication.

1.3.1 Qualitative Synthesis

The corollary of the quantitative systematic review is the qualitative review. Qualitative reviews aim to define themes or constructs that are similar across different studies, such as interviews, focus groups, or surveys. The method of reasoning is inductive rather than deductive, and the result may be the development of a new theory. In health research, qualitative studies of patient groups are extremely important in defining priorities for quantitative research. The techniques are also applied to determine how people deal with difficult aspects of their lives. For example, the stress of frequent euthanasia of animals affects people working in veterinary medicine including animal research, as well as in animal shelters. A qualitative review found that there is no well-defined programme to help employees manage occupational stress associated with caring for animals, that the stresses are similar across occupational groups, and that social stigma associated with euthanasia is a significant contributor to occupational stress. Improving awareness of the positive impact of animal caregiving (e.g. through workplace social support networking) was highly recommended to avoid adverse influences on employee well-being, particularly for those who have difficulty coping and are more likely to leave the field. The unanswered question is whether those who become 'survivors' continue because they become desensitised or because they develop successful coping strategies [30].

These studies follow similar steps as the quantitative systematic review. Acquired information is subjected to thematic review with the aim of developing key quotes, themes, concepts, and metaphors. Findings are coded or classified, compared, and integrated. In health research, qualitative reviews of patient experience are sometimes combined with quantitative systematic review to provide more comprehensive understanding of a body of research [31].

1.4 Systematic Reviews of Animal Studies

Since 1979 when one of the first systematic reviews of animal studies was published [32], the number of systematic reviews of animal studies has grown to 800 per year (Fig. 2) in the journals indexed by PubMed.

Twenty-five years after systematic reviews of human research appeared in journals, it seemed to suddenly emerge that animal researchers published low-quality research. This conclusion was based largely on analysis of randomisation, concealment, and blinding [33, 34, 35]. Opponents of animal research were quick to capitalise on the idea, leading to several articles purporting to be systematic reviews published by authors affiliated with anti-animal research groups.

The application of systematic review methods to animal experiments quickly established that some human clinical trials may have been rushed. A bellwether duo of systematic reviews of the effects of the calcium channel blocker nimodipine on focal cerebral ischaemia, first in humans and subsequently in experimental animals, showed that the animal experiments predicted the failure of nimodipine [36]. Subsequently, animal experiments were shown to have predicted the failure of low-level laser treatment of wounds [37] and treatment of glioma with nitrosourea compounds [38]. Even in vitro studies were criticised for failing to utilise randomisation, blinding, and adequate statistical power [39].

The most common reason cited in support of the claim that animal research was 'flawed' or that 'methodological quality was poor' was the lack of information included in published papers, particularly of randomisation and blinding. Altman and others quickly responded with guidance for animal researchers [40, 41], although published guidelines were not available until 2010 [3, 42]. Rothwell [43] concluded that training of preclinical researchers was necessary, stating:

> Animal studies are vital to advances in therapy, but pre-clinical researchers need better training in the many issues that should be considered in the design and analysis of therapeutic trials in general, and clinicians who recruit patients into trials and ethics committees that review them need to be more questioning of the validity of animal data.

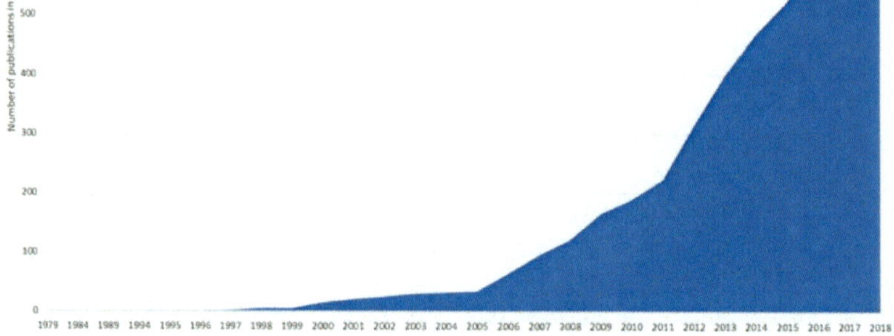

Fig. 2 Number of systematic reviews of animal research indexed in PubMed from 1979 to 2018

1.5 Discipline-Specific Systematic Reviews

Notable among research disciplines which have led the way in conducting research synthesis of preclinical studies is that of stroke. In particular, the Macleod group has generated enthusiasm for research synthesis and led the way, via the CAMARADES collaboration, for others to adapt the procedures to preclinical research.

Other areas of research have adapted systematic reviews to analyse evidence from different streams, such as in vitro, animal, and human research.

- Hoffman et al. [44] explained how toxicology research utilises systematic reviews.
- Vandenberg et al. [45] proposed a framework for reviewing endocrine-disrupting chemicals, citing earlier suggestions for a 'navigation guide' to research synthesis in the environmental health field [46]. The important rationale, as expressed by a report from the UN Environment Programme and the World Health Organization, was to evaluate evidence of associations between exposure to endocrine disruptors and adverse health outcomes in humans. Separate lines of research including biochemical, cell-based, mechanistic, epidemiological, and exposure are all incorporated into the framework.

The chapter co-author has not only collaborated with Macleod but has developed an entire department devoted to the pursuit of systematic reviews in animal research. Training and support are available for anyone interested in learning about the methods.

It is now apparent that evidence-based methodology has arrived in the animal research environment. Systematic reviews are considered to be a prerequisite to human RCTs [47]. All researchers should be familiar with the concept and able to judge the quality of systematic reviews in their field. Undertaking a systematic review requires diligent effort by a team trained in all aspects of the method. Acquiring these skills should form part of the graduate training of all research scientists.

1.6 Umbrella Reviews

As more systematic reviews were written, it became necessary to develop a method for analysing systematic reviews themselves. The term 'umbrella review' (depicted in Fig. 3) refers to the analysis of several systematic reviews in an attempt to compare results and follow a uniform approach for repeating meta-analyses. Ioannidis [48] offered a primer on the complex aspects of umbrella reviews and treatment networks, and Fusar-Poli and Radua [49] summarised key points

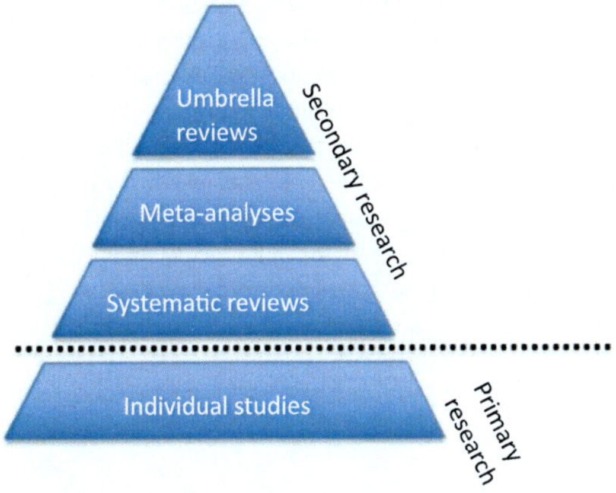

Fig. 3 Hierarchy of evidence synthesis methods [49]

in conducting such reviews. Lamontagne et al. [50] published an umbrella review of preclinical systematic reviews of sepsis therapy.

As with systematic reviews, umbrella reviews should follow a pre-specified (and publicly available) protocol with clearly defined methods. In general, umbrella reviews utilise similar methodology to systematic reviews, with particular care taken to use the same outcome measures and analyse causes of heterogeneity and bias, as well as to publish all the methods used and fully explain the limitations of the review.

2 How Systematic Reviews Inform Preclinical Research

Systematic reviews of animal research have largely utilised human review methodology. Adherence to practices in human evidence-based practice is a common approach to ensure the production of high-quality systematic reviews of animal experiments. Both SYRCLE and CAMARADES have developed tools and guidance for the preclinical field.

Animal research is probably as old as human research and exists largely to understand the mechanisms of physiology and disease as they might be applied to humans. Veterinary research has a similar objective for animal health. A number of systematic reviews of animal research in support of improving veterinary medicine have been conducted, and evidence-based veterinary medicine is well on its way to becoming the norm.

One major difference between animal and human systematic reviews is the large number of reviews, meta-analyses, syntheses and even larger reviews published in the human literature. Preclinical researchers can learn from the experience in the human clinical field. The risks of allowing poorly conducted systematic reviews of animal research to gain traction in the mass media are the criticism from those opposing animal research, the potential for political repercussions, and the loss of support for research which is still not feasible in human subjects.

Table 1 Examples of preclinical reviews of treatment effects

Authors	Topic
Jerndal et al. [52]	Effect of erythropoietin on ischaemic stroke
Hooijmans et al. [53]	Effect of fatty acid supplements on Alzheimer's disease
Gibson and Murphy [54]	Effect of HDAC-inhibiting drugs on acute brain injury
Ker et al. [55]	Effect of beta-2 receptor agonists on traumatic brain injury
Gritsch et al. [56]	Effect of orthodontic loading on dental implants
Lam et al. [46]	Effect of PFOA on foetal growth
Ainge et al. [57]	Effect of maternal high-fat diet on offspring glucose control
Muhlhausler et al. [58]	Effect of maternal fatty acid supplements on fat mass in offspring
Dirx et al. [59]	Effect of energy restriction on mammary tumours
Jamaty et al. [60]	Effect of lipid emulsions in treating poisoning
Lamontagne et al. [50]	Effect of sepsis therapy (umbrella review)
Mapstone et al. [61]	Effect of fluid resuscitation for haemorrhage
Matthan et al. [62]	Effect of fatty acids on cardiac arrhythmia
Percie du Sert et al. [63]	Effect of 5-HT3 receptor agonists on vomiting (ferret model)
Petticrew and Davey Smith [64]	Effect of stress on heart disease in nonhuman primates

Tables 1, 2, and 3 are a small illustrative sample of systematic reviews of preclinical animal studies. Many are the corollary of human drug therapy reviews; others are reviews of various animal models of human conditions. A few address procedures used in animal care and use [51]. Some of these could also be addressed as critically appraised topics (see Sect. 11) for very focused or specific refinements.

Table 2 Systematic reviews of animal models of human conditions

Authors	Human condition modelled
Hainsworth and Markus [65]	Stroke (cerebral small vessel disease)
Bailey et al. [66]	Lacunar stroke (hypertensive rats)
Radde et al. [67], Egan et al. [68]	Alzheimer's disease
Angius et al. [69]	Nerve regeneration on scaffold materials
Ahern et al. [70]	Cartilage defects
Faggion et al. [71]	Dental implant infection
Corpet and Pierre [72]	Colon cancer
De Vries et al. [73]	Articular cartilage tissue engineering

Table 3 Reviews of experimental or standard laboratory animal procedures

Authors	Procedure
Wever et al. [74]	Ischaemic preconditioning for renal ischaemia-reperfusion injury
Wever et al. [51]	Effect of toe or ear clipping on discomfort measures in rodents
Hooijmans et al. [75]	Effect of anaesthetics on tumour metastasis in animal models of cancer
Leenaars et al. [76]	Corticosterone measurement in mice (mapping protocol)
Valentin and Zsoldos [77]	Surface electromyography in large animals
Scotney et al. [30]	Effects of euthanasia/occupational stress on personnel (qualitative review)
Klopfleisch et al. [78]	Effect of biopsy on subsequent metastasis of tumours
LaFollette et al. [79]	'Rat tickling' to increase positive affective state
Lidster et al. [80]	Improving animal welfare in epilepsy research models
Dzikamunhenga et al. [81]	Effect of routine husbandry procedures on pain in neonatal piglets
Laurin et al. [82]	Pooling samples for health surveillance testing in aquatic animals

2.1 The Concept of Validity

All experiments are an attempt to learn about the truth in the real world. How widespread a condition is, whether an intervention can affect a disease course, and how to make a diagnosis are all intertwined in the perception of the validity of an experiment. The two logical parts of validity are *internal* (the extent to which the results represent the truth in the population) and *external* (whether the results can also be applied to similar situations in a different setting).

2.1.1 Internal Validity of Preclinical Experiments

Internal validity involves the conduct of quality scientific research, including appropriate experimental design and analysis, use of valid methods, and detailed reporting of the results. Early publications, such as those published by Kilkenny et al. [3], adapted guidelines from human clinical trials to animal studies, with an emphasis on welfare of the animals and the 3Rs (reduction, replacement, and refinement). Researchers complained that the ARRIVE guidelines were too prescriptive and too focused on animal welfare details and that they increased word limits and page charges assessed by journals. Numerous scientific journals endorsed the guidelines but then failed to enforce them adequately [83]. The ARRIVE guidelines are currently in revision, and others are suggesting a simplified reporting checklist for preclinical research to include randomisation, blinding, sample size estimation, and data handling rules [84]. The US National Institutes of Health posted principles and guidelines for reporting of preclinical research following a workshop in 2014 [85]. The European consortium EQIPD (European Quality in Preclinical Data) WP3 study group was formed to improve and formalise guidelines for designing, conducting, and analysing animal experiments, after an initial systematic review of existing guidelines [86]. A working group of the International Council for Laboratory Animal Science (ICLAS) published the HARRP guidelines, a list of eight requirements for reporting, as an effort to further harmonise the others, hoping to improve uptake by researchers and journal editors worldwide [11].

2.1.2 External Validity of Animal Experiments

External validity, or generalisability, is more challenging: how can we apply information learned from animal models to the care and treatment of human patients? In the field of stroke, despite 13 years of guidance on improving the quality of animal experiments, animal research had not resulted in improvements for human patients [87]. Intuitively obvious reasons, such as the use of young animals to model diseases of the elderly, the presence of co-morbidities in most humans, and the lack of controlled diet and environment in patient populations, have been argued as both beneficial and disastrous for science. Scientists generally attempt to control all variables except the variable of interest, but at some point, this becomes such a reductionist approach that very little of translational use is gleaned from animal studies. The value of stepwise accumulation of knowledge is augmented by the conduct of systematic reviews.

Researchers could be more cautious in understanding and comparing experimental models to human pathological conditions. A more comprehensive knowledge of the biology and characteristics of the animal species may enable researchers to predict species differences in the effect of experimental manipulations. For example, Varga et al. (2015) [88] reviewed rodent models of type II diabetes treated with rosiglitazone and included additional covariates (e.g. method of inducing diabetes, drug administration route, sex of animals, and their diet). They concluded that the most relevant model was streptozotocin administration to rats (most often the Sprague-Dawley strain), with rosiglitazone given by oral gavage. Neither sex nor diet affected the deviation between animal models and human patients. Reliability of animal models can be assessed by assessing their face validity (the pathophysiological similarity to the human disease), construct validity (the method of inducing the disease in animals), and predictive validity (how animals respond to treatment).

A recent clinical trial disaster illustrates the rare but tragic consequences of assuming that experiments in animals will surely predict safety in human beings. TGN-1412 is a superagonist antibody which stimulates T cells. It was tested in rats, macaques, and in vitro human cells. However, when administered to six healthy men in a clinical trial, every one developed cytokine release syndrome, an acute production of pro-inflammatory cytokines which caused multiple organ failure. In the aftermath, the scientist who developed TGN-1412 described three factors contributing to the disaster: (1) mice lived in clean conditions, whereas the humans had developed T_{EM} cells during their lives in typical human environmental conditions; (2) macaque CD4+ cells, in contrast to human CD4+ cells, lose CD28 expression during development into T_{EM} cells; and (3) in vitro testing of human blood cells did not elicit the cytokine response because the T cells were not cultured at sufficiently high cell density [89].

With 20/20 hindsight, it is an easy matter to conclude that researchers should have been more aware of the differences in the animal species and in vitro techniques. The potential for such errors may be widespread throughout the scientific community, unless a wider team of people with expertise in comparative medicine, statistical analysis, and in vitro alternatives to living systems are all included in the decision to proceed to human clinical trials.

2.2 The Value of Systematic Reviews

A properly executed systematic review applies rigorous, transparent methods to evaluate all previously published data using expert judgement. Assignment of quality ratings to animal research reports is critical to the conduct of a proper systematic review. As the number of published systematic reviews of animal research rises, it is incumbent upon the reader to assess the quality of those reviews, which is the objective of this chapter. Readers must develop the ability to look for key indicators of the quality of a systematic review and/or meta-analysis, as the production of such reviews in clinical medicine has reached 'epidemic proportions', while the majority 'are unnecessary, misleading, and/or conflicted' [90].

In 2007, a new tool for appraising the quality of systematic reviews was published, and subsequently updated in 2017. AMSTAR 2 ('assessment of multiple systematic reviews') is a freely available checklist for use in conducting systematic reviews [2] (Box 1). The inter-rater reliability of AMSTAR 2 supports its use as a valid instrument for assessing the methodological quality of systematic reviews [91]. Seven of the 16 items were considered by the developers as critically important for the validity of a systematic review and its conclusions. These items address prior planning, comprehensiveness of the literature search, full justification for excluding studies, assessing and incorporating the risk of bias, use of appropriate meta-analytical statistics, and accounting for small-study publication bias.

Box 1 The questions in the AMSTAR 2 critical appraisal tool for systematic reviews. Items marked with ‡ (2, 4, 7, 9, 11, 13, and 15) are considered critical domains in most situations. If decisions are to be based on the AMSTAR 2 analysis, the team should agree in advance which domains are most important

1. Did the research questions and inclusion criteria for the review include components of PICO(T) (patient/intervention/comparator/outcome/time)?
2. Did the report of the review contain an explicit statement that the review methods were established prior to the conduct of the review, and did the report justify any significant deviations from the protocol?‡
3. Did the review authors explain their selection of the study designs for inclusion in the review?
4. Did the review authors use a comprehensive literature search strategy?‡
5. Did the review authors perform study selection in duplicate?
6. Did the review authors perform data extraction in duplicate?

(continued)

Box 1 (continued)

7. Did the review authors provide a list of excluded studies and justify the exclusions?‡
8. Did the review authors describe the included studies in adequate detail?
9. Did the review authors use a satisfactory technique for assessing the risk of bias in individual studies that were included in the review?‡
10. Did the review authors report on the sources of funding for the studies included in the review?
11. If meta-analysis was performed, did the review authors use appropriate methods for statistical combination of results?‡
12. If meta-analysis was performed, did the review authors assess the potential impact of risk of bias in individual studies on the results of the meta-analysis or other evidence synthesis?
13. Did the review authors account for risk of bias in primary studies when interpreting/discussing the results of the review?‡
14. Did the review authors provide a satisfactory explanation for, and discussion of, any heterogeneity observed in the results of the review?
15. If they performed quantitative synthesis, did the review authors carry out an adequate investigation of publication bias (small-study bias) and discuss its likely impact on the results of the review?‡
16. Did the review authors report any potential sources of conflict of interest, including any funding they received for conducting the review?

If a research team uses AMSTAR 2 to determine how systematic reviews should inform future research, appraisers should agree to the importance of each item in advance. It is discouraged to attempt to assign a total 'score' to individual systematic reviews, as the presence of critical flaw(s) in a review could be averaged out, disguising potentially fatal flaws. Each systematic review should instead be assigned a rating of whether it provides an accurate and comprehensive summary of the results of available studies that address the PICO(T) question:

- *High*: no weaknesses or one non-critical weakness
- *Moderate*: more than one non-critical weakness
- *Low*: one critical flaw with or without non-critical weaknesses
- *Critically low*: more than one critical flaw with or without non-critical weaknesses

3 Procedure for Conducting a Systematic Review

Production of a systematic review may be regarded as one of the initial steps in any research plan, in order to conserve valuable resources, ensure that the planned experiments will fit well into the context of what is already known, and not repeat any previous flaws, particularly with respect to experimental design and reporting. Inherent in the science of systematic reviews is that a team of people with the required expertise must collaborate. The team approach ensures that the systematic review is correctly and rigorously conducted and biases are acknowledged. The method for systematic reviews of human studies has been well-established over many years ([24, 92–96]).

A systematic review requires a great deal of time and effort from a team of experts. It has been estimated that systematic reviews of human studies take on average 67 weeks from start to publication [97], with funded systematic reviews taking nearly twice as long to produce. The standard timeline for Cochrane reviews is at least 12 months [93, 98]. Although systematic reviews require time and effort, they are worth the investment if they are used to support planning of future research. Experts in the field are actively encouraging research funding organisations and government authorities to require (and fund) systematic reviews for preclinical [35] and human RCTs [98].

For more detailed questions which need to be answered during the development of a research programme, a critically appraised topic may be suitable to determine best methods to be used (see Sect. 11). These brief mini-reviews use evidence-based methods to locate and appraise the value of evidence, i.e. for specific experimental protocols, animal care and welfare, and effects of specific interventions on experimental data.

Before committing to the project, conduct a thorough search for both in-progress and completed systematic reviews on similar topics. Previous systematic reviews will likely be found in databases of publications. Searching for similar systematic reviews which have not yet been completed requires more effort, as there is not yet a widely accepted central repository of systematic review protocols.

- SyRF hosts a protocol database (CAMARADES) of preclinical research protocols dating to 2013. This is also an online tool to conduct the entire systematic review.
- SYRCLE's protocol registration database was transferred to PROSPERO in 2018, for systematic reviews relevant to human health. SYRCLE still accepts systematic review protocols related to laboratory animal science and veterinary medicine.
- PROSPERO is funded by the UK National Institute for Health Research and prioritises UK-based registrations. Reviews of animal studies for human health protocols can be filtered in the search engine.

A pilot study is extremely useful during the planning stages and/or just prior to the collection of data. The team must discuss and determine how to use pilot projects: will they be used to refine the main question of the review or to test the forms used to enter data from the selected publications? Both types of pilot study are useful in different ways.

Online training in systematic reviews of human studies is available from numerous sources. Advanced degrees in evidence-based healthcare

are offered by Oxford University, and many institutions offer certificates in the topic, particularly in medicine and nursing. SYRCLE (available for free at https://syrcle.ekphost.nl, login code 'syrcle') offers online training and hands-on workshops on systematic reviews of animal studies and alternatives to animal studies. The UK NC3Rs and CAMARADES groups created the Systematic Review Facility (SyRF) to provide easily accessible sources of support and guidance for systematic reviews of animal studies.

3.1 Key Steps in a Systematic Review

The typical steps involved in conducting a systematic review are listed in Box 2. The strategy for systematic reviews of interventions is consistent. Each step has a great deal of influence on the subsequent ones. The review team must not make the mistake of circling back once the review has been started, i.e. by changing the type of data collected after the search has been completed because it is discovered that something has been missed out. This leads to biased reviews and is a major reason for publishing the review protocol in advance.

Box 2 Typical steps in conducting a systematic review

- Frame the review question in a standardised format (usually as PICO(T): population/intervention/-comparator/outcome/time).
- Publish a structured protocol that clearly sets out the predetermined plan for the review.
- Conduct a comprehensive literature search, with the aim of finding *all* relevant information that can possibly be found.
- Screen the resulting publications using inclusion and exclusion criteria.

(continued)

Box 2 (continued)

- Subject the resulting record set to critical appraisal and data extraction.
- Summarise the information and conduct any pre-planned statistical analysis.
- Detail all evidence in the final review, including an indication of when and under which circumstances the review should be updated.

The following sections detail the steps involved in producing a systematic review of experiments in which interventions (usually drug administration) are conducted on animals and their effect on specific outcomes are measured. Systematic reviews of surgical interventions and diagnostic tests are outside the scope of this text. For essentially any preclinical research question, a systematic review of existing evidence is possible and sensible.

4 Assembling the Research Team

No one can conduct a proper systematic review as an individual. The range of expertise required is too broad and the risk of making biased judgements too high. The leader of the team should be sure that it includes skilled people who will work together on the project. It takes too much effort and time to produce a systematic review to risk doing a poor job by cutting corners.

Broadly, five areas of expertise are required to conduct a systematic review:

- The researcher leads the team and initiates the project.
- Subject matter experts, including researchers in the same field. Laboratory animal veterinarians, veterinary pathologists, imaging specialists, geneticists, cancer specialists, behaviourists, and others may be required to round out the list.
- Information specialists ensure a comprehensive search is conducted.

- Experts in conducting systematic reviews will ensure production of a high-quality review.
- Statistics experts in the relevant area of the review will be needed if a meta-analysis is to be conducted.

Some types of systematic review, such as those involving research of significant public concern, may benefit from including patient representatives, healthcare workers, government representatives, or other stakeholders with an interest in the topic of the review. Borah [97] found that, on average, the number of people on systematic review teams was 5 (with a range of 1–27 and a standard deviation of 3).

4.1 Team Leader

As with any endeavour in research, a passion and energy for the work to be done are required to keep everyone motivated and on task. The team leader asks a great deal of the others, usually as volunteers, and so a diplomatic personality and a willingness to return the favour someday are mandatory. The team leader works closely with the systematic review expert, who advises on how to plan for all phases of the work. The leader also guides the development of the question, as one of the subject matter experts, and additionally does the heavy lifting of organisation, analysis, and presentation of the data.

4.2 Subject Matter Experts

The systematic review expert can help plan the work and coordinate the efforts of the team. Past experience in conducting systematic reviews will ensure that plans and deadlines are reasonable and that the review adheres to expected procedures and culminates in a truly useful publishable product.

To avoid making mistakes by focusing too intensely on the particular animal model while omitting external validity information, an expert in laboratory animal medicine and science can be a valuable member of the team. Lab animal vets can provide context such as comparative biological relevance, differences among animal species and genetic strains, and supportive information on environment, husbandry, and health. For biomedical applications, veterinarians are a vital professional link between animal and human studies, as part of the One Health Initiative.

4.3 Information Specialists

The availability of free online databases can lead to the erroneous assumption that anyone can develop a comprehensive search strategy. To locate all relevant research on the topic of the systematic review, while filtering out irrelevant papers which will waste precious time, requires the professional services of information specialists. In addition to their obvious skills with different databases and search taxonomies, they provide an unbiased view of the question and can provide wider context for the project, as well as identify essential databases for the particular search question.

4.4 Statisticians

For some types of systematic reviews, freely available meta-analysis software, such as RevMan, is often used. However, in preclinical research, statistical methodology needs to be adapted [100]. An expert in preclinical research and systematic review statistics will provide the upfront data collection tools and prevent errors in interpreting the outcome data collected. Some types of preclinical studies utilise complex study design elements, which must be interpreted correctly during the data extraction and analysis steps. These should be subjected to appropriate review in order to ascertain whether systematic bias or error may have occurred [101].

5 Step 1. Ask the Question

The very first question on the AMSTAR 2 checklist is about the question addressed by the review [2]:

> 1. Did the research questions and inclusion criteria for the review include the components of PICO(T)?

This is the most important step, as it sets out the entire project. Correctly formatted questions usually follow the PICO(T) format. The PICO(T) is a guide used to inform the search strategy, inclusion and exclusion criteria, data to be extracted, and result synthesis [45]. Because the original systematic reviews were based on human RCTs, additional progress may result in some alterations as systematic reviews are applied to animal studies. However, adhering to the PICO(T) format is important to keep the review tightly focused on the most important task at hand and to prevent the research team from veering off-target as they discover information that might seem more interesting or relevant. Changing the plan of a systematic review must be avoided if at all possible, just as changing any experiment in midstream is poor scientific practice.

Some systematic reviews are quite broad in scope, for example, seeking to review all animal models of bone research. Others may be quite narrow. A single broad review may include several syntheses, for example, by species of animal, type of tissue or target, type of investigation (development, growth, or repair), type of intervention, and so on. Broad reviews may be more generalisable than narrow reviews but will usually have more heterogeneous results. A single PICO(T) for the overall review may incorporate several PICO(T)s for comparisons [102].

Once the research team is established, a period of brainstorming the question is important to ensure the review is fit for purpose. A systematic review which states that additional topics were added after the project was initiated does not adhere to the strategy and should be seen as poor design. The initial PICO(T) question should be assessed in a very brief pilot study to ensure nothing has been missed out. The pilot study should include a search, inclusion and exclusion criteria, data extraction, quality assessment, and analysis.

5.1 Animal Subjects ('P')

The vast majority of animals used for research are rodents, and the ways in which they differ from humans are obviously central to the concept of translational research. For over 100 years, animals have been kept in controlled environments to minimise the between-subject differences and the confounding factors which plague research with human subjects. Animals bred for research have a defined life history, are similar or even identical genetically, live a consistent lifestyle, and have no co-morbidities. Their lifespans are shorter than that of humans, and their immune exposure is far more limited than that of humans due to their captive housing environment. These practices have been established over many years to ensure that animals are of high quality and healthy with minimal variation. Even lifelong experiments can be accomplished, keeping laboratory rodents in good health as they develop various conditions of normal ageing.

Researchers have been remiss in not reporting more information about the animal subjects of their experiments, resulting in extensive criticism of the quality of animal research. This criticism must be addressed in original research publications before it will influence systematic reviews. As focused as researchers in basic academic research tend to be, it may have seemed acceptable to cut corners when reporting such within-group details as correct nomenclature of genetically modified mice, age and sex of animals, and environment and housing. However, in a systematic review, it is crucial to record as many details as possible. For many years in future, systematic reviewers of animal research will be forced to record and report that the quality of the research was inferior, due almost entirely to lack of complete reporting.

Data extraction protocols should include sufficient information about the subjects of the experiment to assess whether the within-group differences were minimised when the experiment began. Records of randomisation to treatment groups (including the method used), blinding of assessors, and data about relevant aspects of animal husbandry and health must be included.

5.2 Intervention ('I')

While drug interventions are the subject of most systematic reviews, other types of intervention should be included, such as husbandry practices, experimental procedures, genetic manipulation, and methods for inducing animal models of disease. In an expanded statement of a PICO(T) question, the specifics of the intervention should be included, i.e. not simply 'animals given drug XXX' but 'animals given drug XXX at a dose of YYY by subcutaneous injection once daily for ZZZ days'. In environmental health, for example, an exposure of animal foetuses to perfluorooctanoic acid (PFOA) (a chemical in non-stick cookware, now ubiquitous in human blood) defined the intervention in its expanded PICO(T) as 'one or more oral, subcutaneous, or other treatment(s) of any dosage of PFOA or its salts during the time before pregnancy and/or during pregnancy for females or directly to embryos' [46].

Data extraction protocols should include information regarding the exact treatments, timing of intervention, and induction of animal disease model.

5.3 Comparator or Control ('C')

The vast majority of animal experiments include controls, which should be well-described in reports. The concept of which controls actually are best is a matter of some debate. The same is true for comparators in systematic reviews. Many experts advocate using multiple mouse strains or genetic types as controls to increase validity. Genetically modified mice bred in-house should not be compared to a parental strain purchased from a vendor. Sham surgical procedures should be discussed by the review team for their relevance to the final outcome; for example, implantation of a mini-pump to deliver a compound may not require a sham surgical control if the outcome isn't assessed for many weeks and does not involve the possible confounders of anaesthesia, surgical wound healing, or the effect of single housing. As an example of a good statement of the comparator, Lam et al. used 'experimental animals receiving different doses of PFOA or vehicle-only treatment' [46]. Another good example involved omega-3 fatty acids in animal diets; the reviewers made the effort to select comparison diets which were iso-caloric and had minimal differences in the fatty acid composition [62]. A different review of maternal diet omega-3 fatty acids [58] did not specify the comparator in the statement of the aim of the review and, in the Results section, pointed out that the type of diet fed to control animals varied greatly; they concluded that 'it will be important in future studies to select control diets which do not have effects on the outcome measures . . . '. Of these examples, one [46] was able to come to a crisp conclusion that PFOA is known to be toxic based on evidence of decreased foetal growth.

Data extraction protocols should include a description of the controls in detail, including the type of treatment (i.e. placebo, 'gold standard' drug, sham, drug vehicle, untreated tumours, and disease management or endpoints for welfare reasons).

5.4 Outcome ('O')

The outcomes which will be ultimately summarised (and possibly subjected to meta-analysis) are the true nuggets of any systematic review. More than one outcome may be collected, e.g. blood levels of a drug, behavioural test measurements, feed intake, body weight, litter size, tumour growth, infarct size, etc. A clear definition of the outcomes to be collected is an important part of the PICO(T) question, to avoid selection bias. For example, the previously discussed Lam review on PFOA toxicity [46] specified outcomes of body weight during the first 5 days after parturition, total litter weight, and measures of body size. Matthan [62], studying fatty acids and cardiac arrhythmias, collected data on incidence of death, ECG parameters (such as runs of ventricular tachycardia and ventricular fibrillation, amount of current required to induce fibrillation, ventricular premature beats, length of normal sinus rhythm, and arrhythmia score), and infarct size at necropsy. In contrast, a poorly conducted systematic review of dental implants described different outcomes in the results from what was stated in the initial protocol. This failure to follow the initial PICO(T) made it difficult to comprehend the review. The result was the foregone conclusion that there are several animal models using implants in different locations and evaluated by different methods.

Data extraction protocols should ensure that all animals which started in an experiment were accounted for [103]. Outcome measures must include units of measure and original data, if available, or notation of the method of extracting data (e.g. from figures).

5.5 Time ('T')

The dynamic of time in a PICO(T) question is pertinent when there is an important or limited time factor in the experiments to be reviewed. In drug studies, the time of administration is often important, particularly in reference to the occurrence of drug-induced effects. In animal models of disease, investigations of development or ageing, and other dynamic situations, time is a critical factor. In these situations, the appropriate time should be incorporated into the PICO(T) question and followed through the inclusion and exclusion criteria, data extraction, and analysis. Time factors are extremely important in stroke models, for example, when treatments must be given within 1 hour of the stroke to have a positive effect [104, 105]. Timing of therapeutic drug delivery is also important in sepsis [106] and poisoning [60]. Alternatively, the meaning of 'time' in the sense of 'duration of treatment' is important in diseases such as Alzheimer's [53] and studies of the protective value of oestrogen in ischaemic stroke [107].

The time involved in inducing an animal model may have important ramifications. A systematic review of microdialysis to collect levels of the neuroregulator adenosine revealed that the recovery time after the anaesthetic to implant the collecting devices was not reported often enough to conduct a meta-analysis of baseline values; additional animal experiments were therefore going to be required to ascertain this information [36, 108].

6 The Systematic Review Protocol

The second AMSTAR 2 question addresses whether the review was pre-planned in detail [2]:

> 2. Did the report of the review contain an explicit statement that the review methods were established prior to the conduct of the review and did the report justify any significant deviations from the protocol?

A 'yes' answer to this question verifies that the systematic review protocols have been registered and/or published, including the description of the plans for statistical analysis, investigation of causes of heterogeneity, and justification for any deviations from the protocol. Sometimes the answer to this AMSTAR question is 'partial yes' and is acceptable if the authors state that they used a written guide that included a review question, search strategy, inclusion/exclusion criteria, and a risk of bias assessment. The information contained in the protocol is quite useful for preparing the final publication, so it can be regarded as a standard first step in the production of the published review.

Developing the review protocol prior to conducting the review helps avoid bias in the final results. In narrative reviews, selection bias or 'cherry-picking' may mislead the reader and invoke a biased point of view. Systematic reviews are a form of observational research and must therefore follow a predetermined design.

Protocols are often written in a highly structured format using templates from the various online organisations which publish them. SYRCLE and PROSPERO publish animal study protocols online. Protocols must be submitted before commencing data extraction, to reduce potential bias affecting the final product of the review.

Protocols include a method to update progress until final publication. This promotes transparency and holds authors accountable to adhere to the original plan (or fully explain why it had to be changed) and to publish the final result, even if the final answer is along the lines of 'we found no good evidence to address our question'.

SYRCLE proposed a format for preclinical systematic reviews, adapting the fields from the Cochrane standards [109] to conform with preclinical research. It is a 50-item checklist of steps to be undertaken in the review, adding specific details to guide the project. The entire review team should approve the protocol, so it is clear to all what their roles will be.

The first section lists details such as author information, date of registration, and title of the review. Importantly, it also includes the funding source for the review and any potential conflicts of interest of the authors. Next, the background and rationale for the review are briefly presented. The components of the PICO(T) question are listed, and the final question is assembled.

The largest section of a protocol is the Methods section, in which detailed plans are presented. It is divided into six subsections:

1. Searching and study identification
2. Study selection
3. Study characteristics to be extracted (AMSTAR question 3: *Did the review authors explain their selection of the study designs for inclusion in the review?*)
4. Risk of bias assessment
5. Collection of outcome data
6. Data analysis and synthesis

Once a protocol is published on the PROSPERO site, it remains there permanently, along with any updates. When the review is completed and/or published, the relevant dates and links should be updated. If the authors decide to update the review at a later date, the original PROSPERO record is amended and processed as a new review.

7 Step 3. Literature Search

The fourth AMSTAR 2 question relates to the use of appropriate literature searches:

> 4. Did the review authors use a comprehensive literature search strategy?

Searching at least two databases is considered best practice in human systematic reviews. This is not an area on which to scrimp and save resources. Animal studies, particularly those which produced negative results, are likely to be difficult to locate because they may have been reported in abstracts at conferences, combined into larger publications, or not published at all.

At a minimum, reviewers should publish search keywords, databases used, and years covered. The full search strategy, including how it was altered for use in different databases, should be readily available for those who wish to repeat it. In order to improve the search for animal species keywords, SYRCLE published step-by-step search guides and filters for animal studies in PubMed and Embase [42, 110–113]. The search strategies can easily be added to the search for other key topics, thereby increasing the number and scope of results.

7.1 Databases

It is not appropriate to search only one database for a systematic review. Databases are easy to access (certainly by information specialists), and it is well known that they have different areas of coverage depending on the subject matter and journals indexed. Yet reviews that only searched a single database (usually MEDLINE) are not uncommon. Searching one database and leaving out the list of databases searched and the search terminology are cause to question the quality of the review.

7.1.1 MEDLINE, PubMed, and PubMed Central

The US National Library of Medicine made its database, MEDLINE, available for free, at a time when private companies charged fees for access. MEDLINE is the largest and most frequently used source for searching the biomedical literature and is the top database used for systematic reviews in the PROSPERO catalogue [97]. It contains over 30 million citations dating to 1946, indexes 5200 journals, and covers medical and biomedical science topics.

PubMed, also free to use, contains MEDLINE and other types of citations. It includes in-process and ahead-of-print citations, citations from before 1966 which have not been entered in MEDLINE yet, some non-MEDLINE journals which submit full text to PubMed Central (PMC), citations of author manuscripts of NIH-funded researchers, and citations of books in the NCBI Bookshelf. MEDLINE is indexed using MeSH® (Medical Subject Headings), which is updated annually.

PMC was launched in 2000 and is also free. It is an archive of biomedical and life science journal articles and manuscripts submitted according to NIH Public Access Policy. Articles in PubMed may be available for free if the PMC logo is displayed, because PubMed and PMC are linked.

Academic institutions generally provide an interface, such as Ovid, for users to search MEDLINE and other databases.

7.1.2 Embase

Embase, the second most used database in biomedical research [97], was created by a group of Dutch physicians in 1946 (called Excerpta Medica Abstract Journals). It was merged with the Dutch publishing giant Elsevier in 1972. In 2010, Embase expanded its coverage to include all MEDLINE citations. Embase covers areas not incorporated in MEDLINE, such as pharmaceutical, complementary/alternative medicine, prognostic studies, telemedicine, psychiatry, and health technology journals. Over 29 million records are contained in Embase, with 2000 more journals than MEDLINE, particularly European titles. Over 260,000 conference abstracts are included. Interestingly, even in academic medical schools with an Embase subscription, researchers do not appear to replace MEDLINE searching with the larger Embase database [114]. The indexing methods and search terms are very different between the two databases, so searches may retrieve different results when both are searched. Emtree, used to search Embase, was based on MeSH at first but has diverged to include more terms for drugs, diseases, medical devices, and life science concepts. It is updated every 3 months. In general, Embase focuses more upon drugs and chemicals, and MeSH focuses on medicine, dentistry, nursing, and veterinary medicine. The Ovid system can also access Embase, as well as numerous other databases.

7.1.3 Web of Science

Not a literature database, but a citation indexing service, Web of Science selects journals, books, and conference materials for inclusion based on assessment by its editorial team. The selection process involves 24 quality criteria and 4 impact criteria. Its content includes life sciences, biomedical sciences, engineering, social sciences, and arts and humanities. Web of Science consists of its Core Collection and BIOSIS (which covers preclinical and experimental life science research). Resources for examining impact factors include Journal Citation Reports, InCites, and Essential Science Indicators. Following the citation report for individual publications may reveal other records of value in the systematic review and constitutes a form of hand-searching.

7.1.4 Scopus

Scopus, also owned by Elsevier, includes citations and abstracts of scientific journals, trade journals, books, patent records, and conference publications. It includes MEDLINE.

7.1.5 LILACS

LILACS [115] (*Literatura Latino-Americana e do Caribe em Ciências da Saúde*) is a free database of over 800 journals from Latin America and the Caribbean, many of which are not indexed in other databases. Cochrane now requires searching of LILACS for its systematic reviews [116].

7.1.6 CAB Abstracts

The Commonwealth Agricultural Bureaux (CAB) was created in 1947, merging agricultural, mycological, parasitological, and entomological entities. It is owned by a consortium of 49 member countries. Its computerised database was launched in 1973. The name was changed to CAB International, and the head office, database, and journal production were centralised in Oxfordshire, UK, in 1987. Its focus is still agriculture, life sciences, and environmental topics. It indexes some 500,000 journal articles, conference papers, reports, and grey literature, of which 80% are not indexed elsewhere.

7.1.7 Google and Microsoft Academic

These tools find records via web crawling and are not actually searchable databases. Google's search algorithms are proprietary and adapt to individual users or computer IP addresses. Google might reveal grey literature sources and various reports, but the general recommendation is to consider these as methods of searching the grey literature and limit the evaluation to the first 200–300 results [117]. As Internet search engines improve, their use in academic research will no doubt continue to increase.

7.2 Language

The search description should include what languages were included or excluded along with the reasons why (e.g. because the topic of the review was not relevant in a particular country or language area). With freely available online translation software, it is no longer appropriate to exclude publications in unfamiliar languages simply due to lack of translation. Systematic reviews which include only papers in English are therefore of lower quality.

7.3 Search Terms

In the information sciences world, there is a longstanding debate over whether searching the full text of the database records using keywords in a search box is as good as building a search combining subject headings (a 'controlled vocabulary'). It is generally accepted that people these days are accustomed to Google-like keyword searching and find it difficult to use controlled vocabulary to construct a search of an online database [118].

The Medical Subject Headings (MeSH) thesaurus, used by the National Library of Medicine (NLM), is the method used to index publications in MEDLINE. It is updated annually; however, little or no updating of previously indexed papers occurs. It is therefore important to realise that search strategies using terms which are newer than the publication years being searched may not yield correct results. New terms arise in science constantly, so the search strategy must include both recent and older terminologies for relevant topics.

The NLM recommends building a new search using MeSH by selecting and coordinating terms to develop a comprehensive search strategy. A complete set of tutorials is available, providing valuable information on best practices. In addition to learning more about searching the database, the tutorials also provide invaluable advice on writing publications which contain the correct information where it will be found by indexers. For example, indexers look first at a publication's title, abstract, and introduction looking for specific information: the main points of the article, an overview of content, and the authors' statement of purpose. Only techniques and subjects discussed in the Results section will be indexed, leaving out others mentioned in the Background or Materials and Methods sections. Negative findings are indexed only if they are discussed in the Results section. Keywords suggested by the authors are noted only insofar as they may suggest additional indexing terms to consider.

Borah [97] criticised MeSH as being unserviceable for systematic reviews because it returned too many irrelevant articles, the keywords were imprecise and/or overlapping, and there was a long lag time from publication to indexing. Additionally, MeSH terminology is updated frequently, but the database is not back-indexed to include older material.

Entering search terms in the search box is often used in addition to controlled vocabulary terms. This will pick up papers which use different (i.e. older) terms than those included in the MeSH terminology. For example, a systematic review of intracerebral microdialysis included four papers retrieved by hand-searching which would have been found by the search strategy had older synonyms for 'microdialysis' been included (i.e. 'chemitrode', 'dialytrode', 'brain dialysis', 'intracerebral dialysis', 'intracranial dialysis', 'transcranial dialysis', or 'implanted perfused hollow fibre') [108].

The MeSH Publication Type 'systematic review' was added in the 2018 revision, although there were already over 100,000 publications containing these words in the title. Systematic reviews as a publication type are now considered a 'study characteristic' along with case reports, validation studies, and clinical studies; formerly they were considered a subset of the Review publication type.

Occasionally the NLM will update previous index entries with applicable new terms, but not always. Search strategies must take this into account and either develop alternative search terms or conduct hand-searches of the bibliographies of the initial search results to find other relevant papers. In the late 2018, PubMed began to utilise a hybrid approach of assigning MeSH terms by both machine learning and manual rules, in an attempt to speed up the process of indexing publications [119].

Numerous alternatives and aids to searching are available, and although none will replace using a qualified information specialist on the project team, they may be worth investigating. The Polyglot Search Translator, for example, is a free online tool included with the Systematic Review Accelerator supported by Bond University [120]. The user pastes a search strategy for one search engine, such as MEDLINE, into a query box, and the translator automatically creates similar search terms for other databases, such as Ovid MEDLINE, Embase, Web of Science, and Scopus. In an RCT, the creators of Polyglot found that it sped up searches by approximately 30% and made fewer errors [121]. In the environmental health field, a computer programme called SWIFT-Review [122] is available to assist with both formulating the PICO(T) question and prioritising results of literature searches by machine learning.

7.4 Beyond Databases

In order to locate all relevant published evidence, other sources must often be used. Publications might have been missed due to incorrect indexing, inadequate search strategy, or lack of inclusion in the major online databases.

Grey literature searching will help to locate unpublished animal data from postgraduate theses, conference proceedings, and posters and is often overlooked in systematic reviews of animal research. Efforts to assist with searching the grey literature, such as OpenGrey [123], Information Services at the University of Edinburgh [124], and AGRICOLA [125], are potentially valuable sources of information. Searches conducted with Google Search, Google Scholar, and/or Microsoft Academic are considered as grey literature searching.

Hand-searching is usually conducted by going through the bibliographies of publications retrieved in the literature search, searching for additional work which was missed. Other sources to be hand-searched might include proceedings of scientific meetings which contain abstracts or posters, relevant journal issues or supplements, databases of theses and dissertations at various locations, textbooks, or even personal collections of publications belonging to subject matter experts. The Cochrane Register of Studies includes a complete list of some 2500 journals which have been professionally hand-searched for RCTs by information specialists, thus saving time for other groups doing Cochrane reviews [126]. Cochrane provides an online handbook for hand-searchers [127].

The value of hand-searching was reinforced by a Cochrane group which conducted a methodology review to compare electronic and hand-searching of human RCTs. Hand-searching identified 92–100% of the relevant papers, whereas electronic searches retrieved between 42% (when using a 'simple' search strategy) and 80% (when using the Cochrane Highly Sensitive Search Strategy). A combination of hand- and electronic searching was recommended to identify reports of RCTs [128]. Similarly, Craane et al. [129] found 52 publications (75% of the total) in 3 major online databases and added 17 publications (25% of the total) using hand-searching.

8 Screening the Results and Extracting the Data

Questions 5–8 of AMSTAR 2 are:

> 5. Did the review authors perform study selection in duplicate?
>
> 6. Did the review authors perform data abstraction in duplicate?
>
> 7. Did the review authors provide a list of excluded studies and justify the exclusions?
>
> 8. Did the review authors describe the included studies in adequate detail?

The processes of screening and data extraction consist of going through the search results in detail, selecting which papers meet the criteria for inclusion as set out in the protocol, and then collecting the relevant data from each paper. The people conducting this part of the systematic review must be well-versed in the topic and have undergone training and a pilot run prior to the actual process. Because they may ultimately review hundreds of publications, their work must be consistent from start to finish.

Preclinical studies are not generally analysed using Cochrane tools, but the Cochrane site has a wealth of up-to-date information and training material which is relevant for anyone doing evidence-based analyses. Cochrane reviewers utilise a web-based system called Covidence to screen references and extract information, as well as to conduct the risk of bias analysis and prepare the final data for analysis with a companion tool, RevMan [108].

Standard practice is for at least two reviewers to screen the search results and to extract data from the final publications. Inter-rater agreement can easily be calculated or a kappa score if one person conducted the initial review and was checked by a second person. Some process for reaching consensus is required (resolving discrepancies by discussion and/or asking a third reviewer) and should have been explained in the systematic review protocol.

8.1 Screening

A flow diagram showing the number of publications at each step of the process is an important part of the final publication. PRISMA includes a standard for the diagram [12] (Fig. 4). There are four phases of the review:

- Identification of the total number of records retrieved from the search and the number of duplicates removed
- Number of records screened by title and abstract and the number excluded
- Eligible number of full records reviewed and the number and reasons for exclusion
- Number of records included in the final analysis, including those used in qualitative and/or meta-analysis

The efficiency of the search strategy ('yield rate') is the ratio of the number of records meeting inclusion criteria to the number identified during the search. It may seem impressive to depict that over 10,000 papers were retrieved, but if only 10 were used in the final review, the search strategy may have been too broad, causing the review team to waste time looking at titles and abstracts. Extremely low yield rates, on the order of 3% [97], are common.

Once the references have been acquired, the first step is to remove duplicates. A large number of duplicates can indicate that the databases used had significant overlapping content and that perhaps the reviewers would have better used their resources to search conference abstracts, grey literature, or other sources of information. Reviews which only use MEDLINE and Embase (which

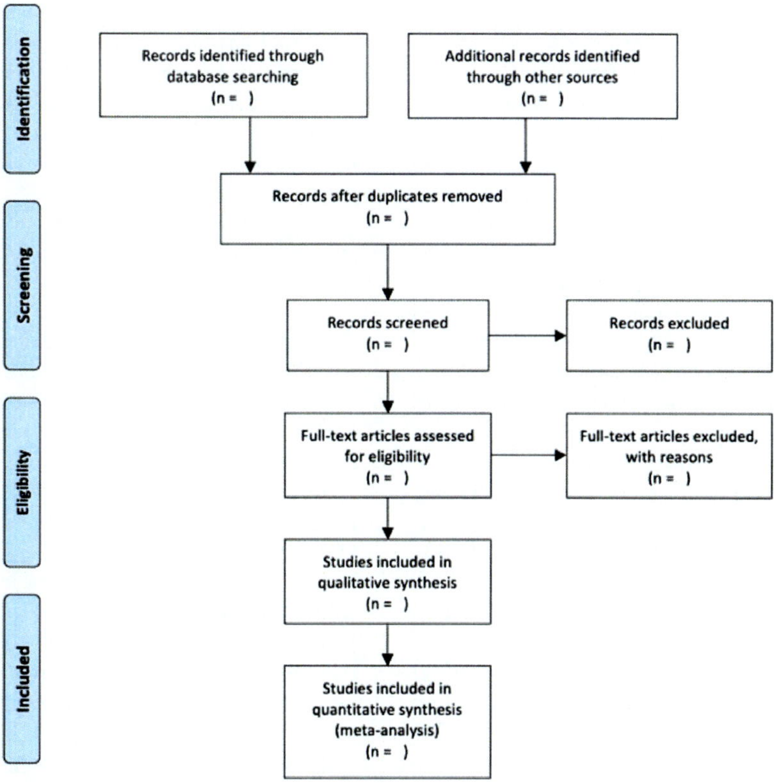

Fig. 4 The PRISMA flow diagram [12]. Creative Commons Attribution License

includes MEDLINE) will generally depict a great deal of duplication.

A more challenging de-duplication task is to determine whether data have been published more than once, for example, in both a conference abstract and a final paper. This may be left to the data extraction phase in order to verify whether duplication of data occurred in multiple publications.

The first phase of reviewing search results is to read the titles and abstracts of the found set. Well-written abstracts such as those written using a structured format [130] should include enough information to make an initial determination of the suitability of the paper. If there is any doubt, the paper continues to the second phase of review, in which the entire paper is analysed. In a third phase, authors of individual papers may be contacted for additional information if required.

AMSTAR 2 steps 7 and 8 require that lists of included and excluded studies be maintained. Reasons for excluding studies must be listed. If excluded studies never appear in the final review, others may find fault with their absence in future reviews, and the impact of their exclusion on the results will be unknown. Exclusion should be based upon inappropriate or irrelevant elements of the PICO(T) question, e.g. because they utilised different animals, interventions or controls, or measured outcomes not included in the systematic review protocol. Exclusions should not be made based on the quality assessment for risk of bias, which is dealt with at a later stage.

The best way to conduct the review is to use a form of some sort to capture each reviewer's decisions on every study. Online tools such as the Systematic Review Facility (SyRF) can be used as a way for reviewers to evaluate records using pre-specified questions. The Systematic Review Toolbox [131] offers a searchable database of tools to support various tasks, including data extraction for text or numerical data. Additional descriptors beyond the basic PICO(T) requirements may be useful later for analysing heterogeneity in the outcomes (e.g. by dose, age, strain, etc.).

Machine learning tools are being developed to screen abstracts and assign a probability that a document should be included, rather than a dichotomous decision. The technique involves using a training set of documents which have been manually labelled for the variable of interest, transforming the documents into number sequences, assigning weights (coefficients) to important words, and 'learning' to distinguish a potentially good document from an irrelevant one. A human reviewer screens a sample of the retrieved documents until a sufficient number has been identified by the software (this is roughly half the found set). The software then offers a ranked set of the remaining documents with those deemed most relevant at the top of the list. Machine learning is under development for preclinical studies and offers a very promising way to decrease the time to screen results. It was 98.7% sensitive and 88.3% specific in one study, which was comparable to dual human screening; however, to date, it is most useful for relatively broad PICO questions [132].

8.2 Data Extraction

Collection of data from the final set of sources must be done by at least two independent people, with any disagreements resolved by a third person. AMSTAR 2 allows for circumstances, such as extraction of data from a sample of studies, with an 80% agreement of two people leading to the remainder of the extraction being conducted by one reviewer.

Automated methods may again come into play when extracting data, e.g. DistillerSR, a fee-based data extraction system [133]. One systematic review of study designs used in preclinical brain trauma/stroke and toxicology research identified 7 of 100 included studies which described using 'factorial' design and suggested that 'split-plot-like design' (or other straightforward phrases) would have been simpler and more accurate for automated searching software [101].

The data extraction form is often quite large. It generally includes the following information: [134]

- Study identification, e.g. title, author, citation, type of publication, source of funding
- Study characteristics, e.g. aim of the study, experimental design, statistical analysis, inclusion/exclusion parameters, details of randomisation and blinding, unit of analysis
- Animal information, e.g. species, age, sex, strain, environment, anaesthesia
- Outcome data, e.g. numerical data including units, qualitative information, length of follow-up or dosing and data collection, number of animals, statistical results such as means and variance, confidence intervals, additional outcomes
- Subgroup data for analysis of heterogeneity
- Risk of bias information

The piloting process should have enabled the review team to define strategies and instructions for extracting data, e.g. deriving numerical data from published graphs, calculating required numerical data from related data reported in the paper, etc.

In addition to extracting data for the main findings of the systematic review, the data required to assess risk of bias can also be extracted at the same time.

9 Risk of Bias

Question 9 of AMSTAR 2 is:

> 9. Did the review authors use a satisfactory technique for assessing the risk of bias in individual studies that were included in the review?

If the response is 'yes', the risk of bias must also have assessed the allocation sequence and verified that the results reported were not biased because of multiple measurements or analysis of specified outcomes.

The assessment of the quality of evidence of a study is not well defined. Published research varies immensely in methodological rigour. Some select the wrong study design for the objective; some do not measure the most appropriate outcomes, use poor statistics, use poor technique in animal procedures, and/or fail to report the experiment completely. Flawed research can result in bias.

Instead of attempting to measure 'quality', systematic reviews usually assess the risk of bias. 'Bias' refers to systematic deviations from the true underlying effect brought about by poor study design or conduct [94]. Differences in study results can often be explained by differing types and amounts of bias in the way the studies were conducted and/or reported.

While there is general agreement on the value of the exercise, there is less agreement on how to do it properly in each area of research and on how to make it more reliable. The methods used vary and include scales, component analysis, and checklists [135].

The Cochrane Collaboration's Risk of Bias Tool was initially developed in 2008 by a group of statisticians, epidemiologists, and expert review authors. The current version, RoB 2 [4], includes five domains of bias used to evaluate the study. Within each of the domains, there are several signalling questions, response options, and risk of bias judgements ('low' or 'high' or 'some'):

1. Bias resulting from the randomisation process: whether the allocation sequence was random and adequately concealed until after the patients were enrolled and assigned to groups and whether baseline differences between groups reveal a possible problem with the randomisation process
2. Bias due to deviations from the intended interventions: whether participants, carers, and others delivering the intervention were aware of the patient's group and whether deviations occurring during the study may have affected the outcome
3. Bias due to missing outcome data: whether outcome data were available for all participants and whether (and in which direction) the missing data would have affected the result
4. Bias in measurement of the outcome: whether the measurement used was appropriate and consistent across all groups and whether the researchers were aware of which intervention had been implemented in individuals they were assessing
5. Bias in selection of the reported result: whether the study followed the protocol and the assessors remained blinded until after analysis and whether the numerical data might have been selected on the basis of the results of either multiple outcomes measured or multiple analyses conducted

The overall risk of bias judgement for a single study is classified as [4]:

1. Low risk of bias: The study is judged to be at low risk of bias for all domains for this result.
2. Some concerns: The study is judged to raise some concerns in at least one domain for this result, but not to be at high risk of bias for any domain.
3. High risk of bias: The study is judged to be at high risk of bias in at least one domain for this result, or the study is judged to have some concerns for multiple domains in a way that substantially lowers confidence in the result.

In preclinical research, the best-known tool for assessing risk of bias originated from SYRCLE [136], based on the Cochrane method and adjusted for differences in study design commonly used in preclinical research. Answers to a series of signalling questions are rated as green, yellow, or red. Bias is reported in the following domains:

1. *Sequence generation* refers to the methods used to assign animals to comparable groups using a chance process. In human RCTs, this usually means employing a computerised randomisation to determine whether patients receive a test treatment or a placebo. In animal

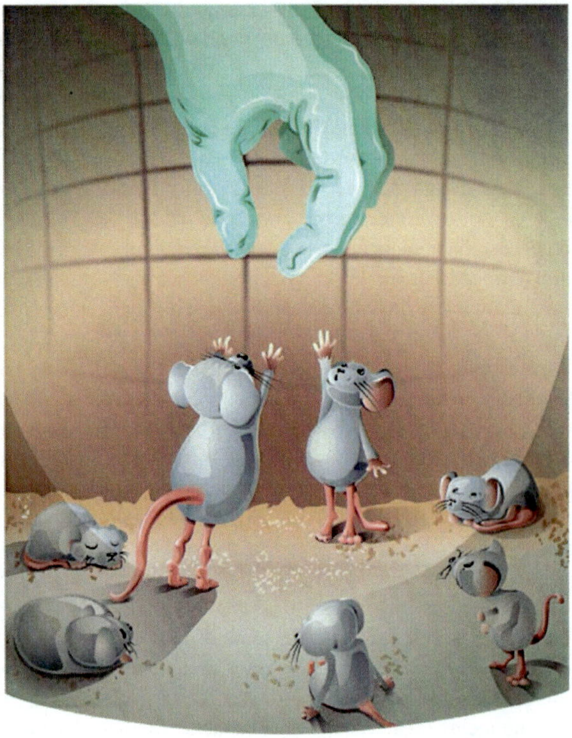

Fig. 5 Simply reaching for the first mouse that can be caught in a cage is not random (V. Altounian/*Science*) [103]. Used with permission

studies, this is also a good practice, as extensively discussed in Bespalov [137]. Simply assigning animals to experimental groups based on location of cages on a rack, on how they were caged on arrival in the facility, or on how easy they were to catch in the cage is not a random sequence generation (Fig. 5). If a particular disease or condition is induced in some of the animals before the experiment, this process should also be randomly allocated.

2. *Baseline characteristics* of the animals may alter experimental responses. If there are similarities in these characteristics (age, weight, sex, genetic strain) or physiological parameters (e.g. serum cholesterol levels), potential pathogens (e.g. *Helicobacter* in rodents), or other characteristics which are relevant to the research area, these should be discussed in advance and tabulated in research publications to demonstrate the regard for selection bias.
3. *Allocation sequence concealment* refers to how the random allocation method was implemented, ensuring that the person who selected animals for each study group was unaware of the treatment the animals would receive.
4. *Random housing location* of animals is a way to prevent performance bias from occurring. For example, light levels in different locations on a large rack of rodent cages may differ. Researchers should also be concerned about noise and movements in the room, vibration or ultrasonic noise from equipment, and location within a facility, i.e. a room located near a loud cage wash area.
5. *Blinding to intervention* of those who cared for and conducted experimental procedures is another way to avoid performance bias. Previous studies have been heavily criticised for not including any information about blinding (and randomisation); current recommendations are

to explain this in more detail than simply stating that 'experimenters were blinded to the treatment conditions'. The type of randomisation and blinding used, tools, stratification variables, and statements about the integrity and directors of the processes should all be reported [137].

6. *Random outcome assessment* during collection of data ensures that detection bias is avoided.
7. *Blinding to outcome* of those who make assessments also avoids detection bias and is again thoroughly discussed in Bespalov [137].
8. *Attrition bias* occurs when animals do not complete an experiment for any reason. All experimental subjects described in the Methods and Materials section must be accounted for in the Results section. For example, failing to report the fate of all animals in an experiment can be considered a form of attrition bias [103]. This is common: 80% of rheumatology papers failed to report it [138], as did 64% of stroke and 73% of cancer papers [139].
9. *Selective outcome reporting* occurs when authors choose which results they include in a publication. It is a form of reporting bias. They may leave out entire outcomes (e.g. because the results did not show statistical significance), report on a selection of subgroups but not all, or present analyses which have been adjusted while omitting to report unadjusted data.

Results of the risk of bias analysis are generally tabulated for each of the studies included in the review, as shown in Fig. 6. Often this detail is left out of the final publication, and a version which combines all studies is published, as shown in Fig. 7 [140].

Whatever the term or method used, appraising the quality of the evidence affects the assessment of internal validity. Studies which are biased or even flawed lead to overestimation or underestimation of the outcome or effect being measured.

Although an overwhelming number of reviews to date have addressed randomisation and

	Random sequence generation (selection bias)	Allocation concealment (selection bias)	Blinding of participants and personnel (performance bias)	Blinding of outcome assessment (detection bias)	Incomplete outcome data (attrition bias)	Selective reporting (reporting bias)
Ader, 1976	?	?	?	?	+	?
Baretto, 2007	?	?	?	?	?	?
Buske-Kirschbaum, 1996	?	?	?	?	+	?
Coover, 1977	?	?	?	?	+	?
Coover, 1980	?	?	?	?	+	?
Davis, 2005	?	?	?	?	+	?
Detke, 1989	?	?	?	?	+	?
Dyck, 1990	?	?	?	?	+	?
Exton, 1995	?	?	?	?	+	?
Golombek, 1994	?	?	?	?	+	?
Graham, 1980	?	?	?	?	+	?
Janz, 1991	?	?	?	?	+	?
Janz, 1996	?	?	?	?	+	?
Kassil, 1998	?	?	?	?	+	?
Kreutz, 1992	?	?	?	?	+	?
Morell, 1988	?	?	?	?	+	?
Natelson, 1984	?	?	?	?	+	?
Onaka, 1998	?	?	?	?	+	?
Pacheco-Lopez, 2004	?	?	?	?	+	?
Rozendaal, 1990	?	?	?	?	?	?
Smotherman, 1980	?	?	?	?	+	?
Smotherman & Levene, 1980	?	?	?	?	+	?
Surwit, 1985	?	?	?	?	+	?
Tencin, 2001	?	?	?	?	+	?
Woods, 1972	?	?	?	?	+	?
Woods, 1977	?	?	?	?	+	?

Fig. 6 Results of the risk of bias assessment using the SYRCLE tool. Green indicates low risk of bias; yellow indicates an unclear risk. Two authors independently assessed the risk for each study; if they disagreed, a third person was consulted [140]

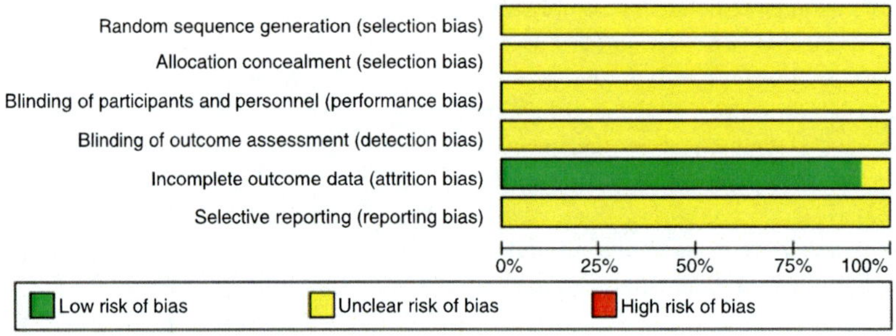

Fig. 7 A diagram of the risk of bias in animal studies, shown as a percentage of the selected studies showing the risk in a green-yellow-red format [140]

blinding problems in preclinical research [33, 52, 55, 68, 141–144], this may indicate that reporting was poor, but does not necessarily cast doubt on the results of the studies. Reviewers must also be acutely aware of unit-of-analysis errors including nested allocation, group allocation, split-plot-like designs, repeated measures, and pseudo-replication. Researchers often utilise these complex study designs. The statistical member of the systematic review team must ensure that the data extraction from complex experimental designs is correctly performed, to avoid missing possible systematic bias or unit-of-analysis errors [101].

Recent initiatives have proposed adapting the GRADE approach for rating outcomes (not studies) in preclinical systematic reviews [9, 10]. Initially developed to facilitate clinical practice guidelines, the GRADE method has been adapted to other uses. GRADE assigns one of four levels of certainty or quality of evidence to an outcome, ranging from 'very low' to 'high'. GRADE uses five domains to rate a particular outcome downwards in quality:

1. *Risk of bias*: a determination of whether the bias is sufficiently high that the confidence in the estimate of treatment effect is less robust.
2. *Imprecision*: certainty is lowered if there were only one or two small studies, yielding a wide 95% confidence interval. Sample size calculations and power of the included studies will affect imprecision.
3. *Inconsistency*: refers to consistency of findings across several studies. Point estimates and 95% confidence intervals are compared between studies to check for overlap. Heterogeneity (measured as I^2 and chi-squared) should be explored if it was part of the protocol; otherwise, the quality of evidence should be rated downwards.
4. *Indirectness*: refers to how similar the experimental animals, interventions, and outcomes are to the human counterparts. The use of several different animal models, surrogate outcomes, and possibly species similarity to humans should be included.
5. *Publication bias*: if this can be inferred from the analysis, it can downgrade the quality of the evidence.

9.1 Including Risk of Bias in the Results

In the systematic review section entitled 'Limitations', review authors discuss all possible limitations of their review, and this is where many decide to touch on the risk that the results were biased due to the assessment described above. After having gone to the effort of appraising the risk of bias in the included publications, it may be difficult to decide how to interpret and present these results in combination with the data analysis. Many authors essentially disregard the entire assessment of bias by stating the obvious:

- *While these findings are encouraging, the risk of bias and heterogeneity limited the strength of our findings . . . .*
- *The majority of studies had an unclear risk of bias . . . .*

A more useful approach is to incorporate the risk of bias with each of the data analysis results. Examples of good practice include statements such as:

- *Comparing treatment A with treatment B, participants who received treatment A may be slightly less depressed after the intervention (MD −2.87, 95% CI −5 to −0.5; 2 studies, 83 participants,* ***low-certainty evidence****) . . .* [145].
- *Reporting of blinded assessment of outcome* ($Q = 33.62$, $df = 1$, $p < 0.007$) *and animal exclusions* ($Q = 28.99$, $df = 1$, $p < 0.007$) *account for a significant proportion of the observed heterogeneity . . .* [146].

Cochrane reviews combine the risk of bias results with the outcomes of each included study. For example, in the forest plot, the included studies can be grouped by their risk of bias (low, some, or high), with individual effect sizes shown for each group and the overall total at the very bottom of the plot. This may illustrate that studies with low risk of bias had more closely clustered outcome measures near the overall mean, while studies with high risk of bias had much larger confidence intervals and tended to favour the intervention more highly (Fig. 2 in [4]).

9.2 Funding Sources

Question 10 of AMSTAR 2 is:

> 10. Did the review authors report on the sources of funding for the studies included in the review?

Several reviews have found that industry-sponsored research tends to exaggerate efficacy and/or minimise harms [147–149]. Such conflicts of interest should be included in publications and form part of the risk of bias analysis, for example, as a subgroup in a meta-analysis.

10 Data Synthesis

At long last, we arrive at what everyone set out to do: analyse results of previous studies to summarise all the best literature and draw conclusions about the body of evidence! Again, the PICO(T) question is used to guide the process. In broad reviews, there may be multiple PICO(T)s for each comparison planned. In some comparisons, tabulation of data may lead to the requirement for statistical meta-analysis.

A systematic review will contain several tables with the relevant information extracted during the previous steps. In contrast to narrative reviews which usually consist of lengthy narrative discussion, the tabular products of a systematic review are all-encompassing and transparent, providing a way of grouping and depicting the results of the review to make them easier to analyse. The table design facilitates a full view of the results so that readers may find good information on a variety of topics. Reviewers must prepare these tables with clarity, transparency, and as much simplicity as possible, to put forth their findings well.

The tables should include the characteristics of the animals, the interventions, the outcomes, and the time factors discovered during the data extraction phase, as well as the risk of bias. Funding source is often also included, particularly for drug intervention studies. Combining the results into several different tables will aid the reader in understanding how the included studies addressed the systematic review question; the tables should not simply be presented in toto and left for the reader to analyse. Review authors will often go through several iterations of the final tables to be included in the published review.

Cochrane [150] suggests a variety of methods for summary and synthesis of information (Table 4).

Table 4 Available methods for summary and synthesis [150]

Methods	Questions addressed	Example plots
Text or table	Narrative summary	Forest plot without a combined effect estimate
Vote counting	Is there any evidence of an effect?	Harvest or effect direction plot
Combine p values	Is there evidence of an effect in at least one study?	Albatross plot
Summary of effect estimates	What is the range and distribution of observed effects?	Box-and-whisker plot, bubble plot
Pairwise meta-analysis	What is the *common* intervention effect (fixed-effect model)? What is the *average* intervention effect (random-effect model)?	Forest plot
Network meta-analysis	Which intervention of multiples is most effective?	Forest plot, network diagram, rankogram plots
Subgroup analysis/meta-regression	What factors modify the magnitude of the intervention effects?	Forest plot, box-and-whisker plot, bubble plot

10.1 Characteristics of Included Studies

The first tables will include characteristics of each included study, including PICO(T) data. In particular, a table of characteristics of the animals tested (the ‘P’) is often missing in preclinical systematic reviews, impairing the ability to generalise to other animals, age groups, sexes, or life histories. Tables 5 and 6 are examples of best practice. In a systematic review of rat tickling as an habituation technique to model positive behavioural affect, one table of study characteristics included characteristics of the rats (the ‘P’ of PICO(T)): number, strain, sex, age, number per cage, and days of acclimation. A second table included columns for interventions (‘I’): method of tickling, durations (total and active tickling), number of sessions, total time per rat, and the type of surface during the tickling [79].

In broad reviews, studies of similar topics may be compared in a matrix format. For example, in a review of animal models of chemotherapy-induced peripheral neuropathy, the reviewers planned to synthesise behavioural outcomes and the effects of drug interventions. This resulted in four data sets: (1) models that reported pain-related behaviours, (2) models that reported other behavioural outcomes, (3) effects of interventions on pain-related behaviours, and (4) effects of interventions on other behavioural outcomes. Each of the data sets was analysed in the synthesis, a 34-page long report with 19 authors [146]. The preponderance of preclinical systematic reviews, however, is more limited in scope.

There will be many different interventions and outcomes in the included studies. Preclinical studies are often criticised for using many different interventions and outcomes, making

Table 5 Table of animal characteristics, extracted from LaFollette et al. (Table 3, [79]). Included studies and dates in the first two columns are used to sort the table. Additional columns include information about the rats and their acclimation to the study. Open-access article under the terms of the Creative Commons Attribution License

Author	Year	N	Strain	Sex	Age, days	No. per cage	Acclimation, days
Boulay	2013	6–16	SD	M	21	4	1
Burgdorf	2001	8–49	LE	M&F	37	1	?
Burgdorf	2009	18–83	LE	M&F	24–126	1	N/A
Cloutier	2012	16, 32	SD	M	35, 57	1	?
Garcia	2015	20, 30	SD	M	40	1	10
Hori	2013a	12	Fisher	M	37.5	1	5
Mallo	2009	62	Wistar	M&F	21	1, 4	0
Paredes-Ramos	2012	20, 30	?	F	31, 92	1	?, 5

Table 6 Example of a table of characteristics of the interventions in studies of rat tickling (Table 1 in [79]). Type = type of tickling (P=Panksepp, PV=Panksepp variation). When articles had two experiments with different values, the values are split by a comma. ? = not reported. Open-access article under the terms of the Creative Commons Attribution License

Author	Year	Type	Total duration, min	Active tickling, min	No. of sessions	Total time per rat, min	Tickling bedding
Boulay	2013	PV	?	0.5	1–6	?	Sawdust
Burgdorf	2001	P	0.5–2	0.15–1	2–5	8–10	None
Burgdorf	2009	P	2	1	5	10	None
Cloutier	2012	P	2	1	15, 17	30, 34	Wood fibre
Garcia	2015	P	2	1	4	8	Wood fibre
Hori	2013a	PV	5	2	1	5	Cloth
Mallo	2009	P	2	1	14	14	None
Paredes-Ramos	2012	PV	6	3	10	60	None

systematic review difficult; this also occurs in systematic reviews of human studies, although to a lesser extent. These may be grouped together into similar types, e.g. by drug used, method of administration, dose, and/or duration. If a disease or condition was induced, the included studies might also be grouped by the timing of disease induction and intervention (i.e. the effect of dietary supplements on development of Alzheimer's disease). The rationale for grouping must be described, as judgement (with the potential for bias) is involved in grouping studies together. This is often the case with grouping by age or weight of the animals, method of administration of a drug, or duration and dose of the intervention. The rat tickling review contained a table of commonly assessed outcomes in tickled vs control rats, i.e. responses to human approach, vocalisations at high or low frequencies, displays of anxiety, and reaction to handling. All in all, the LaFollette systematic review contained seven tables and three figures, combining the results to provide a clear and thorough summary of the effects of the procedure and recommendations for methodology, with caution advised due to inter-individual variation of random-bred rats and generally incomplete reporting quality.

Cochrane reviews involve very detailed analysis of extracted information, which helps to examine and evaluate all of the studies. The review team goes through this exercise in great detail and often discovers new information in the process of combining the results (sorted by PICO(T) elements) in different ways [150]. Systematic reviews of animal models could be more thorough in the analysis, similar to Cochrane reviews.

As with any paper, readers should be alert to whether the results of the systematic review fully support statements in the discussion. Careful reading of the Results section may pick up additional information which should qualify conclusions in the discussion. For example, a review of the effects of a drug on rat foetal weights included two studies showing (study 1) weight increase in rats (unknown number) and (study 2) an increase in hypoxic rats (n = 7) and a *decrease* in non-hypoxic rats (n = 7); yet the abstract and discussion contained the misleading sentence '[Drug XX] *increased* foetal weight in rats'. This is a good example of how a systematic review with tabular results is more difficult to influence with possible author bias.

10.2 Meta-analysis

Questions 11–13 of AMSTAR 2 address the relationship between risk of bias and meta-analysis of results:

> 11. If meta-analysis was performed, did the review authors use appropriate methods for statistical combination of results?
>
> 12. If meta-analysis was performed, did the review authors assess the potential impact of risk of bias

in individual studies on the results of the meta-analysis or other evidence syntheses?

13. Did the review authors account for risk of bias in individual studies when interpreting/discussing the results of the review?

10.3 What Is Meta-analysis?

The full explanation of meta-analysis is beyond the scope of this book. Statistical advice must be sought before commencing a systematic review in which it is anticipated that sufficient data for meta-analysis will result. Meta-analysis, like other topics in biomedical statistics, is an emerging field of endeavour. Simply having access to statistical software does not mean the correct tests are obtained in all cases.

Meta-analysis is a statistical method of combining the results of a number of studies to produce an estimate of the treatment effect (outcome). There are several methods, most of which are ways to calculate a weighted average of the treatment effect estimates from the studies included in the systematic review. The mathematics are not that complicated; selecting the appropriate statistical procedure is more challenging. The result of an inappropriate meta-analysis is a precise but biased estimate of associations. It may be a more valuable service to consider the causes of differences between studies (*heterogeneity*) than to fall prey to the lure of the diamond at the bottom of the forest plot.

Human RCTs often utilise dichotomous outcomes (e.g. mortality, metastasis, hospital discharge). Outcomes are expressed as odds ratios or relative risk. Preclinical studies are usually seeking continuous outcomes, a more complex statistical situation; the standardised mean difference is often utilised.

The inverse variance method is used most often in meta-analyses; Cochrane's own tool (RevMan) implements it. It can be applied to either continuous or dichotomous data. The inputs from continuous outcomes comparing two groups are the means, standard deviations, and sample sizes from each study. If the outcomes were all reported on the same scale, the means are used; if the scales were different, the standardised mean difference (SMD) is calculated. If instead the inputs compared change from a baseline value, a regression model or analysis of covariance (ANCOVA) is used to produce an adjusted estimate of the intervention effect and its standard error. Other types of outcomes (ordinal, measurement scales, counts or rates, time-to-event) are explained in the *Cochrane Handbook* [151].

There are two distinct approaches to inverse variance meta-analysis: fixed effects and random effects. These are summarised below and in Table 7:

- *Fixed-effect* meta-analysis assumes that the true treatment effect is the same in all of the studies; if so, then any variation between the studies is entirely due to sampling variation. The treatment effect is universal, and the meta-analysis provides the best estimate of it. The summary effect calculated by fixed effects is the common effect size. The information about treatment effect is better in large studies, so small studies can be ignored. To test this assumption, a test of heterogeneity between studies is performed. Fixed-effect models are relatively rare in biomedical research; for example, it would be appropriate for a trial in 1000 inbred mice divided into equal-size groups for the sake of the time it takes to test them all. All conditions would be identical, and there is no intent to generalise to the larger population of mice as a whole.
- *Random-effects* meta-analysis assumes that the true treatment effect varies among the studies, so the included studies produce a random sample of treatment effects. The meta-analysis produces a mean effect of treatment, around which the true study effects vary. The summary effect is the estimate of the mean of the treatment effects. Large studies will have more weight than small ones. Random-effects meta-analysis takes heterogeneity into account. Most systematic reviews which conduct meta-analysis utilise the random-effects model, because they summarise a series of studies conducted by different researchers

Table 7 Comparison of fixed-effect and random-effect meta-analyses [152]

	Fixed effect	Random effects (more conservative)
Assumption about the true treatment effect size	*Same in all studies* (tested with chi-squared test of heterogeneity, Q)	*Different in all studies*; therefore we estimate the between-study variance (τ^2)
Cause of variation in between-study treatment effect sizes	Sampling error only (within study)	Sampling error (within study) plus random error (between studies)
Effect of size of study	Large studies heavily weighted Small studies have very small weight	Less influenced by study size, if they are normally distributed estimates
Forest plot: horizontal lines (95% confidence intervals)	Within-study error	Within-study plus between-study error
Forest plot: solid box size (proportional to weight of study)	Wide range of study weights (box sizes)	Weights (box sizes) fall in narrower range Weights will be more balanced
Forest plot: diamond at the bottom of plot	Summary estimate = estimated mean size of effects Centre at vertical line of no treatment effect Width depicts 95% confidence interval	Summary estimate = estimated mean size of effects Centre at vertical line of no treatment effect Width depicts 95% confidence interval
Variance, standard error, and 95% confidence interval	Smaller than random effects Less uncertainty	Larger than fixed effect More uncertainty
Null hypothesis	Summary effect = 0 in every study	Mean of summary effects = 0

under at least slightly different conditions, so it is assumed that there will be error inherent in the mean, and the goal is to generalise to a range of possibilities.

10.4 Heterogeneity

This is question 14 of AMSTAR 2:

> 14. Did the review authors provide a satisfactory explanation for, and discussion of, any heterogeneity observed in the results of the review?

The art of meta-analysis of a set of studies often comes down to how different they were from each other. If all systematic reviews compared the exact same outcome from identical experiments, there would be very few such reviews in the literature, and their generalisability would be inconsequential. Meta-analysis aims to make reasonable estimates of effects using logical combinations of studies. At one end of the spectrum, studies in a found set might all measure body weight in genetically homozygous female mice at the same time point after an identical intervention – a homogeneous group. At the opposite end of the spectrum, studies of the size of solid tumours treated with different anti-cancer drugs in several outbred rat strains would have much wider variation in results – a heterogeneous group. Whether combining studies yields a reasonable estimate of the true effect, or a meaningless set of numbers, depends to a large degree upon the original hypothesis of the systematic review and whether the question asked has relevance to the population of interest. *Heterogeneity* is the variability among studies included in a systematic review.

The use of different experimental methods in preclinical studies is a major source of heterogeneity: different animal strains (which can lead to clinical heterogeneity), interventions given with different methods/doses/times, different controls, and, frequently, different outcomes measured at different times post-treatment (more specifically termed statistical heterogeneity). No statistical magic can atone for all of these differences. The reader must be careful in interpreting the published results and make a wise judgement about whether the meta-analysis was reasonable.

To complicate matters further, the risk of bias must be considered in the meta-analysis. While it would seem logical to use only the studies with the lowest risk of bias, this is rarely an option in preclinical studies due to the overwhelming effects of unknown randomisation or blinding, as well as failing to report data completely. Those attempting to conduct meta-analysis must, at the outset, recognise that the final results will be less than ideal, plan accordingly, and fully describe the limitations of their review.

Statistical testing for the presence of heterogeneity was pioneered by Rebecca DerSimonian and Nan Laird, who published a landmark paper in 1986 [153] cited over 22,000 times. They assigned weights to the component trials to adjust for differences in sample size and methodology. In a set of eight reviews of clinical trials in humans, they noted that the authors had estimated treatment effects of the included trials as if they were constant. DerSimonian and Laird applied a random-effects approach to divide the observed treatment effects into two components: the true treatment effect and the sampling error. True treatment effect (e.g. survival rates of alcoholic hepatitis patients given steroids or control therapy) in each of the separate trials was affected by patient characteristics and other inherent causes of bias. To measure how constant the treatment effect was across different strata (homogeneity), they used the chi^2 statistic (Q), the sum of squares of the treatment effect about the mean. Their formula for estimating between-study variance in random-effect meta-analysis (tau^2) is commonly used in systematic reviews. It is based on Q, the unadjusted weights, and the number of contributing studies [154].

When there are few studies and small sample sizes, the chi^2 and tau^2 tests are interpreted cautiously; values of $p < 0.10$ are usually considered significant. Some statisticians believe that statistical heterogeneity is always present in meta-analyses. A way to improve the interpretation of the meta-analysis is to assume heterogeneity is always present and measure its impact on the results of the analysis. Higgins I^2 statistic represents the percentage of variation between the sample estimates due to heterogeneity (if $I^2 = 0\%$, there is no heterogeneity). It is commonly accepted that values of I^2 are interpreted as follows [151, 155]:

- 0–40%: heterogeneity might not be important.
- 30–60%: may represent moderate heterogeneity.
- 50–90%: may represent substantial heterogeneity.
- 75–100% considerable heterogeneity.

10.4.1 Subgroup Analysis

Subgroup analysis is a method of exploring statistical heterogeneity. Subgroups must have been pre-specified in the protocol of the systematic review and interpreted with caution. Diversity of the animals used in studies is a frequent cause of homogeneity and is one reason for using subgroup analysis. Other subgroups might be sex, location, or types of intervention.

Caution should be used in determining the number of subgroup analyses to conduct, as false-negative and false-positive results are more likely with larger numbers of subgroups.

10.4.2 Sensitivity Analysis

Sensitivity analysis is a method of examining the effect of the decisions made by the review authors on the overall findings of the review. Many such decisions may have been a bit arbitrary, e.g. deciding at what age a mouse becomes an 'adult' for inclusion in the analysis, using data from grey literature, or by imputing data from graphs or incomplete reports. Preclinical reviews often utilise data from studies with 'unclear' risk of bias, another matter of judgement on the part of the review team. In addition, one or two outlying studies with results that greatly conflict with the others may cause heterogeneity. The review team must determine if there is an obvious reason for the conflict before considering removing these studies from the meta-analysis.

To conduct a sensitivity analysis, alternative ranges or values are substituted, and the entire meta-analysis is run again. In some cases, entire 'outlier' or highly biased studies may be removed prior to re-analysing the data. The analysis aims to answer the question: 'Are the findings robust to the decisions made in the process of obtaining them?' [151].

Sensitivity analyses differ from subgroup analyses. They do not compare results in different subgroups, rather they develop different ways to estimate the outcomes of interest, which are then discussed and presented with great caution.

10.5 Forest Plot

As its name suggests, the forest plot (sometimes called a *blobbogram*) looks a bit like a tree structure. Figure 8 is an example of a forest plot showing the results of a meta-analysis of the effects of giving antenatal corticosteroids to women at risk of preterm birth. In this report, the studies are ranked by weight. The components of the forest plot are:

- The solid vertical line, placed at the null effect, representing no association between the intervention and the outcome or between interventions.
- The horizontal axis showing the scale for the statistic; it may be many different things including odds ratio (OR), relative risk (RR), absolute risk reduction (ARR), standardised mean difference (SMD), or others. Usually a text entry clarifies how to interpret the results to the right or left of the line of null effect (i.e. favouring corticosteroids or control). In the figure, the Risk Ratio (RR) is plotted on a semi-log scale, so the point estimate is in the centre of the 95% confidence interval. Arrows at the end of some horizontal lines indicate they go beyond the limits on the axis, to keep the plot to a reasonable size.
- Rows (usually a single study per row) representing a single study in the included set.
  - The size of the solid box indicates the study's outcome and the weight of the study in this meta-analysis.
  - The horizontal line represents the boundaries of the 95% confidence interval (or similar measure of spread). If the horizontal line crosses over the vertical line, the result was not statistically significant (in the figure, only two studies were significant). If there is little overlap of the lines across all the studies shown, heterogeneity is likely present.
- The solid diamond represents the treatment effect (its size) and confidence intervals (its width) of the combined studies above it. Because it does not cross the vertical line of null effect, the improved result in corticosteroid-treated patients was statistically significant at the 5% level.
- Two columns depicting the number of patients, both with the outcome (*n*) and the total in the group (*N*).
- The numerical results of the individual studies (RR in this plot) listed at the far right, with the total results at the bottom of the column.

At the bottom of the plot are the results of the test for heterogeneity of the included studies:

- Heterogeneity test: $tau^2 = 0.05$; $chi^2 = 21.30$, $df = 14$, $p = 0.09$, and $I^2 = 34\%$. This indicates that there was heterogeneity in the population. The results of this heterogeneity test (indicated by the low p value of the chi^2 test) would therefore have required use of random-effects meta-analysis.
- Test for overall effect: $Z = 2.99$ ($p = 0.0028$). This should agree with the inference from the 95% confidence interval (RR = 0.72, 95% CI 0.58 to 0.89).
- Test for subgroup differences: not applicable because of the I^2 value.

Overall, this forest plot and associated meta-analysis would be interpreted as follows:

- Perinatal deaths decreased by 28% when at-risk mothers were treated with corticosteroids (RR 0.72, 95% CI 0.58 to 0.89; 6729 participants in 15 studies; moderate-quality evidence).
- The result illustrates the power of meta-analysis; despite 13 of the 15 studies failing to show a treatment benefit, the meta-analysis showed a clear benefit for neonatal infants.

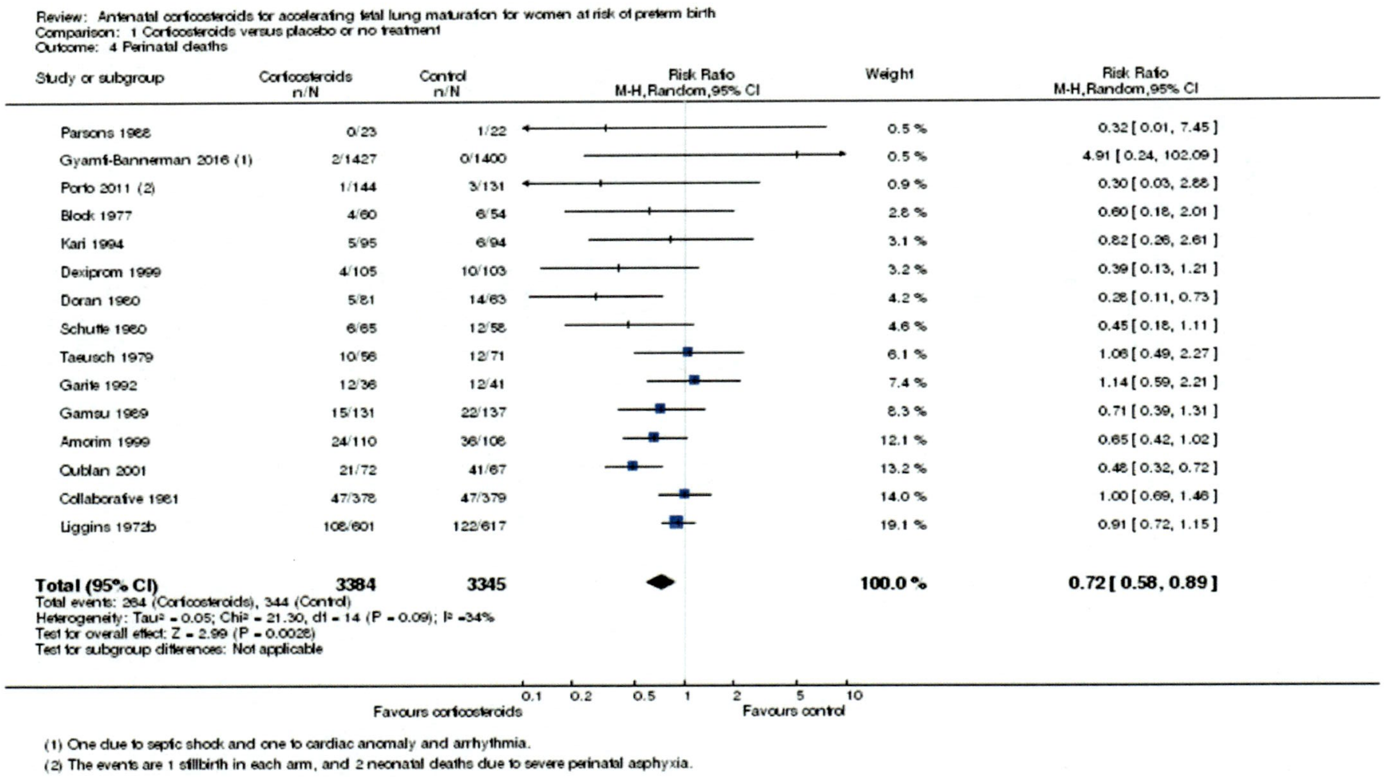

Fig. 8 Forest plot depicting the effect of antenatal corticosteroid treatment on perinatal mortality [156]

10.6 Publication Bias and the Funnel Plot

Question 15 of AMSTAR 2 relates to publication bias:

> 15. If they performed quantitative synthesis did the review authors carry out an adequate investigation of publication bias (small study bias) and discuss its likely impact on the results of the review?

Publication bias (a measure of the likelihood that experimental results were not published because the findings are either 'negative' or disagree with the overarching goals of the research) is by definition extremely difficult to assess. The extent of publication bias in preclinical research is largely unknown; estimates are 50% in a survey of Dutch researchers [157] and 42% in a random sample of animal study protocols at two German medical schools [158]. This is in agreement with estimates of the numbers of human clinical trials which go unpublished [159].

Methods to estimate publication bias include Egger's test for funnel plot asymmetry, the Fail-Safe number, and the trim-and-fill method. Egger's test is the most commonly used [9].

The funnel plot is a dot plot of the effect size (horizontal axis) vs the precision (often standard error) (vertical axis) (see Fig. 9). Larger studies appearing at the top of the plot generally have smaller effect size, while smaller studies have larger effect sizes, giving an inverted funnel-shaped appearance to the plot symbols. Lines are added to indicate a triangle in which 95% of the studies are expected to fall if heterogeneity or selection bias is unimportant. If the symbols in the plot are missing in one area causing asymmetry in the funnel plot shape, it may be assumed that these 'missing' points represent studies which were not found during the literature search, possibly because they generated results which were 'negative'. To apply a more rigorous analysis to funnel plots, various statistical methods have been developed, the most common of which is the Egger's linear regression method. This method is intended to capture the amount of bias in the funnel plot and works with a range of study sizes. Imputing the missing studies is often done using a method referred to as 'trim and fill'. One first removes the most extreme values from the smaller studies and then re-calculates the effect size, continuing one at a time until the funnel plot is symmetrical about the central axis. The removed studies are then added back, with a 'mirror image' calculated for each one to fill in the missing studies. The result is an adjusted effect size and a rough estimate of how many studies are 'missing'. The adjusted effect may be similar to the original one, or it may shift the magnitude of the effect size or even cast doubts on the effect size entirely.

11 Critically Appraised Topics (CATs)

While a systematic review is the best approach to determine the evidence for important questions such as which animal model to use and how

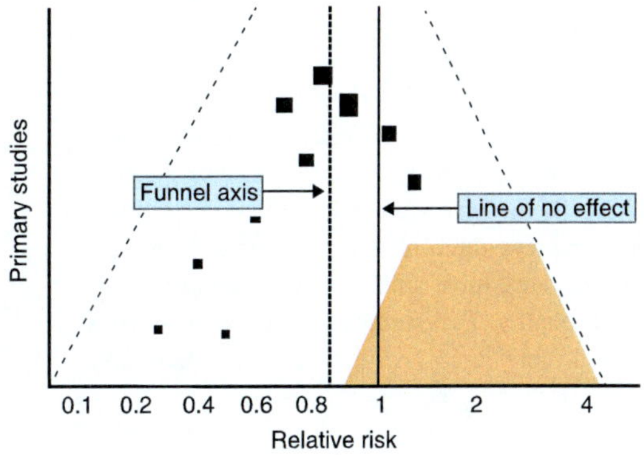

Fig. 9 A diagram of a funnel plot [160]. Larger studies are shown as larger squares; their weight causes them to lie closer to the central vertical axis. Smaller studies (smaller boxes) lie further from the centre. The coloured area contains no studies, which may be due to publication bias

it compares with a human condition, preclinical research incorporates dozens of technical details which must be worked out during the preparation of an experimental plan. Highly focused decisions, i.e. route of drug administration, effect of analgesics or anaesthetics upon the outcome measure, environmental factors, and experimental methods, can be made using the critically appraised topic (CAT).

CAT methodology is similar to that of the systematic review but provides a short summary of the most up-to-date evidence of information retrieved using structured searches. CATs differ from systematic reviews in being less time-consuming and more narrowly focused. The population studied is often more narrowly defined, the intervention is restricted to a single variable, and the outcome might concentrate only on fixed-term effects. As in the systematic review, the PICO(T) question is essential to the success of the entire venture.

In human and veterinary medicine, CATs are a valuable tool in clinical practice. Several groups have created online CAT libraries to appraise evidence on current clinical issues. The CATs often include both animal and human studies in the results. Libraries include the CAT Bank [161], BestBETS [162], BestBETS for Vets [163], and many others. A new journal, *Veterinary Evidence*, encourages submission of 'knowledge summaries' for publication [164]. Berdoy and Repp [165] proposed the creation of an online service specifically for CATs relevant to 3Rs methodology in animal research, which has not yet been realised.

In preclinical research, CATs could be used to assess numerous topics and help improve the quality and design of animal studies. As an example from human medicine, a CAT was written to determine whether emergency cooling for people with heat stroke differed between men and women, a simple sex difference question [166]. Of the nine studies identified in the literature review, three reported differences by sex. Two of these three studies were rated as moderate in quality. Two studies reported that females cooled more rapidly with an average effect size of 2.4 (range 0–3.9). In another CAT from the same journal, non-invasive methods of quantifying scapular movement for shoulder problems, along with estimates of the inter-rater reliability, were summarised [167]. This CAT resembles a typical 3Rs approach to determining which method of measurement might be both effective and non-invasive.

11.1 Method of Producing a Critically Appraised Topic

Four steps are used to structure a CAT:

1. Write a focused, answerable question in PICO(T) format.
2. Search for best available evidence in at least one database.
3. Appraise the evidence critically for validity and relevance.
4. Interpret and apply the results to preclinical research.

11.1.1 PICO(T) Question

The format for the question in a CAT is the same as in a systematic review, but the question is usually much more narrow and tightly focused on a particular area. Otherwise, the CAT would be too difficult to complete in a short period of time. Examples of questions from published CATs include the following:

- In a patient with an immunobullous disorder, is transportation of the skin biopsy in normal saline adequate for direct immunofluorescence analysis? [168]
- Is CCNU (lomustine) valuable for treatment of cutaneous epitheliotropic lymphoma in dogs? [169]
- For a healthy individual, are proprioceptive neuromuscular facilitation stretching programmes more effective in immediately improving hamstring flexibility when compared with static stretching programmes? [170]

In the authors' experience, the CAT process is a preferred substitute when answering questions arising from daily practice as laboratory animal veterinarians. A worked example is illustrated here to aid readers in preparing CATs in their own investigative areas.

Pinworms (most often *Syphacia muris*) are not uncommon in laboratory rats, despite efforts to keep pathogenic organisms out of animal facilities. Pinworm eggs are quite sticky and resistant to common disinfection efforts and can therefore be introduced not only when new animals are brought to a facility but possibly by contact with pet rodents at home or even (theoretically) by stepping into the faeces of wild rodents and carrying the eggs into the facility on the shoes. When pinworms are diagnosed on routine health screening, researchers can become alarmed at the suggestion that they will be eradicated using the anthelmintic fenbendazole as a feed additive. The test case to be used here is one in which pinworms have been found in an animal facility and a researcher conducting behavioural studies in young rats is concerned about the effect of treatment upon ongoing studies. The PICO(T) question might therefore be:

> Does oral fenbendazole affect behavioural parameters in rats?

The elements of the PICO(T) question would be:

- Population: laboratory rats, all sexes, ages, and strains
- Intervention: administration of fenbendazole by the oral route, including in the feed
- Outcome: physiological measures including weight, growth rates, and feed intake; behavioural measures in any common behavioural test
- Comparator: rats not treated with fenbendazole
- Time: not relevant

11.1.2 Literature Search

If evidence can be found from up-to-date evidence guidelines or systematic reviews, the search can be considerably shortened, particularly if the patient group in the CAT is the same. For human-based questions, the Cochrane summaries are often the easiest to locate and the highest-quality reviews. Other sources include the TRIP database [171], DARE [172], and the ACP [173] Journal Club. Topic-specific databases in many human medical areas are also excellent sources of high-level evidence, i.e. the Global Resource of Eczema Trials [174].

In preclinical research, because the above-named sources do not yet exist, restricting the search to one or two databases (i.e. Web of Science and MEDLINE) is considered acceptable [175]. Often the services of an information specialist are not utilised, unless the project leader is unable to find sufficient evidence via the usual methods. However, some libraries make the services of an information specialist available at no cost, which surely will improve the quality of the search. As for systematic reviews, the search strategy, date searched, and results are included in the final CAT in such a way that future updates are easily accomplished.

In our pinworm example, search terms were developed in the PubMed MeSH thesaurus. The terms included those related to fenbendazole, *rats* as a MeSH term, and *behavior*. The PubMed searches therefore included the following:

1. Rats [MeSH Terms]: 1,605,522 hits
2. Behavior [MeSH Terms] OR animal behavior [MeSH Terms]: 1,794,426 hits
3. Fenbendazole [MeSH Terms]: 790 hits
4. #1 and #2 and #3: 3 hits

Since only three hits resulted when restricting the search to MeSH terms only, the same keywords were used without MeSH restrictions:

1. Rats [All fields]: 1,684,519 hits
2. Behavior [All fields] OR animal behavior [All fields]: 3,943,776 hits
3. Fenbendazole [All fields]: 1182 hits
4. #1 and #2 and #3: 8 hits

Simply typing the phrase *rats and fenbendazole and behavior* into the search box in PMC yielded 140 hits. The reason for this is found by examining the details in the search box in the sidebar. This 'bashing' approach causes PMC to automatically build the following search:

("rats"[MeSH Terms] OR "rats"[All Fields])

AND

("fenbendazole"[MeSH Terms] OR "fenbendazole"[All Fields])

AND

("behaviour"[All Fields] OR "behavior"[MeSH Terms] OR "behavior"[All Fields])

The combination of the [All Fields] and [MeSH Terms] components greatly broadens the search, but does not necessarily yield relevant results. For example, publications in other species and non-behavioural studies were returned. The term 'behaviour' often referred to pharmacokinetic behaviour of a compound rather than to animal behaviour.

Repeating the above search but exchanging the term 'animal behavior' for 'behavior' produced 11 hits in PMC, most of which were conference abstracts not meeting the inclusion criteria, and a single hit in PubMed.

Web of Science was also searched using the terms *rats*, *fenbendazole*, and *behavior*, yielding six results, of which none were different from the PubMed searches.

Google Scholar was searched using the same three terms, and the first four pages were examined. This produced a new reference [176] and one dissertation [177], along with duplicates from other searches.

Once the search has been conducted, hand-searching is often fruitful, although time-consuming. In the pinworm CAT, using the PubMed 'similar articles' links in the sidebar yielded no further publications. Similarly, the publications which were deemed to be relevant were reviewed, but no further publications of interest were suggested.

Grey literature was searched using OpenGrey, the Czech National Repository of Grey Literature, the Edinburgh Research Archive, AGRICOLA (USDA National Agricultural Library), and WorldWideScience. There were numerous hits on the terms *fenbendazole* and of course *rat* and *behavior* and a few on *pinworm*. The AGRICOLA search found a previously missed publication [178]; hand-searching yielded two additional publications [179, 180] on the possible teratogenic effects of other benzimidazole anthelmintics, but none of these addressed behavioural alterations. A narrative review concluded that fenbendazole was the recommended treatment for pinworms in rodents due to its 'lack of documented interference with research, its large margin of safety, and its ovicidal, larvicidal, and adulticidal effects' [181].

Taken together, the searches yielded a total of eight references which met the inclusion criteria [176, 177, 179, 182–186].

After reviewing the results in full, four publications were deemed appropriate for data extraction [177, 183, 184, 186]. Four were excluded because no behavioural tests were performed [176, 178, 179, 182]; one was excluded because there was only a personal communication that there was 'no change in experimental parameters related to the use of ... the diet' [185].

11.1.3 Evidence Appraisal

Inclusion criteria for a CAT are usually much more restrictive than for a systematic review, in line with the size of the project and scope of the PICO(T) question. This should make the evidence gathering and appraisal process much easier than for a full systematic review.

First the abstracts are checked and those which obviously do not meet the criteria are excluded. For the remainder, full publications should be retrieved. The PICO(T) helps define the data to be extracted, along with technical details of the publication (authors, year, journal information).

In the pinworm example, review of the references yielded the following information:

- Non-pinworm-infected Sprague-Dawley rats were continuously fed fenbendazole-medicated chow (vs controls fed a different non-medicated chow formulation) from before mating (parents) until the resulting progeny was tested. This is far longer than the typical treatment regime. Maternal weights and water consumption were similar between groups (17 fenbendazole-treated vs 11 controls), and there was no evidence of pup malformations or mortality. The fenbendazole-treated pups were slower to be able to right themselves at postnatal day (PND) 5 and ran more slowly on a wheel during the first 5 minutes of the day's procedure (18–24 rats per group). There were no differences in negative geotaxis response, time in a digging maze, or performance in a Morris water maze [183].

- Extending from the Barron study, Keen et al. studied 24 adult male Sprague-Dawley rats in a naturally infected colony (presumably *Syphacia obvelata*). They found no differences between fenbendazole-treated rats and non-medicated rats in a testing paradigm involving stimulus-evoked head entry into a food cup in a variety of timings between stimulus and response. There was no difference in body weights [184].
- Non-pinworm-infected adult male Sprague-Dawley rats (n = 24) ate similar amounts of fenbendazole-medicated and control non-medicated feed but exhibited a preference for non-medicated feed when they had a choice of both [186].
- Sprague-Dawley rats in maternal deprivation experiments were tested in open-field apparatus for measurement of rearing, line crossing, locomotion, and stereotypic behaviours. Fenbendazole-medicated feed given in an alternating cycle for 18 weeks was given, with testing performed after washout. There were no differences between experimental groups on the treatment regime for the longest and shortest time periods, and group body weights were similar [177].

11.1.4 Risk of Bias Assessment

Using the SYRCLE risk of bias tool, Table 8 was constructed. Risk of bias was unclear in all areas except baseline data and attrition bias, both of which were low bias. Reporting of blinding and randomisation was largely absent, and when it was mentioned, it was only as a single word in

Table 8 Risk of bias of four references

Signal question	Barron (2000)	Vento (2008)	Keen (2005)	Morgan (2003)
Was allocation sequence adequately generated and applied?	Unclear; not stated	Unclear; not stated	Unclear; not stated	Unclear; not stated
Were groups similar at baseline?	Unclear; not stated	Yes	Yes	Yes
Was allocation to groups adequately concealed?	Unclear; not stated	Unclear; not stated	Unclear; not stated	Unclear; not stated
Were cages located at random sites in the room?	Unclear; not stated	Unclear; not stated	Unclear; not stated	Yes, weekly rotation
Were caregivers/investigators blinded to treatment groups?	Unclear; 2 different diets were used	Unclear; not stated	Unclear; not stated	Unclear; not stated
Were rats selected randomly for outcome assessment?	Unclear; not stated	Unclear; not stated	Unclear; not stated	Yes
Was the outcome assessor blinded?	Unclear; not stated	Unclear; not stated	Unclear; not stated	Partially
Were all animals included in the analysis?	Unclear; not stated	Unclear; not stated	Unclear; not stated	Yes
Was it clear that the paper included all expected outcomes?	Yes, but animal numbers not reported, only statistical variance	Yes	Yes	Yes

Yes = low risk of bias; no = high risk of bias; unclear = unclear risk of bias the text. All three papers were published prior to the ARRIVE guidelines. The quality of the evidence is relatively poor by modern standards, due more to lack of reporting than to obvious errors in conducting the research.

11.1.5 Interpretation

There is very limited and poor-quality evidence for the effect of fenbendazole on rats. Rats consume fenbendazole-medicated feed as normal, although if given a choice would prefer non-medicated feed. There is no evidence of foetal or neonatal abnormality when fenbendazole is administered to pregnant dams. Behavioural effects are limited to slow righting reflexes during the first week of life and a slower initial pace on a running wheel. Stimulus-response activities, negative geotaxis, digging, and performance in the Morris water maze are not affected. In another study, open-field behaviours were not affected. Taken together, the limited available evidence suggests that fenbendazole-medicated feed has minimal if any behavioural effects upon laboratory rats and no effect on weight gain in rat pups.

12 Conclusion

The competent preparation of systematic reviews and critically appraised topics are essential to provision of high-quality, objective, and critical overviews of the available scientific evidence. Ultimately, this will benefit animals, humans, and science.

References

1. Shea BJ, Grimshaw JM, Wells GA, et al. Development of AMSTAR: a measurement tool to assess the methodological quality of systematic reviews. BMC Med Res Methodol. 2007;7:10. https://doi.org/10.1186/1471-2288-7-10.
2. Shea BJ, Reeves BC, Wells G, et al. AMSTAR 2: a critical appraisal tool for systematic reviews that include randomised or non-randomised studies of healthcare interventions, or both. BMJ. 2017;358:j4008. https://doi.org/10.1136/bmj.j4008.
3. Kilkenny C, Browne WJ, Cuthill IC, Emerson M, Altman DG. Improving bioscience research reporting: the ARRIVE guidelines for reporting animal research. PLoS Biol. 2010;8:e1000412. https://doi.org/10.1371/journal.pbio.1000412.
4. Sterne JAC, Savović J, Page MJ, et al. RoB 2: a revised tool for assessing risk of bias in randomised trials. BMJ. 2019;366:l4898. https://doi.org/10.1136/bmj.l4898.
5. National Centre for the Replacement Refinement Reduction of Animals in Research. The CAMARADES/NC3Rs Systematic Review Facility (SyRF). https://www.nc3rs.org.uk/camaradesnc3rs-systematic-review-facility-syrf, 4 June 2020.
6. Group CONSORT. CONSORT: Transparent reporting of trials. http://www.consort-statement.org/, 4 June 2020.
7. Medicine UOOCFSI. EQUATOR Network: Enhancing the Quality and Transparency of Health Research. Oxford: https://www.equator-network.org/, 7 June 2020.
8. Guyatt GH, Oxman AD, Vist GE, et al. GRADE: an emerging consensus on rating quality of evidence and strength of recommendations. BMJ. 2008;336:924–6. https://doi.org/10.1136/bmj.39489.470347.AD.
9. Wei D, Tang K, Wang Q, et al. The use of GRADE approach in systematic reviews of animal studies. Journal of Evidence-Based Medicine. 2016;9:98–104. https://doi.org/10.1111/jebm.12198.
10. Hooijmans CR, De Vries RBM, Ritskes-Hoitinga M, et al. Facilitating healthcare decisions by assessing the certainty in the evidence from preclinical animal studies. PLOS ONE. 2018;13:e0187271. https://doi.org/10.1371/journal.pone.0187271.
11. Osborne N, Avey MT, Anestidou L, Ritskes-Hoitinga M, Griffin G. Improving animal research reporting standards: HARRP, the first step of a unified approach by ICLAS to improve animal research reporting standards worldwide. EMBO Rep. 2018;19 https://doi.org/10.15252/embr.201846069.
12. Moher D, Liberati A, Tetzlaff J, Altman DG, PRISMA G. Preferred reporting items for systematic reviews and meta-analyses: the PRISMA statement. J Clin Epidemiol. 2009;62:1006–12. https://doi.org/10.1016/j.jclinepi.2009.06.005.
13. Research NIFH. PROSPERO: International prospective register of systematic reviews. https://www.crd.york.ac.uk/prospero/, 5 June 2020.
14. RadboudUMC. Systematic Review Center for Laboratory Animal Experimentation (SYRCLE). https://www.radboudumc.nl/en/research/departments/health-evidence/systematic-review-center-for-laboratory-animal-experimentation, 7 June 2020.
15. Cochrane AL. Effectiveness and efficiency: random reflections on health services. Nuffield Trust. 1972;1

16. Daniels M, Hill AB. Chemotherapy of pulmonary tuberculosis in young adults; an analysis of the combined results of three Medical Research Council trials. Br Med J. 1952;1:1162–8. https://doi.org/10.1136/bmj.1.4769.1162.
17. Cochrane AL. Effectiveness and efficiency: random reflections on health services, vol. 1: The Nuffield Provincial Hospitals Trust; 1972.
18. Thomas H. Medical research in the Rhondda valleys. Postgrad Med J. 1999;75:257–9. https://doi.org/10.1136/pgmj.75.883.257.
19. Chalmers I, Hedges LV, Cooper H. A brief history of research synthesis. Eval Health Prof. 2002;25:12–37. https://doi.org/10.1177/0163278702025001003.
20. Pearce SC. Breakthroughs in statistics. In: Kotz S, Johnson NL, editors. . New York: Springer; 1992.
21. Mulrow CD. The medical review article: state of the science. Ann Intern Med. 1987;106:485–8.
22. Chalmers I, Eakin M, Keirse MJNC. Effective care in pregnancy and childbirth. Oxford: Oxford University Press; n.d.
23. Van der Mierden S, Tsaioun K, Bleich A, Leenaars CHC. Software tools for literature screening in systematic reviews in biomedical research. ALTEX 2019;36:508–17.
24. Egger M, Smith GD, Altman DG. Systematic reviews in health care: meta-analysis in context. 1st ed. London: BMJ Books; 2001. p. 487.
25. Kirkwood BR, Sterne JAC. Chapter 32: Systematic reviews and meta-analysis. Essential Medical Statistics. Malden, Mass.: Blackwell Science; 2003. p. 371–387.
26. Greenberg SA. How citation distortions create unfounded authority: analysis of a citation network. BMJ. 2009;339:b2680. https://doi.org/10.1136/bmj.b2680.
27. Greenberg SA. Understanding belief using citation networks. J Eval Clin Pract. 2011;17:389–93. https://doi.org/10.1111/j.1365-2753.2011.01646.x.
28. Sena ES, Briscoe CL, Howells DW, Donnan GA, Sandercock PAG, Macleod MR. Factors affecting the apparent efficacy and safety of tissue plasminogen activator in thrombotic occlusion models of stroke: systematic review and meta-analysis. J Cereb Blood Flow Metab. 2010;30:1905–13. https://doi.org/10.1038/jcbfm.2010.116.
29. Chalmers I, Bracken MB, Djulbegovic B, et al. How to increase value and reduce waste when research priorities are set. Lancet. 2014;383:156–65. https://doi.org/10.1016/S0140-6736(13)62229-1.
30. Scotney RL, McLaughlin D, Keates HL. A systematic review of the effects of euthanasia and occupational stress in personnel working with animals in animal shelters, veterinary clinics, and biomedical research facilities. J Am Vet Med Assoc. 2015;247:1121–30. https://doi.org/10.2460/javma.247.10.1121.
31. Garside R. Systematic review and synthesis of qualitative research. In: Ziebland S, Coulter A, Calabrese JD, Locock L, editors. Understanding and using health experiences. Oxford: Oxford University Press; 2013. p. 104–15.
32. Wegener K. Systematic review of thorotrast data and facts: animal experiments. Virchows Arch A Pathol Anat Histol. 1979;381:245–68.
33. Macleod MR, Fisher M, O'Collins V, et al. Good laboratory practice: preventing introduction of bias at the bench. Stroke. 2009;40:e50-2. https://doi.org/10.1161/STROKEAHA.108.525386.
34. Pound P, Bracken MB. Is animal research sufficiently evidence based to be a cornerstone of biomedical research. BMJ. 2014;348:g3387. https://doi.org/10.1136/bmj.g3387.
35. Hooijmans CR, Ritskes-Hoitinga M. Progress in using systematic reviews of animal studies to improve translational research. PLoS Med. 2013;10:e1001482. https://doi.org/10.1371/journal.pmed.1001482.
36. Horn J, de Haan RJ, Vermeulen M, Luiten PGM, Limburg M. Nimodipine in animal model experiments of focal cerebral ischemia: a Systematic review. Stroke 2001;32:2433–2438. https://doi.org/10.1161/hs1001.096009.
37. Lucas C, Criens-Poublon LJ, Cockrell CT, de Haan RJ. Wound healing in cell studies and animal model experiments by low level laser therapy; were clinical studies justified? A systematic review. Lasers in medical science. 2002;17:110–34.
38. Amarasingh S, Macleod MR, Whittle IR. What is the translational efficacy of chemotherapeutic drug research in neuro-oncology? A systematic review and meta-analysis of the efficacy of BCNU and CCNU in animal models of glioma. J Neuro-Oncol. 2009;91:117.
39. Galley HF. Systematic skepticism. Crit Care Med. 2003;31:1284–5.
40. Festing MF, Altman DG. Guidelines for the design and statistical analysis of experiments using laboratory animals. ILAR J. 2002;43:244–58. https://doi.org/10.1093/ilar.43.4.244.
41. Altman DG. Improving design and analysis of research: lessons from clinical research. Altern Lab Anim. 2004;32:31–9.
42. Hooijmans CR, Leenaars M, Ritskes-Hoitinga M. A gold standard publication checklist to improve the quality of animal studies, to fully integrate the Three Rs, and to make systematic reviews more feasible. Altern Lab Anim. 2010;38:167–82.
43. Rothwell PM. Clinical trials are too often founded on poor quality pre-clinical research. J Neurol. 2005;252:1115.
44. Hoffmann S, de Vries RBM, Stephens ML, et al. A primer on systematic reviews in toxicology. Arch Toxicol. 2017;91:2551–75. https://doi.org/10.1007/s00204-017-1980-3.

45. Vandenberg LN, Ågerstrand M, Beronius A, et al. A proposed framework for the systematic review and integrated assessment (SYRINA) of endocrine disrupting chemicals. Environ Health. 2016;15:74. https://doi.org/10.1186/s12940-016-0156-6.
46. Lam J, Koustas E, Sutton P, et al. The Navigation Guide – evidence-based medicine meets environmental health: integration of animal and human evidence for PFOA effects on fetal growth. Environ Health Perspect. 2014;122:1040–51. https://doi.org/10.1289/ehp.1307923.
47. Mignini LE, Khan KS. BMC medical research methodology methodological quality of systematic reviews of animal studies: a survey of reviews of basic research. BMC Medical Research Methodology. 2006;6:10. https://doi.org/10.1186/1471-2288-6-10.
48. Ioannidis JPA. Integration of evidence from multiple meta-analyses: a primer on umbrella reviews, treatment networks and multiple treatments meta-analyses. CMAJ. 2009;181:488–93.
49. Fusar-Poli P, Radua J. Ten simple rules for conducting umbrella reviews. Evid Based Ment Health. 2018;21:95–100.
50. Lamontagne F, Briel M, Duffett M, et al. Systematic review of reviews including animal studies addressing therapeutic interventions for sepsis. Crit Care Med. 2010;38:2401–8.
51. Wever KE, Geessink FJ, Brouwer MAE, Tillema A, Ritskes-Hoitinga M. A systematic review of discomfort due to toe or ear clipping in laboratory rodents. Lab Anim. 2017;51:583–600.
52. Jerndal M, Forsberg K, Sena ES, et al. A systematic review and meta-analysis of erythropoietin in experimental stroke. J Cereb Blood Flow Metab. 2010;30:961–8.
53. Hooijmans CR, Pasker-De Jong PCM, de Vries RBM, Ritskes-Hoitinga M. The effects of long-term omega-3 fatty acid supplementation on cognition and Alzheimer's pathology in animal models of Alzheimer's disease: a systematic review and meta-analysis. J Alzheimers Dis. 2012;28:191–209.
54. Gibson CL, Murphy SP. Benefits of histone deacetylase inhibitors for acute brain injury: a systematic review of animal studies. J Neurochem. 2010;115:806–13.
55. Ker K, Perel P, Blackhall K. Beta-2 receptor antagonists for traumatic brain injury: a systematic review of controlled trials in animal models. CNS Neurosci Ther. 2009;15:52–64.
56. Gritsch K, Laroche N, Morgon L, et al. A systematic review of methods for tissue analysis in animal studies on orthodontic mini-implants. Orthod Craniofac Res. 2012;15:135–47.
57. Ainge H, Thompson C, Ozanne SE, Rooney KB. A systematic review on animal models of maternal high fat feeding and offspring glycaemic control. Int J Obes. 2011;35:325–35.
58. Muhlhausler BS, Gibson RA, Makrides M. The effect of maternal omega-3 long-chain polyunsaturated fatty acid (n-3 LCPUFA) supplementation during pregnancy and/or lactation on body fat mass in the offspring: a systematic review of animal studies. Prostaglandins Leukotrienes & Essential Fatty Acids. 2011;85:83–8.
59. Dirx MJ, Zeegers MP, Dagnelie PC, van den Bogaard T, van den Brandt PA. Energy restriction and the risk of spontaneous mammary tumors in mice: a meta-analysis. Int J Cancer. 2003;106:766–70.
60. Jamaty C, Bailey B, Larocque A, Notebaert E, Sanogo K, Chauny JM. Lipid emulsions in the treatment of acute poisoning: a systematic review of human and animal studies. Clinic Toxicol. 2010;48:1–27.
61. Mapstone J, Roberts I, Evans P. Fluid resuscitation strategies: a systematic review of animal trials. Journal of Trauma-Injury Infection & Critical Care. 2003;55:571–89.
62. Matthan NR, Jordan H, Chung M, Lichtenstein AH, Lathrop DA, Lau J. A systematic review and meta-analysis of the impact of omega-3 fatty acids on selected arrhythmia outcomes in animal models. Metab Clin Exp. 2005;54:1557–65.
63. Percie du Sert N, Rudd JA, Apfel CC, Andrews PL. Cisplatin-induced emesis: systematic review and meta-analysis of the ferret model and the effects of 5-HT3 receptor antagonists. Cancer Chemotherapy & Pharmacology. 2011;67:667–86.
64. Petticrew M, Davey Smith G. The monkey puzzle: a systematic review of studies of stress, social hierarchies, and heart disease in monkeys. PLoS ONE [Electronic Resource]. 2012;7:e27939.
65. Hainsworth AH, Markus HS. Do in vivo experimental models reflect human cerebral small vessel disease? A systematic review. J Cereb Blood Flow Metab. 2008;28:1877–91.
66. Bailey EL, McCulloch J, Sudlow C, Wardlaw JM. Potential animal models of lacunar stroke: a systematic review. Stroke. 2009;40:e451–8.
67. Radde R, Duma C, Goedert M, Jucker M. The value of incomplete mouse models of Alzheimer's disease. Eur J Nucl Med Mol Imaging. 2008;35:S70–4.
68. Egan K, Sena E, Vesterinen H, MacLeod M. Transgenic mouse models of Alzheimer's disease – a systematic review and meta-analysis. Neurodegener Dis. 2011;8
69. Angius D, Wang H, Spinner RJ, Gutierrez-Cotto Y, Yaszemski MJ, Windebank AJ. A systematic review of animal models used to study nerve regeneration in tissue-engineered scaffolds. Biomaterials. 2012;33:8034–9.
70. Ahern BJ, Parvizi J, Boston R, Schaer TP. Preclinical animal models in single site cartilage defect testing: a systematic review. Osteoarthr Cartil. 2009;17:705–13.
71. Faggion CM Jr, Chambrone L, Gondim V, Schmitter M, Tu YK. Comparison of the effects of treatment of peri-implant infection in animal and human studies: systematic review and meta-analysis. Clin Oral Implants Res. 2010;21:137–47.

72. Corpet DE, Pierre F. Point: from animal models to prevention of colon cancer. Systematic review of chemoprevention in min mice and choice of the model system. Cancer Epidemiology Biomarkers and Prevention. 2003;12:391–400.
73. de Vries RB, Buma P, Leenaars M, Ritskes-Hoitinga M, Gordijn B. Reducing the number of laboratory animals used in tissue engineering research by restricting the variety of animal models. Articular cartilage tissue engineering as a case study. Tissue Eng Part B Rev. 2012;18:427–35. https://doi.org/10.1089/ten.TEB.2012.0059.
74. Wever KE, Menting TP, Rovers M, et al. Ischemic preconditioning in the animal kidney, a systematic review and meta-analysis. PLoS ONE [Electronic Resource]. 2012;7:e32296.
75. Hooijmans CR, Geessink FJ, Ritskes-Hoitinga M, Scheffer GJ. A systematic review of the modifying effect of anaesthetic drugs on metastasis in animal models for cancer. PLoS One. 2016;11:e0156152. https://doi.org/10.1371/journal.pone.0156152.
76. Leenaars CHC, van der Mierden S, Durst M, et al. Measurement of corticosterone in mice: a protocol for a mapping review. Lab Anim. 2020;54:26–32. https://doi.org/10.1177/0023677219868499.
77. Valentin S, Zsoldos RR. Surface electromyography in animal biomechanics: a systematic review. J Electromyogr Kinesiol. 2016;28:167–83. https://doi.org/10.1016/j.jelekin.2015.12.005.
78. Klopfleisch R, Sperling C, Kershaw O, Gruber AD. Does the taking of biopsies affect the metastatic potential of tumours? A systematic review of reports on veterinary and human cases and animal models. Vet J. 2011;190:e31–42.
79. LaFollette MR, O'Haire ME, Cloutier S, Blankenberger WB, Gaskill BN. Rat tickling: a systematic review of applications, outcomes, and moderators. PLoS One. 2017;12:e0175320. https://doi.org/10.1371/journal.pone.0175320.
80. Lidster K, Jefferys JG, Blümcke I, et al. Opportunities for improving animal welfare in rodent models of epilepsy and seizures. J Neurosci Methods. 2016;260:2–25. https://doi.org/10.1016/j.jneumeth.2015.09.007.
81. Dzikamunhenga RS, Anthony R, Coetzee J, et al. Pain management in the neonatal piglet during routine management procedures. Part 1: a systematic review of randomized and non-randomized intervention studies. Anim Health Res Rev. 2014;15:14–38. https://doi.org/10.1017/S1466252314000061.
82. Laurin E, Thakur K, Mohr PG, et al. To pool or not to pool? Guidelines for pooling samples for use in surveillance testing of infectious diseases in aquatic animals. J Fish Dis. 2019;42:1471–91. https://doi.org/10.1111/jfd.13083.
83. Baker D, Lidster K, Sottomayor A, Amor S. Two years later: journals are not yet enforcing the ARRIVE guidelines on reporting standards for pre-clinical animal studies. PLoS Biol. 2014;12:e1001756.
84. Landis SC, Amara SG, Asadullah K, et al. A call for transparent reporting to optimize the predictive value of preclinical research. Nature. 2012;490:187–91. https://doi.org/10.1038/nature11556.
85. National Institutes of Health. Principles and Guidelines for Reporting Preclinical Research. 2014. https://www.nih.gov/research-training/rigor-reproducibility/principles-guidelines-reporting-preclinical-research, 5 June 2020.
86. Vollert J, Schenker E, Macleod M, et al. Protocol for a systematic review of guidelines for rigour in the design, conduct and analysis of biomedical experiments involving laboratory animals. BMJ Open Science. 2018;2:e000004. https://doi.org/10.1136/bmjos-2018-000004.
87. Pound P, Ritskes-Hoitinga M. Is it possible to overcome issues of external validity in preclinical animal research? Why most animal models are bound to fail. J Transl Med. 2018;16:304. https://doi.org/10.1186/s12967-018-1678-1.
88. Varga OE, Zsíros N, Olsson IA. Estimating the predictive validity of diabetic animal models in rosiglitazone studies. Obes Rev. 2015;16:498–507. https://doi.org/10.1111/obr.12278.
89. Hünig T. The storm has cleared: lessons from the CD28 superagonist TGN1412 trial. Nat Rev Immunol. 2012;12:317–8. https://doi.org/10.1038/nri3192.
90. Ioannidis JP. The mass production of redundant, misleading, and conflicted systematic reviews and meta-analyses. Milbank Q. 2016;94:485–514. https://doi.org/10.1111/1468-0009.12210.
91. Lorenz RC, Matthias K, Pieper D, et al. A psychometric study found AMSTAR 2 to be a valid and moderately reliable appraisal tool. J Clin Epidemiol. 2019;114:133–40. https://doi.org/10.1016/j.jclinepi.2019.05.028.
92. Greenhalgh T. How to read a paper: the basics of evidence-based practice, vol. 229: Wiley-Blackwell; 2001.
93. Higgins JPT, Green S. Preparing a Cochrane review. In: Higgins JPT, Green S, editors. Cochrane handbook for systematic reviews of interventions version 5.1.0 [updated March 2011]. Chichester, West Sussex: Wiley; 2011.
94. Centre for Reviews and Dissemination. Systematic reviews: CRD's guidance for undertaking reviews in health care. York: University of York; 2009.
95. Straus SE, Glasziou P, Richardson WS, Haynes RB. Evidence-based medicine: how to practice and teach it. Edinburgh: Churchill Livingston Elsevier; 2011.
96. Sargeant JM, O'Connor AM. Introduction to systematic reviews in animal agriculture and veterinary medicine. Zoonoses Public Health. 2014;61(Suppl 1):3–9. https://doi.org/10.1111/zph.12128.
97. Borah R, Brown AW, Capers PL, Kaiser KA. Analysis of the time and workers needed to conduct systematic reviews of medical interventions using data from the PROSPERO registry. BMJ Open.

2017;7:e012545. https://doi.org/10.1136/bmjopen-2016-012545.
98. Jones AP, Conroy E, Williamson PR, Clarke M, Gamble C. The use of systematic reviews in the planning, design and conduct of randomised trials: a retrospective cohort of NIHR HTA funded trials. BMC Med Res Methodol. 2013;13:50. https://doi.org/10.1186/1471-2288-13-50.
99. CAMARADES. SyRF Protocol Database. http://syrf.org.uk/protocols/, 5 June 2020.
100. Hooijmans CR, IntHout J, Ritskes-Hoitinga M, Rovers MM. Meta-analyses of animal studies: an introduction of a valuable instrument to further improve healthcare. ILAR J. 2014;55:418–26. https://doi.org/10.1093/ilar/ilu042.
101. O'Connor AM, Totton SC, Cullen JN, et al. The study design elements employed by researchers in preclinical animal experiments from two research domains and implications for automation of systematic reviews. PLoS One. 2018;13:e0199441. https://doi.org/10.1371/journal.pone.0199441.
102. Thomas J, Kneale D, McKenzie JE, Brennan SE, Bhaumik S. Chapter 2: determining the scope of the review and the questions it will address. In: Higgins JPT, Thomas J, Chandler J et al., editors. Cochrane Handbook for Systematic Reviews of Interventions. 2019.
103. Couzin-Frankel J. When mice mislead. Science. 2013;342 https://doi.org/10.1126/science.342.6161.922.
104. Willmot M, Gray L, Gibson C, Murphy S, Bath PM. A systematic review of nitric oxide donors and L-arginine in experimental stroke; effects on infarct size and cerebral blood flow. Nitric Oxide. 2005;12:141–9.
105. Macleod MR, O'Collins T, Horky LL, Howells DW, Donnan GA. Systematic review and meta-analysis of the efficacy of melatonin in experimental stroke. J Pineal Res. 2005;38:35–41.
106. Li Y, Sun JF, Cui X, et al. The effect of heparin administration in animal models of sepsis: a prospective study in Escherichia coli-challenged mice and a systematic review and metaregression analysis of published studies. Crit Care Med. 2011;39:1104–12.
107. Gibson CL, Gray LJ, Murphy SP, Bath PM. Estrogens and experimental ischemic stroke: a systematic review. J Cereb Blood Flow Metab. 2006;26:1103–13.
108. van der Mierden S, Savelyev SA, IntHout J, de Vries RBM, Leenaars CHC. Intracerebral microdialysis of adenosine and adenosine monophosphate – a systematic review and meta-regression analysis of baseline concentrations. J Neurochem. 2018;147:58–70. https://doi.org/10.1111/jnc.14552.
109. de Vries RBM, Hooijmans CR, Langendam MW, et al. A protocol format for the preparation, registration and publication of systematic reviews of animal intervention studies. Evidence-based Preclinical Medicine. 2015;2:e00007. https://doi.org/10.1002/ebm2.7.
110. Hooijmans CR, Tillema A, Leenaars M, Ritskes-Hoitinga M. Enhancing search efficiency by means of a search filter for finding all studies on animal experimentation in PubMed. Lab Anim. 2010;44:170–5. https://doi.org/10.1258/la.2010.009117.
111. de Vries RB, Hooijmans CR, Tillema A, Leenaars M, Ritskes-Hoitinga M. A search filter for increasing the retrieval of animal studies in Embase. Lab Anim. 2011;45:268–70. https://doi.org/10.1258/la.2011.011056.
112. Leenaars M, Hooijmans CR, van Veggel N, et al. A step-by-step guide to systematically identify all relevant animal studies. Laboratory animals. 2012;46:24–31. https://doi.org/10.1258/la.2011.011087.
113. de Vries RB, Hooijmans CR, Tillema A, Leenaars M, Ritskes-Hoitinga M. Updated version of the Embase search filter for animal studies.[letter]. Lab Anim. 2014;48(1):88.
114. Lam MT, De Longhi C, Turnbull J, Lam HR, Besa R. Has Embase replaced MEDLINE since coverage expansion. J Med Libr Assoc 2018;106:227–234. https://doi.org/10.5195/jmla.2018.281.
115. BIREME/PAHO/WHO. Latin American and Cariggean Health Sciences Literature (LILACS). https://lilacs.bvsalud.org
116. McLean F. Several databases give free access now. BMJ. 2002;324:790. https://doi.org/10.1136/bmj.324.7340.790/a.
117. Haddaway NR, Collins AM, Coughlin D, Kirk S. The role of Google Scholar in evidence reviews and its applicability to grey literature searching. PLoS One. 2015;10:e0138237. https://doi.org/10.1371/journal.pone.0138237.
118. Gross T, Taylor AG, Joudrey DN. Still a lot to lose: the role of controlled vocabulary in keyword searching. Cataloging & classification quarterly. 2015;53:1–39.
119. Marshall IJ, Wallace BC. Toward systematic review automation: a practical guide to using machine learning tools in research synthesis. [editorial]. Syst Rev. 2019;8(1):163.
120. Bond University Institute for Evidence-Based Healthcare Systematic Review Accelerator. http://sr-accelerator.com/#/
121. Clark JM, Sanders S, Carter M, et al. Improving the translation of search strategies using the Polyglot Search Translator: a randomized controlled trial. J Med Libr Assoc. 2020;108:195–207. https://doi.org/10.5195/jmla.2020.834.
122. Sciome Software. SWIFT Review. 2019. https://www.sciome.com/swift-review/. Last accessed 25 June 2021.
123. OpenGrey. http://www.opengrey.eu/
124. University of Edinburgh. https://www.ed.ac.uk/information-services/library-museum-gallery/finding-resources/library-databases/databases-subject-a-z/grey-literature
125. AGRICOLA. https://agricola.nal.usda.gov/

126. Cochrane Register of Studies. Cochrane Central Register of Controlled Trials (CENTRAL) Handsearched Jouranls List. http://crso.cochrane.org/HandsearchedJournals.php
127. US Cochrane Center. Training manual for handsearchers. In: Dickersin K, Larson K. 2002. p. 81. https://methods.cochrane.org/irmg/sites/methods.cochrane.org.irmg/files/public/uploads/handsearcher_training_manual.pdf, 5 June 2020.
128. Hopewell S, Clarke M, Lefebvre C, Scherer R. Handsearching versus electronic searching to identify reports of randomized trials. Cochrane Database Syst Rev. 2007 MR000001. https://doi.org/10.1002/14651858.MR000001.pub2
129. Craane B, Dijkstra PU, Stappaerts K, De Laat A. Methodological quality of a systematic review on physical therapy for temporomandibular disorders: influence of hand search and quality scales. Clin Oral Investig. 2012;16:295–303. https://doi.org/10.1007/s00784-010-0490-y.
130. NIH National Library of Medicine. Structured Abstracts. 2018. https://www.nlm.nih.gov/bsd/policy/structured_abstracts.html, 5 June 2020.
131. Marshall C. Systematic review toolbox. 2015. http://systematicreviewtools.com/, 5 June 2020.
132. Bannach-Brown A, Przybyła P, Thomas J, et al. Machine learning algorithms for systematic review: reducing workload in a preclinical review of animal studies and reducing human screening error. Systematic Rev. 2019;8:23. https://doi.org/10.1186/s13643-019-0942-7.
133. Evidence Partners. DistillerSR. 2020. https://www.evidencepartners.com/. Last accessed 25 June 2021.
134. University of York. Systematic reviews: CRD's guidance for undertaking reviews in health care. York: Centre for Reviews and Dissemination; 2009.
135. Armijo-Olivo S, Stiles CR, Hagen NA, Biondo PD, Cummings GG. Assessment of study quality for systematic reviews: a comparison of the Cochrane Collaboration Risk of Bias Tool and the Effective Public Health Practice Project Quality Assessment Tool: methodological research. J Eval Clin Pract. 2012;18:12–8. https://doi.org/10.1111/j.1365-2753.2010.01516.x.
136. Hooijmans CR, Rovers MM, de Vries RBM, Leenaars M, Ritskes-Hoitinga M, Langendam MW. SYRCLE's risk of bias tool for animal studies. BMC Med Res Methodol. 2014;14:43. https://doi.org/10.1186/1471-2288-14-43.
137. Bespalov A, Wicke K, Castangé V. Blinding and randomization. In: Bespalov A, Michel M, Steckler T, editors. Handbook of experimental pharmacology, volume 257: good research practice in non-clinical pharmacology and biomedicine. Cham: Springer; 2019.
138. Ting KH, Hill CL, Whittle SL. Quality of reporting of interventional animal studies in rheumatology: a systematic review using the ARRIVE guidelines. Int J Rheum Dis. 2015;18:488–94. https://doi.org/10.1111/1756-185X.12699.
139. Holman C, Piper SK, Grittner U, et al. Where have all the rodents gone? The effects of attrition in experimental research on cancer and stroke. PLoS Biol. 2016;14:e1002331. https://doi.org/10.1371/journal.pbio.1002331.
140. Skvortsova A, Veldhuijzen DS, Kloosterman IEM, et al. Conditioned hormonal responses: A systematic review in animals and humans. Frontiers in Neuroendocrinology. 2019;52:206–18. https://doi.org/10.1016/j.yfrne.2018.12.005.
141. Macleod MR, van der Worp HB, Sena ES, Howells DW, Dirnagl U, Donnan GA. Evidence for the efficacy of NXY-059 in experimental focal cerebral ischaemia is confounded by study quality. Stroke. 2008;39:2824–9. https://doi.org/10.1161/STROKEAHA.108.515957.
142. Henderson VC, Kimmelman J, Fergusson D, Grimshaw JM, Hackam DG. Threats to validity in the design and conduct of preclinical efficacy studies: a systematic review of guidelines for in vivo animal experiments. PLoS Medicine. 2013;10 https://doi.org/10.1371/journal.pmed.1001489.
143. Hirst JA, Howick J, Aronson JK, et al. The need for randomization in animal trials: an overview of systematic reviews. PloS one. 2014;9:e98856. https://doi.org/10.1371/journal.pone.0098856.
144. Provencher S, Archer SL, Ramirez FD, et al. Standards and Methodological Rigor in Pulmonary Arterial Hypertension Preclinical and Translational Research. Circ Res. 2018;122:1021–32. https://doi.org/10.1161/CIRCRESAHA.117.312579.
145. Lai NM, Chang SMW, Ng SS, Tan SL, Chaiyakunapruk N, Stanaway F. Animal-assisted therapy for dementia. Cochrane Database Syst Rev. 2019;2019 https://doi.org/10.1002/14651858.CD013243.pub2.
146. Currie GL, Angel-Scott HN, Colvin L, et al. Animal models of chemotherapy-induced peripheral neuropathy: A machine-assisted systematic review and meta-analysis. PLOS Biology. 2019;17:e3000243. https://doi.org/10.1371/journal.pbio.3000243.
147. Abdel-Sattar M, Krauth D, Anglemyer A, Bero L. The relationship between risk of bias criteria, research outcomes, and study sponsorship in a cohort of preclinical thiazolidinedione animal studies: a meta-analysis. Evid Based Preclin Med. 2014;1:11–20. https://doi.org/10.1002/ebm2.5.
148. Bero L, Anglemyer A, Vesterinen H, Krauth D. The relationship between study sponsorship, risks of bias, and research outcomes in atrazine exposure studies conducted in non-human animals: Systematic review and meta-analysis. Environ Int. 2016;92-93:597–604. https://doi.org/10.1016/j.envint.2015.10.011.
149. Wareham KJ, Hyde RM, Grindlay D, Brennan ML, Dean RS. Sponsorship bias and quality of randomised controlled trials in veterinary medicine. BMC Vet Res. 2017;13:234. https://doi.org/10.1186/s12917-017-1146-9.

150. McKenzie JE, Brennan SE, Ryan RE, Thomson HJ, Johnston RV. Chapter 9: summarizing study characteristics and preparing for synthesis. In: Higgins JPT, Thomas J, Chandler J et al., editors. Cochrane Handbook for Systematic Reviews of Interventions. 2019.
151. Deeks JJ, JPT H, Altman Douglas G. Chapter 10: Analysing data and undertaking meta-analysis. In: Higgins JPT, Thomas J, Chandler J, Cumpston M, Li T, Page MJ, Welch VA, editors. Cochrane handbook for Systematic reviews of interventions, version 6.0. 2019.
152. Borenstein M, Hedges LV, Higgins JPT, Rothstein HR. Chapter 13: fixed-effect versus random-effects models. Introduction to meta-analysis. Chichester: John Wiley & Sons; 2009.
153. DerSimonian R, Laird N. Meta-analysis in clinical trials. Control Clin Trials. 1986;7:177–88. https://doi.org/10.1016/0197-2456(86)90046-2.
154. Kirkwood BR, Sterne JAC. Chapter 36: measurement error: assessment and implications. Essential medical statistics. Oxford: Blackwell Science; 2003. p. 429–46.
155. Sedgwick P. How to read a forest plot in a meta-analysis. BMJ. 2015;351:h4028. https://doi.org/10.1136/bmj.h4028.
156. Roberts D, Brown J, Medley N, Dalziel SR. Antenatal corticosteroids for accelerating fetal lung maturation for women at risk of preterm birth. Cochrane Database of Systematic Reviews. 2017https://doi.org/10.1002/14651858.CD004454.pub3
157. ter Riet G, Korevaar DA, Leenaars M, et al. Publication bias in laboratory animal research: a survey on magnitude, drivers, consequences and potential solutions. PLoS One. 2012;7:e43404. https://doi.org/10.1371/journal.pone.0043404.
158. Wieschowski S, Biernot S, Deutsch S, et al. Publication rates in animal research. Extent and characteristics of published and non-published animal studies followed up at two German university medical centres. PLoS One. 2019;14:e0223758.
159. Glasziou P, Chalmers I. Can it really be true that 50% of research is unpublished? 2017. http://blogs.bmj.com/bmj/2017/06/05/paul-glasziou-and-iain-chalmers-can-it-really-be-true-that-50-of-research-is-unpublished/
160. Suchmacher M, Geller M. Chapter 13. Systematic reviews and meta-analyses. In: Suchmacher M, Geller M, editors. Practical biostatistics: a user-friendly approach for evidence-based medicine. Amsterdam: Elsevier; 2012. p. 159–66.
161. Renaissance School of Medicine at Stony Brook University. CAT Bank. https://renaissance.stonybrookmedicine.edu/pedrescurriculum/cat-bank. Accessed 17 Feb 2021.
162. Mackway-Jones K. BestBETs: Best Evidence Topics. Manchester UK: Manchester Royal Infirmary; 2020. https://bestbets.org/, 5 June 2020
163. University of Nottingham Centre for Evidence-Based Veterinary Medicine. BestBETs for Vets. 2021. https://bestbetsforvets.org. Accessed 17 Feb 2021.
164. Veterinary Evidence. Veterinary evidence. London: RCVS Knowledge; 2020. https://veterinaryevidence.org/index.php/ve/index, 5 June 2020.
165. Berdoy M, Repp CR. A proposed higher education institution-based Three Rs advisory service. Altern Lab Anim. 2004;32(Suppl 2):9–11. https://doi.org/10.1177/026119290403202s04.
166. Boehm KE, Miller KC. Does gender affect rectal temperature cooling rates? A critically appraised topic. J Sport Rehabil. 2019;28:522–5. https://doi.org/10.1123/jsr.2018-0081.
167. Silverson O, Cascia N, Hettrich CM, Hoch M, Uhl T. Reliability of clinical assessment methods to measure scapular upward rotation: a critically appraised topic. J Sport Rehabil. 2019;28:650–5. https://doi.org/10.1123/jsr.2018-0012.
168. Patel AN, Simpson RC, Cohen SN. In a patient with an immunobullous disorder, is transportation of the skin biopsy in normal saline adequate for direct immunofluorescence analysis? A critically appraised topic. Br J Dermatol. 2013;169:6–10. https://doi.org/10.1111/bjd.12198.
169. Laprais A, Olivry T. Is CCNU (lomustine) valuable for treatment of cutaneous epitheliotropic lymphoma in dogs? A critically appraised topic. BMC Vet Res. 2017;13:61. https://doi.org/10.1186/s12917-017-0978-7.
170. Hill KJ, Robinson KP, Cuchna JW, Hoch MC. Immediate effects of proprioceptive neuromuscular facilitation stretching programs compared with passive stretching programs for hamstring flexibility: a critically appraised topic. J Sport Rehabil. 2017;26:567–72. https://doi.org/10.1123/jsr.2016-0003.
171. Trip Database Ltd. TRIP database. 2020. https://www.tripdatabase.com/, 5 June 2020.
172. University of York Centre for Reviews and Dissemination. DARE: Database of Reviews of Effects. 2020. https://www.crd.york.ac.uk/CRDWeb/. Accessed 17 Feb 2021.
173. American College of Physicians. The ACP Journal Club. 2020. https://www.acpjournals.org/journal/aim/acpjc/purpose-and-procedure. Accessed 17 Feb 2021.
174. University of Nottingham Centre of Evidence Based Dermatology. Global Resource for Eczema Trials (GREAT). 2017. http://www.greatdatabase.org.uk/GD4/Home/Index.php, 5 June 2020.

175. Callander J, Anstey AV, Ingram JR, Limpens J, Flohr C, Spuls PI. How to write a critically appraised topic: evidence to underpin routine clinical practice. Br J Dermatol. 2017;177:1007–13. https://doi.org/10.1111/bjd.15873.
176. Johnston NA, Bieszczak JR, Verhulst S, Disney KE, Montgomery KE, Toth LA. Fenbendazole treatment and litter size in rats. J Am Assoc Lab Anim Sci. 2006;45:35–9.
177. Morgan CJ. The effects of early maternal deprivation on adult behavior in Sprague Dawley rats [dissertation]. New York, NY: City University of New York; 2003.
178. Cristòfol C, Navarro M, Franquelo C, et al. Disposition of netobimin, albendazole, and its metabolites in the pregnant rat: developmental toxicity. Toxicol Appl Pharmacol. 1997;144:56–61. https://doi.org/10.1006/taap.1997.8114.
179. Villar D, Cray C, Zaias J, Altman NH. Biologic effects of fenbendazole in rats and mice: a review. J Am Assoc Lab Anim Sci. 2007;46:8–15.
180. Yoshimura H. Teratogenic evaluation of triclabendazole in rats. Toxicology. 1987;43:283–7. https://doi.org/10.1016/0300-483x(87)90087-4.
181. Pritchett KR, Johnston NA. A review of treatments for the eradication of pinworm infections from laboratory rodent colonies. Contemp Top Lab Anim Sci. 2002;41:36–46.
182. Coghlan LG, Lee DR, Psencik B, Weiss D. Practical and effective eradication of pinworms (Syphacia muris) in rats by use of fenbendazole. Lab Anim Sci. 1993;43:481–7.
183. Barron S, Baseheart BJ, Segar TM, Deveraux T, Willford JA. The behavioral teratogenic potential of fenbendazole: a medication for pinworm infestation. Neurotoxicol Teratol. 2000;22:871–7. https://doi.org/10.1016/s0892-0362(00)00102-1.
184. Keen R, Macinnis M, Guilhardi P, Chamberland K, Church R. The lack of behavioral effects of fenbendazole: a medication for pinworm infection. Contemp Top Lab Anim Sci. 2005;44:17–23.
185. Barlow SC, Brown MM, Price HV. Eradication of Syphacia muris from food-restricted rats without environmental decontamination. Contemp Top Lab Anim Sci. 2005;44:23–5.
186. Vento PJ, Swartz ME, Martin LB, Daniels D. Food intake in laboratory rats provided standard and fenbendazole-supplemented diets. J Am Assoc Lab Anim Sci. 2008;47:46–50.

Planning Animal Experiments

Adrian J. Smith

Abstract

Despite efforts to improve the planning of animal experiments by better reporting, there is still great room for improvement. Many scientists appear to be unaware of the impact which apparently insignificant routines in an animal facility can have on their experiments, and they rely upon the facility staff to take care of these. The same applies to the more mundane aspects of their research such as handling, injection techniques and blood sampling. The aim of this chapter is to demonstrate the need for close collaboration between scientists and facility staff from day 1 of the planning process. This collaboration will have a win-win effect: improving experimental design, implementing the three Rs, optimising animal welfare and safeguarding all of those affected, directly or indirectly, by the research. The chapter underlines the importance of advice and checklists for planning animal research and testing, such as those embodied in the PREPARE guidelines.

The views expressed in this chapter are the author's, and not necessarily those of Norecopa.

A. J. Smith (✉)
Norecopa, Oslo, Norway
e-mail: adrian.smith@norecopa.no

Keywords

Planning · Quality · Validity · Animal · Research · Experiments · Three Rs · Three Ss · PREPARE · ARRIVE

1 Introduction

The ethics of animal experimentation have been debated for many years, but recently their scientific quality and validity have also come under increasing scrutiny, not least from scientists themselves. Studies of papers reporting animal experiments have revealed alarming deficiencies in the information provided [1, 2], even in journals which have endorsed guidelines for reporting animal research [3]. A Swiss study in 2016 of the impact of the ARRIVE guidelines [4], which were published in 2010, indicates that journal endorsement alone has not ensured widespread compliance: half of the researchers using journals which had endorsed ARRIVE had never even heard of the guidelines [5].

There is also widespread concern about the lack of reproducibility and translatability of laboratory animal research [6–9], which contributes to the failure of drugs tested on animals in human trials [10]. In addition, there are concerns about publication bias (the under-reporting of negative results) and sex bias (an overuse of male animals

© Springer Nature Switzerland AG 2021
J. M. Sánchez Morgado, A. Brønstad (eds.), *Experimental Design and Reproducibility in Preclinical Animal Studies*, Laboratory Animal Science and Medicine 1,
https://doi.org/10.1007/978-3-030-66147-2_11

in research). Karp and Reavey point to the over-representation of male animals in many experiments, with advice on how to remedy this situation [11]. Many mouse phenotypes are influenced by the animal's sex [12], and it has been demonstrated that male and female mice react differently to pain [13]. There is evidence of widespread poor experimental design, incorrect use of statistical analyses and under-reporting of the use of analgesics in surgical research [14–16]. Endorsement of reporting guidelines has not yet improved the reporting quality of papers in terms of animal welfare, analgesia or anaesthesia [17]. Pressures to publish, leading to poorly planned experiments performed in haste, should be avoided, but the publication of negative or non-replicable results should not be suppressed, since this is important information for future experiments and reduces publication bias [18]. Likewise, the fact that a protocol was publishable previously does not necessarily mean that it still has sufficient quality to be repeated. All of these weaknesses have serious ethical implications, since they can lead to wasted funding, false hopes for patients, wastage of animal lives, unnecessary suffering and avoidable repetition of experiments. Many of these are discussed in other chapters in this book.

Many scientists have demanded reduced waste when planning experiments involving animals [19–21]. The process of increasing the quality of animal experiments must begin with better planning, from day 1. This is also an important step in the implementation of the three Rs (replacement, reduction and refinement) of Russell and Burch [22]. As will be seen later, attention to detail at all stages is vital to this process, although it is often underestimated by scientists, who tend to assume that the animal facility will take care of the details. Scientists should, however, be deeply concerned about details, even if they are not their primary responsibility, since even small practical details can cause omissions or artefacts that can ruin experiments which in all other respects have been well-designed. Lack of attention to detail can also generate health risks for all those directly or indirectly involved, including other animals in the facility.

2 Attempts to Improve Animal Experimentation by Better Reporting

Concerns about the scientific quality of animal experiments are not new. Many guidelines have been written on how to report animal experiments, based upon the hope that scientists will then understand the need for better planning of subsequent experiments [4, 23–30]. Today, the best known reporting guidelines are ARRIVE [4], which have been endorsed by over 1000 journals and recently updated [31].

Reporting guidelines such as ARRIVE are undoubtedly an important part of quality assurance of scientific research and improved communication between researchers. However, there are a large number of additional items to be considered when planning animal research, which are rarely described in scientific papers – partly for reasons of space and partly because they are assumed (rightly or wrongly) to be part of the day-to-day responsibility of the work of the animal house, rather than the scientist's domain. However, even if these are indeed the responsibility of the animal facility, it is important that the scientists are aware of them, since they may have a large impact on study quality, animal welfare and health and safety. Animal welfare is important, not just because we have a moral duty towards animals, but also because "happy animals give better science" [32]. Animals that are in harmony with their surroundings will give more correct scientific data if stress is prevented, and it will be easier to detect a treatment effect if baseline levels of parameters affected by stress are lower.

Therefore, planning and reporting guidelines should be viewed as two complementary resources. Importantly, experiments (rather like a loaf of bread) cannot be improved by describing them after they have been created: the only solution is to change the ingredients and the conditions under which they are made. This chapter will focus on practical ways of improving the scientific validity of animal experiments by better planning, which in the process will also improve animal welfare, address important health and safety issues, and further implement a "culture of care" in the animal facility.

3 Common Weaknesses in Animal Experiments

Experience suggests that there are a number of factors which are not offered sufficient attention when animal research is planned. These include, but are not limited to, the following:

- Poor literature searches
- Lack of humane endpoints
- Poor experimental design
- Vague distribution of work and costs between the scientists and the animal facility
- Insufficient evaluation of the facility's competence and infrastructure
- Too little attention to transport and acclimation
- Ignoring health risks for all involved
- Lack of standard procedures for necropsy
- Poor planning of waste disposal
- Little discussion about the fate of the animals

Paradoxically, there already exist good guidelines for addressing these topics, so the main effort must be to ensure their implementation. The laboratory animal community itself has produced guidelines for topics such as harm-benefit assessment, study design, capture, transport, breeding, housing, identification and marking, administration of substances, blood sampling, surgery, anaesthesia and analgesia, humane endpoints and humane killing. In addition, there are a large number of guidance documents from the EU Commission, which have been endorsed by the Member States. These include guidelines for education, for training and competence and for the housing, care and use of research animals [33]. For example, Appendix 1 of the Guidance on Project Evaluation and Retrospective Assessment contains pre-formulated questions for building a project application template, including harm-benefit assessment. Some of these topics will be addressed later in this chapter or are discussed in other chapters.

4 PREPARE Before You ARRIVE

Unlike the large number of reporting guidelines, there exist relatively few guidelines for planning experiments. The Strategic Planning Poster from FRAME (Fund for the Replacement of Animals in Medical Experiments) is an example of one of these, providing a flowchart with general advice on planning animal research [34]. There are also a number of very specific guidelines for certain types of research, such as Australian guidance for osteoarthritis research [35] and the reports from the STAIR conferences for stroke models [36].

A set of general planning guidelines, called PREPARE (Planning Research and Experimental Procedures on Animals: Recommendations for Excellence), was published in 2018 to fill the need for detailed advice, complementary to reporting guidelines such as ARRIVE [37]. The guidelines are web-based [38]. A comparison between ARRIVE and PREPARE is also available [39].

The PREPARE guidelines are designed to be applicable to *all* types of animal research and testing, including field studies. They also many contain topics concerning the management and quality control of animal facilities, since in-house experiments are totally dependent upon this. PREPARE seeks therefore to address the needs of all the stakeholders in animal research: the animals, their caretakers and animal technologists, technical staff, scientists and designated responsible persons, including named veterinarians, training and competency officers and facility managers. PREPARE should also prove helpful for those evaluating proposals for animal studies, such as funding bodies, animal welfare committees, ethical review boards, national committees and regulatory authorities.

The PREPARE guidelines consist of two elements:

4.1 The PREPARE Checklist

First of all, PREPARE contains a 2-page checklist consisting of 15 topics translated into (at present) 25 languages [40]. The topics are divided arbitrarily into three sections, corresponding roughly to their chronological order:

Formulation of the study

1. Literature searches
2. Legal issues
3. Ethical issues, harm-benefit assessment* and humane endpoints
4. Experimental design and statistical analysis

Dialogue between scientists and the animal facility

5. Objectives and timescale, funding and division of labour
6. Facility evaluation*
7. Education and training*
8. Health risks, waste disposal and decontamination*

Methods

9. Test substances and procedures
10. Experimental animals
11. Quarantine and health monitoring*
12. Housing and husbandry
13. Experimental procedures
14. Humane killing, release, reuse or rehoming*
15. Necropsy

The topics with an asterisk are examples of ones which are not often highlighted in reporting guidelines such as ARRIVE, but which are important to consider when *planning* experiments.

Some overlap is bound to exist between the topics, and they may be addressed in any order, since the aim of PREPARE is to discuss and resolve any questions connected to *all* these topics *before* the experiment is commenced (Fig. 1).

Scientists may be quick to point out that several of the elements on the PREPARE checklist are primarily the responsibility of the animal facility, rather than themselves, since they determine the quality and standards of the facility as a whole. However, a research project often raises questions which are not covered sufficiently by the facility's existing routines. These include research activities which have potential health and safety risks. Early and open dialogue between the facility and research group, to create a good atmosphere for collaboration, is therefore essential. For example, if a facility cannot safely conduct an experiment without structural changes or investment in new equipment, the facility should raise the issue at an early stage, however tempting it may be to start collaboration on a prestigious project. Animal welfare and ethics committees can also be a useful forum for some of this dialogue [41].

Scientists may query the need to go through a long checklist every time they plan an animal experiment, and indeed not every item will be equally important each time. Experienced scientists will be acquainted with many of the topics already. However, a checklist is always useful, for two reasons:

1. It encourages close contact with the animal facility from day 1 of planning, which ensures that the staff who will be involved are involved. They will be able to give good advice about the details of the experiment, long before it is performed, and they know the strengths and weaknesses of the facility.
2. Items may get forgotten if a checklist is not used. The importance of checklists can be illustrated by the fact that even experienced pilots use many of them, even on routine flights.

4.2 The PREPARE Website of Resources

Importantly, there is much more to PREPARE than the checklist. On the PREPARE website [38], there are sections for each of the topics on the checklist. These provide explanations of the topics, and links to quality-controlled guidelines on each topic, produced by international experts. Advice is given on topics such as housing and husbandry, injection volumes, blood sampling, anaesthesia and analgesia, humane endpoints and experimental design.

PREPARE

norecopa

The PREPARE Guidelines Checklist

Planning Research and Experimental Procedures on Animals: Recommendations for Excellence

Adrian J. Smith[a], R. Eddie Clutton[b], Elliot Lilley[c], Kristine E. Aa. Hansen[d] & Trond Brattelid[e]

[a]Norecopa, c/o Norwegian Veterinary Institute, P.O. Box 750 Sentrum, 0106 Oslo, Norway; [b]Royal (Dick) School of Veterinary Studies, Easter Bush, Midlothian, EH25 9RG, U.K.; [c]Research Animals Department, Science Group, RSPCA, Wilberforce Way, Southwater, Horsham, West Sussex, RH13 9RS, U.K.; [d]Section of Experimental Biomedicine, Department of Production Animal Clinical Sciences, Faculty of Veterinary Medicine, Norwegian University of Life Sciences, P.O. Box 8146 Dep., 0033 Oslo, Norway; [e]Division for Research Management and External Funding, Western Norway University of Applied Sciences, 5020 Bergen, Norway

PREPARE[1] consists of planning guidelines which are complementary to reporting guidelines such as ARRIVE[2].
PREPARE covers the three broad areas which determine the quality of the preparation for animal studies:

1. **Formulation of the study**
2. **Dialogue between scientists and the animal facility**
3. **Quality control of the components in the study**

The topics will not always be addressed in the order in which they are presented here, and some topics overlap. The PREPARE checklist can be adapted to meet special needs, such as field studies. PREPARE includes guidance on the management of animal facilities, since in-house experiments are dependent upon their quality. The full version of the guidelines is available on the Norecopa website, with links to global resources, at **https://norecopa.no/PREPARE**.
The PREPARE guidelines are a dynamic set which will evolve as more species- and situation-specific guidelines are produced, and as best practice within Laboratory Animal Science progresses.

Topic	Recommendation
	(A) Formulation of the study
1. Literature searches	☐ Form a clear hypothesis, with primary and secondary outcomes. ☐ Consider the use of systematic reviews. ☐ Decide upon databases and information specialists to be consulted, and construct search terms. ☐ Assess the relevance of the species to be used, its biology and suitability to answer the experimental questions with the least suffering, and its welfare needs. ☐ Assess the reproducibility and translatability of the project.
2. Legal issues	☐ Consider how the research is affected by relevant legislation for animal research and other areas, e.g. animal transport, occupational health and safety. ☐ Locate relevant guidance documents (e.g. EU guidance on project evaluation).
3. Ethical issues, harm-benefit assessment and humane endpoints	☐ Construct a lay summary. ☐ In dialogue with ethics committees, consider whether statements about this type of research have already been produced. ☐ Address the 3Rs (replacement, reduction, refinement) and the 3Ss (good science, good sense, good sensibilities). ☐ Consider pre-registration and the publication of negative results. ☐ Perform a harm-benefit assessment and justify any likely animal harm. ☐ Discuss the learning objectives, if the animal use is for educational or training purposes. ☐ Allocate a severity classification to the project. ☐ Define objective, easily measurable and unequivocal humane endpoints. ☐ Discuss the justification, if any, for death as an end-point.
4. Experimental design and statistical analysis	☐ Consider pilot studies, statistical power and significance levels. ☐ Define the experimental unit and decide upon animal numbers. ☐ Choose methods of randomisation, prevent observer bias, and decide upon inclusion and exclusion criteria.

Topic	Recommendation
	(B) Dialogue between scientists and the animal facility
5. Objectives and timescale, funding and division of labour	☐ Arrange meetings with all relevant staff when early plans for the project exist. ☐ Construct an approximate timescale for the project, indicating the need for assistance with preparation, animal care, procedures and waste disposal/decontamination. ☐ Discuss and disclose all expected and potential costs. ☐ Construct a detailed plan for division of labour and expenses at all stages of the study.
6. Facility evaluation	☐ Conduct a physical inspection of the facilities, to evaluate building and equipment standards and needs. ☐ Discuss staffing levels at times of extra risk.
7. Education and training	☐ Assess the current competence of staff members and the need for further education or training prior to the study.
8. Health risks, waste disposal and decontamination	☐ Perform a risk assessment, in collaboration with the animal facility, for all persons and animals affected directly or indirectly by the study. ☐ Assess, and if necessary produce, specific guidance for all stages of the project. ☐ Discuss means for containment, decontamination, and disposal of all items in the study.
	(C) Quality control of the components in the study
9. Test substances and procedures	☐ Provide as much information as possible about test substances. ☐ Consider the feasibility and validity of test procedures and the skills needed to perform them.
10. Experimental animals	☐ Decide upon the characteristics of the animals that are essential for the study and for reporting. ☐ Avoid generation of surplus animals.
11. Quarantine and health monitoring	☐ Discuss the animals' likely health status, any needs for transport, quarantine and isolation, health monitoring and consequences for the personnel.
12. Housing and husbandry	☐ Attend to the animals' specific instincts and needs, in collaboration with expert staff. ☐ Discuss acclimatization, optimal housing conditions and procedures, environmental factors and any experimental limitations on these (e.g. food deprivation, solitary housing).
13. Experimental procedures	☐ Develop refined procedures for capture, immobilisation, marking, and release or rehoming. ☐ Develop refined procedures for substance administration, sampling, sedation and anaesthesia, surgery and other techniques.
14. Humane killing, release, reuse or rehoming	☐ Consult relevant legislation and guidelines well in advance of the study. ☐ Define primary and emergency methods for humane killing. ☐ Assess the competence of those who may have to perform these tasks.
15. Necropsy	☐ Construct a systematic plan for all stages of necropsy, including location, and identification of all animals and samples.

References

1. Smith AJ, Clutton RE, Lilley E, Hansen KEA & Brattelid T. PREPARE:Guidelines for Planning Animal Research and Testing. *Laboratory Animals*. 2017. DOI: 10.1177/0023677217724823.
2. Kilkenny C, Browne WJ, Cuthill IC *et al.* Improving Bioscience Research Reporting. The ARRIVE Guidelines for Reporting Animal Research. *PloS Biology*. 2010; DOI: 10.1371/journal.pbio.1000412.

Further information
https://norecopa.no/PREPARE / post@norecopa.no / @norecopa

Fig. 1 The PREPARE checklist. (Reprinted with permission from *Laboratory Animals* (Ref. [37]))

The PREPARE website is updated frequently as new guidelines and relevant scientific papers appear. More species- and situation-specific guidance is still urgently needed in connection with animal research, especially within areas that are outside mainstream laboratory animal use, such as field studies and fish welfare.

4.2.1 An Example of the Use of PREPARE

In connection with an experiment involving the intravenous injection of a radioactive isotope in mice, scientists might want to focus particularly on the following items, all of which are highlighted in the PREPARE checklist:

- Literature searches to find refinements of the technique.
- Legal issues, including regulations on the use of radioactivity.
- The division of labour between the research group and animal facility. Specifically, this would involve who is to give the injections, which is particularly important if they are to be given at weekends as well.
- An evaluation of the facility, to see if it has the infrastructure to handle radioactive isotopes.
- An evaluation of staff skills, to determine whether they need extra training and/or authorisation before the experiment can start.
- A discussion of how to house the animals, where to perform the procedures and how to conduct necropsies on radioactive carcases.
- An analysis of the potential health risks, all the way through to safe waste disposal and decontamination of the rooms used for housing, procedures and necropsy.

5 Involvement of Facility from Day 1

Scientists should be encouraged to recognise that it is in their own interests to liaise closely with the animal facility from as early a stage as possible. This has a number of advantages, the most important of which is that it prevents scientists from spending time developing a protocol which is unrealistic, either because of constraints at the facility (lack of competence or infrastructure) or because the envisaged procedures are unrealistic or overtly stressful for the animals.

The animal technicians who will be involved in an experiment should be invited to the earliest meetings between the scientists and facility, since it is often only at these meetings that the overall and long-term societal benefits of the project are described. Realisation of these aims will help those at the facility to understand the need for the immediate harms they may witness on the animals in the experiments. Animal care staff, who are likely to be inherently sceptical to many protocols, particularly if they involve pain or suffering, have the right to ask basic questions about the rationale behind animal research. They may also have fears about their own personal safety, particularly if microorganisms, isotopes or x-rays are to be used. While precautions may be second nature to a microbiologist, they are not necessarily so to a caretaker, who is primarily focused on animal welfare. Any concerns they may have will decrease their motivation, making them assume a more passive role in the experiments, rather than being active and creative. Motivated animal care staff, who may well have witnessed similar procedures before on the same or other species, will be eager to share their experience, think laterally and work hard to optimise their quality of the research. Many have also a large network and can ask colleagues at other facilities for advice. Importantly, animal care staff may also find it easier than other scientific staff to ask the fundamentally important and justifiable questions about the planned research: whether it is warranted, the likely level of harm and realistic short- or long-term benefits.

Scientists should therefore feel a moral duty to inform all those involved, early in the process.

In summary, the technicians should be consulted from day 1:

- They have a right to know and will be more motivated.
- They know the possibilities, and limitations, in the animal facility.
- They often possess a large range of practical skills and are good at lateral thinking.
- They know the animals best.
- The animals know them best.
- Lack of involvement creates anxiety, depression and opposition to animal research, as well as limiting creativity which might improve the experiments.

Animal care technicians should also be the primary authors of standard operating procedures that describe the functions they perform. These drafts should then be controlled and authorised by more senior staff.

6 Culture of Care: Essential for Good Planning

Optimal planning of a complex process like an animal experiment demands close cooperation between all parties, with mutual respect and trust for the competencies these possess. A good working relationship will help the process of identifying best practice, preventing weaknesses and dividing labour and costs between the parties. The term culture of care is now being used in the laboratory animal community to indicate *a commitment to improving animal welfare, scientific quality, care of the staff and transparency for the stakeholders*. An International Culture of Care Network [42] has been established to accelerate progress in this area.

The concept (referred to as a *climate* of care) is mentioned in Recital 31 of the EU Directive 2010/63 [43], which states:

> Animal-welfare considerations should be given the highest priority in the context of animal keeping, breeding and use. Breeders, suppliers and users

should therefore have an animal-welfare body in place with the primary task of focusing on giving advice on animal-welfare issues. The body should also follow the development and outcome of projects at establishment level, foster a climate of care and provide tools for the practical application and timely implementation of recent technical and scientific developments in relation to the principles of replacement, reduction and refinement, in order to enhance the life-time experience of the animals.

The EU Commission has produced several guidance documents, endorsed by the competent authorities of the Member States, which provide more practical guidance on how a culture of care can be established and nurtured [33]. The culture of care network referred to above contains several more resources.

An open and friendly work environment will also benefit the planning of animal research because it encourages what has become known as a *culture of challenge* [44]. This concept refers to the state in which co-workers, at any level in the institution, feel able to question plans or decisions, without risking reprisals. This is particularly important for junior staff. It may also be expressed as "looking for the acceptable, rather than choosing the accepted". Any question about current routines which invokes the answer "because we've always done it that way", or "as often as necessary", is a good starting point for a constructive discussion which in many cases will lead to improvements in the protocol. Culturing an atmosphere of care, with the freedom to challenge current policies, is an important part of creating a happy working environment [45].

Ways of recognising and nurturing this behaviour include the establishment of an institutional or national 3R prize [46] and annual 3R symposia where advances are highlighted.

7 The Three Ss

Although the 3R tenet has come to dominate the way in which the laboratory animal community plans animal research, many will find it useful also to consider the 3S concept attributed to Professor Carol Newton (1925–2014). Newton herself never published this concept, but it was mentioned by Dr. Harry Rowsell in the proceedings of a symposium in Washington, D.C., in 1976 [47], where Newton was present. According to Rowsell, the three Ss stand for:

- Good science
- Good sense
- Good sensibilities

The concept was not enlarged upon in the proceedings. In an attempt to provide publicity to the concept, Smith and Hawkins [48] have published a paper where they offer their own interpretation. The Norecopa website has a collection of resources related to the 3Ss [49].

Good Science It is naturally the aim of all scientists. As Carol Newton pointed out in her own presentation at the symposium [50], "experiments should be designed to reduce the effect of certain uncontrollable sources of variation, to permit effective techniques to be used in their analysis, and in general to obtain the most information with greatest certainty in the shortest time using the fewest subjects". However, as mentioned above, there are currently serious concerns about the quality of experimental design, statistical analysis, reporting and peer review [51–53].

Good Sense It refers undoubtedly to common sense, which should be followed if there are no clear scientific paths to follow. As Carol Newton said in her presentation, "One certainly must remain mindful of the risk that the 'correct' model is not among those being considered". In practice, when focusing on a biological system or mechanism of interest, it is essential that the researcher critically reflects on the models and approaches that have traditionally been used in the field, ensuring that "the Right animal is used for the Right Reason" (the three Rs of Harry Rowsell, [54]).

Extrapolation from humans to animals, and vice versa, must always be performed with caution when planning animal experiments. For example, the great differences in metabolic rate between animals of varying sizes make it essential to use allometric scaling when calculating a suitable dose for novel species [55]. Common sense is also essential when designing experiments. Translatability can be poor if drugs are administered to animals by routes which are not commonly used in humans, such as intraperitoneal injection.

Good Sensibilities It refers to the capacity to respond to emotions or events. Empathy for animals is a prerequisite for the reduction of suffering and creation of a "life worth living" [56]. Carol Newton reiterated the 3R principle when she said experimentation on intact animals should be resorted to "only when necessary and by designing experiments as effectively as possible" [50]. Critical anthropomorphism [57] is part of this: assuming that interventions that would cause pain or distress to humans may also cause other vertebrate animals to suffer is a good starting point. This is part of the culture of care referred to earlier.

It is worth noting that both good sense and good sensibilities will further good science, just as the three Rs promote both better science and animal welfare.

8 Contingent Suffering

An important part of planning animal experiments is avoidance of contingent suffering: pain and distress not caused by the procedure itself, but by the animals' experience of their situation. Contingent suffering has the potential to cause as much, if not more, suffering than the experimental procedures themselves, as well as the capacity to confound the science.

Examples of this type of suffering include transport stress, intensive housing and husbandry conditions, concurrent disease and social interactions [58]. For example, it has been reported that single-housed male mice show symptoms of what in humans would be characterised as depression [59]. Likewise, mice picked up by their tails demonstrate higher anxiety levels than those handled in tunnels or picked up by the cup of the hand [60–62]. Gentle handling and conditioning of laboratory animals, although time-consuming, is an important element of preparation for an animal experiment, not only because it creates more mutual confidence but because the reference data collected from the animals will more closely reflect correct background levels of their parameters measured. Conditioning mice to daily handling for just a few minutes for a week has been shown to reduce stress and anxiety [63]. Many species respond well to clicker training [64], so that they learn to associate rewards with the procedure.

Contingent suffering is also part of the cumulative severity which animals experience and therefore becomes an important part of the harm-benefit assessment which many countries demand before a research protocol is approved.

9 Simple Procedures?

Scientists are frequently unaware of the stress on animals caused by routine procedures which they assume to be innocuous. This potential for stress includes the processes of capture, handling and immobilisation, injections, methods for marking and techniques for blood sampling. These procedures are clearly more stressful for wild or partially domesticated animals, but even in tame individuals, they may cause unwanted side effects. For example, the mere volume of an injection or of a blood sample may cause harm or distress, particularly in small animals. There exist a wide range of guidelines for such procedures [65], and these should be followed closely. Since many aspects of laboratory animal science are still in their infancy, there is often a need to discuss plans with colleagues. Scientists should be made aware of the specialist sources of information, which they are unlikely to know about. These include not only journals within laboratory animal science but also email discussion fora such as CompMed, VOLE and LAREF [66].

Scientists should be encouraged to ask themselves critical questions, such as how much blood they really need for an analysis, rather than requesting amounts at the upper end of published limits. Blood loss may cause changes to the animal's physiological or immunological state long before this is easily recognisable.

10 Health Risks

A surprisingly large number of categories of personnel can come into direct or indirect contact with an animal experiment, the buildings or waste products from these. Many of these people often possess a number of features which increase their health risks.

They may:

- Enter the facility outside normal working hours, when advice on hazards may not be readily available.
- Not understand messages left in the facility, especially if scientific jargon is used. Special consideration should be paid to employees with other native languages.
- Have little knowledge of animal research, scientific method and the need for controlled experiments.
- Have no intrinsic concern of potential health hazards unless these are pointed out to them. Ironically, the cleaner and tidier an animal facility appears to be, the less likely they are to be fearful of such hazards.
- Have not been health-screened before entering the facility. Those predisposed for allergy or asthma are particularly at risk when working with animals or handling waste products.
- Be planning a family. Early embryonic development and spermatogenesis are known to be at risk upon exposure to ionising radiation and chemicals, including volatile anaesthetics.

This means that the animal facility must have a policy that informs these people before they enter the period of risk. Since many of the most serious birth defects occur before a woman is aware that she is pregnant, and the process of spermatogenesis takes several months, precautions to avoid health risks must be discussed and routines implemented on a continual basis. More guidance is available on the PREPARE website [67].

11 Special Considerations for Farm Animals and Field Research

Farm animals play an important part in animal research. They are used both to increase our understanding of their own species (or related ones) and as models of human disease. Much of the knowledge that we have gained by keeping them as production animals can be put to good use when planning research, but there are a number of other important factors that also need to be considered. Studies on farm animals can be some of the most demanding experiments to perform, and it is vital that scientists and the animal facility liaise closely together from day 1 of planning [68].

Some, but by no means all, of the challenges include:

- Challenges with capture, restraint and handling
- Health status, acquisition, transport and acclimation to new buildings
- Quarantine and adaptation to new feeding regimes
- Establishment of new social groups
- Provision of sufficient space for exercise, sampling, anaesthesia and necropsy
- Ventilation issues
- The differences in practices between traditional farm work and those used in controlled studies in a laboratory environment
- Health, safety and general hygiene
- Waste disposal
- Containment of pathogens
- Identification of sufficient numbers of staff who are familiar with, and competent to handle, farm animal species

Many of these issues are exacerbated by the sheer size of the animals or cadavers.

An international consensus meeting on the care and use of agricultural animals in research in 2012 addressed many of these issues, both related to the use of farm animals in traditional laboratory animal facilities and to animal research performed under farm conditions [69]. An extensive list of guidelines for farm animal research is available [70].

Similar issues apply to field research, where lack of attention to detail can have even more serious consequences if the absence of a vital piece of equipment or drug is first discovered in the field.

Norecopa has arranged two international consensus meetings on the care and use of animals in field research [69], and a list of guidelines for field research is available [71].

12 Contract Between the Animal Facility and the Research Group

An animal experiment will involve extra work for the facility in which it is carried out. Some of this work will be routine, but some will involve procedures which the staff do not perform regularly and for which they may need special training. In both cases, the work will result in extra costs in the form of staff time and equipment. In addition, much of this work will take place after the scientists have left the building, as the staff clear up, dispose of waste material and decontaminate the rooms used. The division of these costs and labour must be discussed at an early stage, to avoid conflicts between the two parties after the event. A complicating factor may be that many of these procedures must take place at weekends or on public holidays, when the regular, experienced staff are not available.

Importantly, it is vital that agreement is reached, and documented, on which parameters are to be recorded during the experiment and by whom.

A simple contract should be drawn up between the animal facility and research group, indicating the parameters to be recorded during the experiment and who is responsible for the data collection. The contract should also indicate how the expenses are to be shared between the two parties. A copy of the completed contract is kept by both parties and serves as a checklist and reminder of who is responsible for what. An example of a contract based upon the PREPARE guidelines is given on the website [72].

This avoids unpleasant discussions after the experiment, for example, when a paper has been submitted to a journal which asks for more details. If the research group cannot provide the information the journal requests, for example, room temperature during the experiment, it may be difficult to publish the study, wasting human resources, animal lives and research funds.

13 The AAALAC International Template

Quality assurance of animal experiments cannot occur in isolation from the animal facility in which they are performed. Poor routines in the facility will influence the quality for the research results, however well the animal procedures are planned. Both the facility and scientists should be aware of the principles of quality assurance and, at the least, the most critical factors in the facility which will influence their results.

The organisation AAALAC International [73] offers an accreditation scheme for laboratory animal facilities. As part of the process of applying for accreditation, a facility must create a programme description, which gives details of how it relates to four main areas of concern:

- Institutional policies on animal care and use
- Animal environment, housing and management
- Veterinary care
- Physical plant (the infrastructure of the facility)

AAALAC provides a detailed template for production of the programme description. This template is freely available on AAALAC's website [74] and can be used by anyone as a checklist for the quality of a facility, even if they are not planning to apply for accreditation. The quality of the services offered by a facility will improve significantly by working through the template and addressing areas where the current routines are suboptimal. The initial production of a complete programme description involves a great deal of work, but once this is done, the document can easily be updated regularly, as new procedures are introduced.

Importantly, this work will reveal the need for standard operating procedures (SOPs) for critical operations and for some means of reminding the facility when procedures which are not performed regularly (such as service of machinery) are due. A master plan for the facility (see below) is a good way of resolving the latter issue.

14 Master Plan

Both planning an animal experiment and management of an animal facility involve the performance of a series of important elements over a prolonged timescale. To avoid forgetting these procedures, it is essential to have some kind of overview, or master plan, which specifies which tasks are to be performed and when. Such a plan helps to ensure that procedures are carried out at the designated intervals and is particularly useful for operations which are not performed frequently and which therefore tend to get forgotten. Examples of these are service and calibration of equipment, testing of backup systems and health monitoring of animals. The frequency of many of these tasks must be discussed with other staff members and equipment suppliers, all of which contributes to higher standards in the animal facility. A master plan for an animal experiment has the same advantages and is a good starting point for fruitful discussions about the work ahead.

Since a master plan is designed to be a practical aid, care should therefore be taken to ensure that it is perceived as such by all staff members. A pragmatic approach should be used to the intervals designated to each operation: if these intervals prove in practice to be wrong (too frequent or infrequent), they should be adjusted immediately. Used in this manner, a master plan will be seen by staff members as a valuable tool, rather than an additional administrative burden.

Often the most effective means of using a master plan is to create one on paper. It is then easy to display the plan and discuss it around a table at a staff meeting. Sheets designed for planning staff vacation work well for this purpose.

The items on the plan are written in the left-hand column, and open circles are placed in the columns for weeks where the procedure is to be performed. Staff enter their initials in the open circle when the operation has been completed. It is then easy to see who has performed the tasks, in case there is a need to discuss the procedures with the last person who performed them. The open circles can be erased or moved laterally if the facility wishes to alter the frequency of events, for example, as experience is gained in performing the task, or if too many tasks have been scheduled for a particular week. A master plan of this type functions therefore not only as a reminder of tasks to be performed but also as simple yet effective documentation of a large number of procedures.

The contents of a master plan for a facility, and the frequency of the procedures on it, must be tailor-made to the individual institution, after a risk analysis of its operations, infrastructure and location. Standard operating procedures (SOPs) should be written for the procedures themselves. This will also help in deciding how many procedures can practicably be performed in any 1 week. A master plan for an animal study should follow the same principles.

Typical procedures for a master plan include the following activities, but this list is neither exhaustive nor necessarily relevant for all facilities:

1. Cleaning of animal rooms
2. Cleaning of procedure rooms
3. Cleaning of storage and waste disposal rooms
4. Cleaning of personnel areas
5. Service and calibration of equipment (e.g. weighing scales, washing machines, sterilisers, anaesthetic machines, imaging equipment and laboratory instruments)
6. Maintenance of fridges, freezers and washing machines
7. Maintenance of fire safety equipment
8. Fire safety rounds and fire drill
9. Assessment of utilities (water, electricity, other services)

10. Test of backup systems
11. Test of alarm systems, security and emergency procedures
12. Control of medicine, feed and equipment stores
13. Control of animal emergency medication and equipment
14. Health checks and vaccination of staff
15. Control of first aid equipment and routines
16. Education and training of staff and revision of CVs
17. Membership of organisations and evaluation of the facility's library
18. Staff meetings and individual discussions
19. Evaluation of the facility's SOPs
20. Evaluation of the facility's waste disposal system
21. Risk assessment of the facility
22. Evaluation of the facility's health and safety programme
23. Evaluation of the facility's internal control system
24. Evaluation of the facility's contingency plan
25. Evaluation of the facility's master plan

15 Quality Assurance

The only justification for the use of animals in procedures which cause them pain, distress, suffering or lasting harm is that the data obtained from the experiments has value and benefit, either to humans, animals or the environment. If the quality of this data is questionable, then so is the experiment.

The widely accepted principles of quality assurance should therefore be applied, both by the facility and scientists, when planning animal experiments. The critical points in the experiment should be identified and extra attention paid to ensuring their quality. In addition, great effort should be made to assess the impact and effectiveness of each step in the experiment, with a view to improving its quality the next time it is performed.

This process generates an upward spiral of quality, each procedure improving every time it is performed. Realisation of this becomes a major inspirational factor for all those concerned, not least the technicians who have least to gain from an animal experiment, since they rarely become co-authors, but witness at close quarters the animals' reactions to the procedures.

Attention to detail and focus on quality will also help to reveal latent weaknesses in experimental design or facility management which, under special conditions, may cause dramatic treatment effects, poor animal welfare or facility accidents. These latent weaknesses may, individually, be incapable of causing significant problems, but if several of these occur simultaneously, they may precipitate a more dramatic event, a phenomenon known as the Swiss cheese effect [75].

Reason [76] hypothesised that most accidents can be traced to one or more of four failure domains: organisational influences, supervision, preconditions and specific acts. Failures may be "latent" (the first three domains), lying dormant for days, weeks or months until they contribute to the accident, or "active" events that can be directly linked to an accident, such as a mistake made when administering a treatment.

It should come as no surprise that it is important to consider these failure domains in connection with animal experiments. Animals are complex organisms, and our knowledge of the interactions between their organ systems and treatments is still rudimentary. This creates both *known unknowns* and *unknown unknowns* (elements in the Johari window, [77]). Many of the effects of these will not be visible (if at all) until the experiment is performed. For this reason, it is crucial when planning animal experiments to analyse, as far as possible, the consequences of every procedure in the protocol. Attention to detail and to apparently insignificant issues is therefore paramount. This will improve the internal scientific validity of the experiment, even if its external validity (the translational value from an animal species to humans, which is a recurring weakness of animal experimentation) cannot be totally resolved [78].

16 Conclusions: Application of the 3Rs and 3Ss at All Stages

In summary, the principles of replacement, reduction and refinement, and good science, good sense and good sensibilities should be addressed at all stages of the planning process. This includes, but is not restricted to:

- Breeding of the animals to be used
- Transport of the animals from their breeding site to the place of use
- Acclimation to the new environment and staff after transportation
- Choice of procedures, including:
  - Dose
  - Method of administration
  - Methods of data collection
- Consideration of the use of pilot studies on a small number of animals, to test the treatment effect

Søren Kierkegaard (1813–1855) stated:

> It is perfectly true, as philosophers say, that life must be understood backwards.
>
> But they forget the other proposition, that it must be lived forwards. [79]

References

1. Kilkenny C, Parsons N, Kadyszewski E, et al. Survey of the quality of experimental design, statistical analysis and reporting of research using animals. PLoS One. 2009;4:e7824. https://doi.org/10.1371/journal.pone.0007824.
2. Smith JA, Birke L, Sadler D. Reporting animal use in scientific papers. Lab Anim. 1997;31:312–7.
3. Avey MT, Moher D, Sullivan KJ, et al. The devil is in the details: incomplete reporting in preclinical animal research. PLoS One. 2016;11:e0166733. https://doi.org/10.1371/journal.pone.0166733.
4. Kilkenny C, Browne WJ, Cuthill IC, et al. Improving bioscience research reporting: the ARRIVE guidelines for reporting animal research. PLoS Biol. 2010;8:e1000412. https://doi.org/10.1371/journal.pbio.1000412.
5. Reichlin TS, Vogt L, Wurbel H. The researchers' view of scientific rigor-survey on the conduct and reporting of in vivo research. PLoS One. 2016;11:e0165999. https://doi.org/10.1371/journal.pone.0165999.
6. Begley CG, Ellis LM. Drug development: raise standards for preclinical cancer research. Nature. 2012;483:531–3. https://doi.org/10.1038/483531a.
7. Garner JP. The significance of meaning: why do over 90% of behavioral neuroscience results fail to translate to humans, and what can we do to fix it? ILAR J. 2014;55:438–56. https://doi.org/10.1093/ilar/ilu047.
8. Howells DW, Sena ES, Macleod MR. Bringing rigour to translational medicine. Nat Rev Neurol. 2014;10:37–43. https://doi.org/10.1038/nrneurol.2013.232.
9. van der Worp HB, Howells DW, Sena ES, et al. Can animal models of disease reliably inform human studies? PLoS Med. 2010;7:e1000245. https://doi.org/10.1371/journal.pmed.1000245.
10. Prinz F, Schlange T, Asadullah K. Believe it or not: how much can we rely on published data on potential drug targets? Nat Rev Drug Discov. 2011;10:712. https://doi.org/10.1038/nrd3439-c1.
11. Karp NA, Reavey N. Sex bias in preclinical research and an exploration of how to change the status quo. Br J Pharmacol. 2018; https://doi.org/10.1111/bph.14539.
12. Karp NA, Mason J, Beaudet AL, Benjamini Y, Bower L, Braun RE, et al. Prevalence of sex dimorphism in mammalian phenotypic traits. Nat Commun. 2017;8:15475. https://doi.org/10.1038/ncomms15475.
13. Sorge RE, Mapplebeck JCS, Rosen S, Beggs S, Taves S, Alexander JK, et al. Different immune cells mediate mechanical pain hypersensitivity in male and female mice. Nat Neurosci. 2015;18:1081–3.
14. Enserink M Sloppy reporting on animal studies proves hard to change. Science 29. 2017;357(6358):1337–8. https://doi.org/10.1126/science.357.6358.1337.
15. Wallach JD, Boyack KW, JPA I. Reproducible research practices, transparency, and open access data in the biomedical literature, 2015–2017. PLoS Biol. 2018; https://doi.org/10.1371/journal.pbio.2006930.
16. Bradbury AG, Eddleston M, Clutton RE. Pain management in pigs undergoing experimental surgery: a literature review (2012–14). Br J Anaesth. 2016;116:47–5. https://doi.org/10.1093/bja/aev301.
17. Leung V, Rousseau-Blass F, Beauchamp G, Pang DSJ ARRIVE has not ARRIVEd: support for the ARRIVE (Animal Research: Reporting of *in vivo* Experiments) guidelines does not improve the reporting quality of papers in animal welfare, analgesia or anesthesia 2018; PLoS One https://doi.org/10.1371/journal.pone.0197882.
18. van Assen MALM, van Aert RCM, Nuitjen MB, Wicherts JM Why publishing everything is more effective than selective publishing of statistically significant results. 2014; PLoS One, doi:https://doi.org/10.1371/journal.pone.0084896.
19. Chalmers I, Bracken MB, Djulbegovic B, et al. How to increase value and reduce waste when research priorities are set. Lancet. 2014;383:156–65. https://doi.org/10.1016/s0140-6736(13)62229-1.

20. Macleod MR, Michie S, Roberts I, et al. Biomedical research: increasing value, reducing waste. Lancet. 2014;383:101–4. https://doi.org/10.1016/s0140-6736(13)62329-6.
21. Munafò MR, Nosek BA, Bishop DVM, et al. A manifesto for reproducible science. Nat Hum Behav 2017; 1: 0021. Perspective. https://doi.org/10.1038/s41562-016-0021
22. Russell WMS, Burch RL. The principles of humane experimental technique. Wheathampstead: Universities Federation for Animal Welfare; 1959.
23. Ellery AW. Guidelines for specification of animals and husbandry methods when reporting the results of animal experiments. Lab Anim. 1985;19:106–8.
24. Öbrink KJ, Försöksdjurs-kunskap WM. Refinement, reduction, replacement. Lund: Studentlitteratur AB; 1996.
25. Smith JA, Birke L, Sadler D. Reporting animal use in scientific papers. Lab Anim. 1997;31:312–7.
26. Öbrink, Rehbinder. Animal definition: a necessity for the validity of animal experiments? Lab Anim. 2000;34:121–30.
27. Hooijmans CR, Leenaars M, Ritskes-Hoitinga M. A gold standard publication checklist to improve the quality of animal studies, to fully integrate the three Rs, and to make systematic reviews more feasible. Altern Lab Anim. 2010;38:167–82.
28. Brattelid T, Smith AJ. Guidelines for reporting the results of experiments on fish. Lab Anim. 2000;34:131–5.
29. Institute for Laboratory Animal Research NRC. Guidance for the description of animal research in scientific publications. Washington, DC: National Academies Press; 2011.
30. Altman DG, Simera I, Hoey J, et al. EQUATOR: reporting guidelines for health research. Lancet. 2018;371:1149–50. https://doi.org/10.1016/s0140-6736(08)60505-x.
31. Percie du Sert N, Hurst V, Ahluwalia A, et al. The ARRIVE guidelines 2.0: updated guidelines for reporting animal research. PLoS Biol. 2020;18(7):e3000410. https://doi.org/10.1371/journal.pbio.3000410.
32. Poole T. Happy animals make good science. Lab Anim. 1997;31:116–24.
33. Guidance documents to fulfil the requirements under the Directive 2010/63/EU. http://ec.europa.eu/environment/chemicals/lab_animals/pubs_guidance_en.htm
34. Strategic Planning for Research Programmes. https://frame.org.uk/resources/research-planning/
35. Smith MM, Clarke EC, Little CB. Considerations for the design and execution of protocols for animal research and treatment to improve reproducibility and standardization: DEPART well-prepared and ARRIVE safely. Osteoarthr Cartil. 2017; https://doi.org/10.1016/j.joca.2016.10.016.
36. STAIR Consensus Conferences. http://www.thestair.org
37. Smith AJ, Clutton RE, Lilley E, Hansen KEA, Brattelid T. PREPARE: Guidelines for planning animal research and testing. Lab Anim. 2018;52(2):135–41. https://doi.org/10.1177/0023677217724823.
38. PREPARE https://norecopa.no/PREPARE
39. Relationship between PREPARE and ARRIVE. https://norecopa.no/PREPARE/comparison-with-arrive
40. PREPARE checklist https://norecopa.no/PREPARE/prepare-checklist
41. What is Ethical Review? https://science.rspca.org.uk/sciencegroup/researchanimals/ethicalreview
42. Culture of care https://norecopa.no/coc
43. Directive 2010/63/EU of the European Parliament and of the Council of 22 September 2010 on the Protection of Animals Used for Scientific Purposes. http://eur-lex.europa.eu/LexUriServ/LexUriServ.do?uri=OJ:L:2010:276:0033:0079:en:PDF
44. Louhimies, S Refinement facilitated by the Culture of Care. In Proceedings of the EUSAAT 2015-Linz 2005 Congress, Linz, Austria, 20–23 September 2015; Vol 4, p. 154. http://eusaat-congress.eu/images/2015/Abstractbook_EUSAAT_2015_Linz_2015.pdf
45. Maestre FT. Seven steps towards health and happiness in the lab. Nature. 2018; https://doi.org/10.1038/d41586-018-07514-7. https://www.nature.com/articles/d41586-018-07514-7
46. Norecopa's 3R Prize. https://norecopa.no/about-norecopa/3r-prize
47. Rowsell HC. The ethics of biomedical experimentation. In: The future of animals, cells, models, and systems in research, development, education, and testing. Washington, DC: National Academy of Sciences; 1977. p. 267–85.
48. Smith AJ, Hawkins P. Good Science, Good Sense and Good Sensibilities: The Three Ss of Carol Newton. Animals. 2016;6(11):70. https://doi.org/10.3390/ani6110070.
49. The Three S's. https://norecopa.no/3S
50. Newton CM. Biostatistical and biomedical methods in efficient animal experimentation. In: The Future of Animals, Cells, Models, and Systems in Research, Development, Education, and Testing: National Academy of Sciences, Washington, DC; 1977. p. 152–69.
51. AMS; BBSRC; MRC; Wellcome Trust. Reproducibility and reliability of biomedical research: improving research practice. Symposium report, 2015.
52. Eisen JA, Ganley E, CJ MC. Open science and reporting animal studies: Who's accountable? PLoS Biol. 2014;12 https://doi.org/10.1371/journal.pbio.1001757.
53. Newton DP. Quality and peer review of research: an adjudicating role for editors. Account Res. 2010;17:130–45.
54. Rowsell HC, AA MW. The right animal for the right reason. In: Proceedings of the Canadian Association for Laboratory Animal Science 1978–1979, Canadian Association for Laboratory Animal Science Conven-

tion, Ottawa, ON, Canada, 28 August–1 September 1978. Calgary: CALAS National Office; 1978. p. 211–20.
55. Morris TH. Dose estimation among species. In: Hawk CT, Leary SL, Morris TH, editors. Formulary for laboratory animals. 3rd ed. Ames: Blackwell Publishing.
56. Mellor D. Updating animal welfare thinking: moving beyond the "Five Freedoms" towards "a Life Worth Living". Animals. 2016;6 https://doi.org/10.3390/ani6030021.
57. Morton DB, Berghardt GM. Smith JA animals, Science, and ethics—section III. Critical anthropomorphism, animal suffering, and the ecological context. Hast Cent Rep. 1990;20:S13–9.
58. Klein HJ, Bayne KB. Establishing a culture of care, conscience, and responsibility: addressing the improvement of scientific discovery and animal welfare through science-based performance standards. ILAR J. 2007;48:3–11.
59. Kalliokoski O, Teilmann AC, Jacobsen KR, Abelson KSP, Hau J. The Lonely Mouse – Single Housing Affects Serotonergic Signaling Integrity Measured by 8-OH-DPAT-Induced Hypothermia in Male Mice. PLoS One. 2014; https://doi.org/10.1371/journal.pone.0111065.
60. Jennings M, et al. Refining rodent husbandry: the mouse. Lab Anim. 1998;32:233–59.
61. Hurst JL, West RS. Taming anxiety in laboratory mice. Nat Methods. 2010;7(10)
62. Gouveia K, Hurst JL. Reducing mouse anxiety during handling: effect of experience with handling tunnels. PLoS One. 2013;8:1–8.
63. Fridgeirsdottir GA, Hillered L, Clausen F. Escalated handling of young C57BL/6 mice results in altered Morris water maze performance. Uppsala J Med Sci. 2014;119:1–9.
64. Leidinger C, Herrmann F, Thone-Reineke C, Baumgart N. Baumgart J introducing clicker training as cognitive enrichment for laboratory mice. Jove. 2017;121:1–12.
65. Guidelines for animal research. https://norecopa.no/search?fq=type:%22Guidelines%22&fq=db:%223r%22&sort=name_s%20asc&q=*
66. Email discussion lists of relevance to laboratory animal science. https://norecopa.no/more-resources/email-discussion-lists
67. Health risks, waste disposal and decontamination. https://norecopa.no/prepare/8-health-risks-waste-disposal-and-decontamination
68. Farm animals. https://norecopa.no/farm-animals
69. Meetings within laboratory animal science and alternatives. https://norecopa.no/meetings
70. Example guidelines for housing, handling, dosing and sampling in farm animals. A list produced by Dr. Penny Hawkins, Research Animals Department, RSPCA https://norecopa.no/media/6362/guidelines.pdf
71. Guidelines for wildlife research https://norecopa.no/search?q=*&fq=cat:%22Wildlife%22&fq=type:%22Guidelines%22&fq=db:%223r%22.
72. Division of labour, costs and responsibility. https://norecopa.no/prepare/5-objectives-and-timescale-funding-and-division-of-labour/division-of-labour-costs-and-responsibility
73. AAALAC International. https://www.aaalac.org
74. Program Description. https://www.aaalac.org/program-description/
75. The Swiss cheese model. https://en.wikipedia.org/wiki/Swiss_cheese_model
76. Reason J. Human error: models and management. BMJ. 2000;320(7237):768–70.
77. Johari window. https://en.wikipedia.org/wiki/Johari_window
78. Pound P, Ritskes-Hoitinga M. Is it possible to overcome issues of external validity in preclinical animal research? Why most animal models are bound to fail. J Transl Med. 2018;16:304. https://doi.org/10.1186/s12967-018-1678-1.
79. Søren Kierkegaard. https://en.wikiquote.org/wiki/Søren_Kierkegaard